Jodi J. DeLuca
130-C Blue Heron Drive
Daytona Beach, FL 32119

FUNDAMENTALS OF
PSYCHIATRY

FUNDAMENTALS OF PSYCHIATRY

Robert J. Waldinger, M.D.

McLean Hospital
Belmont, Massachusetts

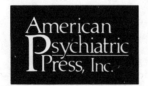

1400 K Street, N.W.
Washington, DC 20005

Note: The author has worked to ensure that all information in this book concerning drug dosages, schedules, and routes of administration is accurate at the time of publication and consistent with standards set by the United States Food and Drug Administration and the general medical community. As medical research and practice advance, however, therapeutic standards may change. For this reason, and because human and mechanical errors sometimes occur, we recommend that readers follow the advice of a physician directly involved in their care or the care of a member of their family.

Books published by the American Psychiatric Press, Inc., represent the views and opinions of the individual authors and do not necessarily reflect the policies and opinions of the Press or the American Psychiatric Association.

Cover design by Dovecote Studios
Text design by Richard E. Farkas
Typeset by Mid-Atlantic Photo Composition
Printed by RR Donnelley & Sons Co.

Library of Congress Cataloging in Publication Data

Waldinger, Robert J., 1951–
  Fundamentals of psychiatry.

  Includes bibliographies and index.
  1. Psychiatry—Methodology. I. Title. [DNLM: 1. Interview, Psychological—methods. 2. Mental Disorders. 3. Personality Assessment. 4. Psychotherapy. WM 100 W163f]
RC437.5.W325   1986   616.89   86-3327
ISBN 0-88048-208-7

CONTENTS

Part IV

INTRODUCTION

This is a book of basics. It was written for professionals who are trying to make sense out of their first encounters with people who are emotionally disturbed. The book is an introduction to the practice of mental health care and, as such, assumes no prior knowledge of the field.

I wrote this book because I wished it had been written for me. When I was a medical student, I was skeptical of psychiatry with all of its jargon, and I was bewildered by the complicated illnesses and profound emotional distress that I encountered during my first experience in mental health care. At the local bookstore, I found quite a few massive comprehensive textbooks and many excellent books devoted to particular areas of psychopathology. But what I wanted was one short book that would give me the basics—that would provide me with an introduction to topics such as schizophrenia and ECT, transference and tranquilizers—and that would do so in plain English. That is what this book is meant to do.

The book grew out of my experiences as a teacher on a team made up of trainees in psychology, social work, nursing, rehabilitation counseling, and psychiatry. While it was clear that people in each of these disciplines brought unique perspectives to their work and served special functions on our multidisciplinary team, everyone needed the same core of clinical knowledge in order to work effectively with clients in emotional distress. Moreover, I discovered that people in other fields are eager to learn about mental illness. Professionals in law and law enforcement, education, primary care medicine, and other forms of social service are often the first to see people who are badly in need of mental health care. These professionals commonly play a central role in helping people find proper treatment, and they therefore require basic tools for understanding the emotional problems they encounter in the course of their work.

The first goal of this book is to provide those tools in chapters that you can read and refer to quickly when you need essential information. Then, when you have time, you can do further reading to pursue in more detail those areas that particularly interest you.

A second goal of the book is to help you make sense of your own reactions to what you see clinically, because your feelings about clients and their problems often provide you with crucial diagnostic information. And the experience of working with people who are in emotional pain can be grueling, particularly when you are new at it. In order to be of help to other people, you have to take care of yourself— and that means paying attention to your own reactions to clinical work and knowing when to get emotional support from friends, colleagues, and supervisors. Throughout these chapters, I have tried to help you focus on yourself as well as your clients.

The book is laid out in four major sections. Chapters 1 through 4 are designed to give you the basic skills with which to carry out a diagnostic evaluation. Chapters 5 through 10 cover particular mental disorders and the disorders of children and adolescents, while Chapters 11 through 14 address some areas that are of clinical concern to everyone who works in mental health care. Finally, Chapters 15 and 16 describe psychotherapies and somatic therapies, respectively.

Because this text is *not* encyclopedic, much has been left out. However, it *will* provide you with a place to start. If these chapters help to make psychiatry more accessible to you and prompt you to delve further into the field, then the book will have accomplished its purpose.

ACKNOWLEDGMENTS

Many generous and capable people contributed to the writing of this book. I am indebted to my teachers and colleagues at McLean Hospital, who advised me on the early drafts of this manuscript:

Jonathan O. Cole, M.D.
Robert Fein, Ph.D.
Arlene Frank, Ph.D.
Shirley Goldstein, M.S.W.
Phyllis Kayne, R.N.
Cynthia N. Kettyle, M.D.
Benjamin Liptzin, M.D.
Margaret McKenna, M.D.
Arthur Rosenberg, Esq.
Alan F. Schatzberg, M.D.
Sharon R. Weinstein, M.D.
Roger Weiss, M.D.

Carolyn B. Robinowitz, M.D., Deputy Medical Director of the American Psychiatric Association, offered valuable perspectives on medical student education. I owe special thanks to Diane Mosbacher, M.D., Ph.D., who somehow found the time and energy during her fourth year of medical school to examine the entire text from a student's vantage point. She heightened my awareness of many social and political issues relevant to clinical care, and she helped me to free the text of some of its cumbersome jargon.

John G. Gunderson, M.D., provided me with a place to work and secretarial support in the Psychotherapy Department at McLean Hospital. He also prodded me when my pace slowed and brought his considerable clinical expertise to bear on many parts of the manuscript. Phillip Isenberg, M.D., Director of Residency Education at McLean Hospital, helped me to conceptualize the textbook and to maintain its focus on the needs of beginning students. Evelyn Stone shepherded the book through each stage of development. Without her knowledge of psychiatric publications and her constant willingness to listen and advise, the book would not have been realized.

Frances MacNeil did the lion's share of the typing of the manuscript and remained helpful and supportive through many long and choppy drafts. Amy Shaughnessy, David Andrews, and Tim Clancy of the American Psychiatric Press, Inc., worked tirelessly to make the book more comprehensible to those with no background in the field and managed to take some of the rough edges off my prose.

Jennifer Stone, M.A., provided important perspectives on work with children. And—more to the point—her optimism, patience, and unflagging moral support were essential in enabling me to finish this project.

For all of their assistance and encouragement, I am very grateful.

Part I

INTRODUCTION

The problems that people bring to mental health professionals run the gamut from memory loss to marital difficulties, from palpitations to hallucinations. The first section of this book is designed to acquaint you with the basic tools used to approach this vast array of problems.

The primary diagnostic tool available to mental health professionals is the clinical interview. Chapter 1 presents the fundamentals of interviewing technique, discusses how good interviewing differs from everyday conversation, and reviews some of the more common problems encountered by interviewers, particularly those with limited experience.

Chapter 2 is a brief summary of the fundamentals of psychodynamic psychology, presented in an attempt to demystify such basic psychodynamic concepts as the id, ego, and superego and the unconscious mind. This chapter will also introduce you to the stages of human development and the idea of psychological conflict and defense—concepts that can be invaluable to you in understanding what people tell you about themselves and their past.

Chapter 3 focuses specifically on how to interview and evaluate a client, because that is usually the first task confronting the student in a mental health care setting. This chapter outlines the aspects of a person's life you will need to explore as part of an initial evaluation, and it provides examples of interview questions that will help you to gather this information.

Chapter 4 complements Chapter 3 in that it describes the mental status examination, which is a fundamental part of every assessment of mental health. In addition to describing the exam and offering suggestions for the best way to conduct it, Chapter 4 is designed to serve as a glossary, defining many of the terms used to label the symptoms of mental disorders. It is important that you become familiar with these terms so that you use them correctly in your work.

These first four chapters serve as a prelude to the rest of the book. Once you have grasped the essentials of interviewing, psychodynamics, and the process of doing an evaluation, you will be prepared to take a closer look at specific mental disorders and the methods we have for understanding and treating them.

CHAPTER 1

The Clinical Interview: Fundamentals of Technique

An interview is, in essence, a conversation. So a chapter on interviewing technique may seem a waste of time. After all, most of us are well practiced in everyday conversation. However, the clinical interview is a very particular kind of conversation and differs from daily discourse in many important respects. These differences are subtle, and interviewing is a skill that takes time and practice to master. The concepts discussed below are important tools in all human service professions. The basic principles of clinical interviewing apply equally to evaluating an adolescent's academic crisis, working with a distraught couple in the midst of a divorce, or embarking on long-term individual psychotherapy. This chapter places particular emphasis on how to interview a new client as part of a diagnostic evaluation, because that is usually one of the first tasks assigned to a student in a mental health care setting.

The aim of interviewing is not simply to gather information about someone's past, but to arrive at an empathic understanding of how that person feels. Such understanding is essential to accurate diagnosis and effective treatment, and the success of the interview hinges on its development. The more sensitive you are as an interviewer, the greater will be your grasp of your client's problems, and the easier it will be for clients to elaborate on the nature of their pain. Emotional distress is often quite isolating, and the experience of sharing one's

3

problems with a concerned listener can be enormously relieving. In a sense, the initial interview is actually the start of treatment.

To evaluate effectively, you must discover as much as you can about how your client's mind works. During the interview, people will offer many clues, both in what they tell you (the *content* of the interview) and in how they tell it (the *process* of the interview).

Being aware of the process of the interview is essential to understanding someone's problems. But process is much more difficult to focus on than content, because most of us are not accustomed to doing so. Attending to process means listening with a "third ear," mentally stepping back from a conversation and watching it even while you participate. It means taking note of how people speak, what topics they bring up and in what order, which subjects they emphasize and which they avoid, how they sit or gesture, what responses they elicit from you, and how they make you feel. This style of listening does not come naturally to most of us, because in everyday conversation we focus on the content of what is said, and think about process only when there is some obvious discrepancy between the two (such as when a friend screams at you, "I am not angry!"). Paying attention to process is hard work, but it is a skill worth developing. Through process, people will give you a glimpse of how they cope with their world and how they approach new relationships. Consider the following case example:

> A young man has just been fired from his most recent job, and complains to you that he is "depressed" because he cannot get along with a series of "difficult" employers. He also notes that his romantic relationships have never worked out, "because women just don't understand me." In your interview, you find that he drones on and on about minute details of his work as an actuary. He becomes frustrated and momentarily angry whenever you attempt to introduce a new topic, saying, "I'll get to that—but first let me finish my story." When you ask about his feelings of depression, he invariably changes the subject back to his work. At the end of the interview, you find that you have gathered little information about his life, or about the specific problems that brought him to see you. You also find yourself feeling angry and impatient with him. The content of the interview is of little help to you. However, your attention to the process of the interview provides you with a glimpse of this man's difficulties. He has rigidly insisted on imposing his own order on your meeting, and he has avoided any subject that might arouse unpleasant feelings. You might infer that his inflexibility and need to flee from emotion hamper both his relationships with women and his ability to work with employers. You might also infer that he makes other people feel angry and impatient with him, just as he has done with you.

Clearly, clients must be given the opportunity to show you the processes by which they form a relationship. They will do this in even a single interview, provided that you give them the freedom to do so. The interviewer who subjects the client to an endless stream of specific questions will never gather this kind of information. This interviewer will not learn, for example, how the person handles silences or sadness. What's more, the interviewer who tends to talk a lot leaves less time to listen and will likely lose touch with his or her own feelings about the client. Therefore, you should try to be as nondirective as possible. Guide people only when they seem to stray from the themes that are relevant to the interview. Obviously, this is not always an easy task, especially for the neophyte interviewer.

Your first goal is to stay out of the way, so that the client can talk and you can listen. You must begin by taking steps to create an atmosphere that is conducive to free-flowing conversation.

SETTING THE TONE

Place

In order to devote your full attention to the work at hand, you and your client must be physically at ease. Choose a quiet place for the interview where you are likely to have as few interruptions as possible. Ideally, this will be a place where you cannot be overheard, so that the client will feel free to discuss confidential matters, and so that noises will not distract either of you.

Meeting the Client

You may be the first person to whom your client has come for help. New clients almost certainly will be anxious about talking to a stranger. They are likely to be worried by their symptoms and apprehensive about what your assessment will be. They may feel embarrassed about personal matters that must be discussed in the interview. Thus, clients are made vulnerable not only by the problems for which they seek help, but also by the very nature of the encounter with you. To minimize these natural feelings on the part of new clients, you must make a special effort to put them at ease and treat them with particular courtesy.

Upon meeting each new client, shake hands and introduce yourself. It is always appropriate to use formal address (Mr., Ms., Mrs.), both as a courtesy to the client and as part of professional decorum. Initially, you may be tempted to put yourself and your clients on a first-name basis, but this usually hinders, rather than helps, a professional therapeutic relationship. After all, since this is your first encounter, the client has not previously granted you the privilege of using his or her first name, and your doing so will seem presumptuous. Moreover, in using familiar forms of address, you convey the impression that the interview is something other than a professional encounter. Since clients are about to reveal intimate information about themselves, your professional attitude will be reassuring to them. You can convey warmth and concern without using terms that imply that you are close friends. Of course, children and adolescents are exceptions to this rule, as it is customary to call them by their first names in business as well as in social settings.

Invite your client to sit down. If the client is offered a choice of seats, note whether he or she sits near to or far from you. Chairs should be arranged comfortably for conversation. And you should sit so as to feel physically relaxed. If you are comfortable, you will be better able to listen, and your relaxed appearance will help put the client more at ease.

Initiate and maintain eye contact, but don't overdo it. A fixed stare is bound to disquiet your client. You will find that varied eye contact will be most effective in establishing rapport. Take notes if you feel comfortable doing so. Should the client ask about your note taking, you should explore his or her concerns about the confidentiality of your meetings, and you can use the opportunity to reassure the client that privacy will be respected.

Time

Let the client know at the outset how much time there is to talk. Traditionally, psychotherapy interviews last 45 to 50 minutes. Of course, some evaluation interviews require more time than this (such as an emergency room consultation), while very agitated clients may not tolerate a meeting lasting longer than a few minutes.

Be prompt for any arranged meeting with a client. If you must be late for a first meeting, an apology is in order. If you are late for subsequent meetings, you should listen for the client's reaction (anger, hurt, relief). You should also examine your own feelings if you are repeatedly late for meetings with a particular client; uncharacteristic lateness on your part may be a reflection of unresolved problems between yourself and the client (such as when a client makes you feel helpless or incompetent).

Note how the client uses time. For example, some clients will arrive far in advance of their appointments. Others will arrive late, and you will want to pay close attention to lateness as a possible indication that your client has some feeling about meeting with you that he or she is not directly expressing (e.g., anger at you, or fear of discussing a painful subject in the interview). When clients arrive late and apologize, do not reassure them that lateness is "OK." Instead, inquire about the circumstances. Obviously, lateness is sometimes unavoidable, especially for someone trying to find the way to an unfamiliar location. But often excuses will be vague ("I forgot to set my alarm clock," "I was engrossed in work and forgot the time") and indicate a lack of attention on the client's part or ambivalence about seeing you. So you may want to ask, "How did you feel about coming today?" to elicit the client's feelings about the interview. Remember: if people truly want to be on time, they can almost always manage. Be sure to end the session on time regardless of when it began, so that your clients will see that it is not in their interest to arrive late.

Defining the Goals of the Interview

A simple statement at the beginning about the length and purpose of the interview will set the stage for your evaluation. Be sure your client understands from the outset the reason for your meeting (e.g., to evaluate the problems brought to you by the client and to determine what interventions, if any, would be of help). Discuss how many meetings the client will have with you, and whether you are likely to continue seeing the client when the evaluation is finished or refer the client to someone else for treatment. This is especially important if you are spending a short period of time in a hospital or outpatient clinic as part of your training. Your clients will develop feelings for you (often, feelings of attachment and trust) as they tell you about their lives and problems. They must be prepared to lose their relationship with you when your work together is finished or when you leave this particular assignment.

YOUR INTERVIEWING STYLE: HELPING YOUR CLIENT TELL YOU WHAT IS WRONG

All of us are likely to have preconceived notions about mental health professionals. Stereotypically, they are cold and distant people who never speak during encounters except to ask a question and who remain unmoved by a client's distress. Yet, working with people who are in pain and emotional distress can be a very moving experience. In your first few interviews, you may feel as if you were having an intimate discussion with a close friend.

A good clinical interview is not a cold interrogation, nor is it a friendly chat, for neither style offers the client the security and the freedom to speak openly about intimate problems. Effective interviewing is not stilted or artificial; in fact, it may even sound like everyday conversation. But interviewing differs from daily discourse in that it is specifically designed to give the client as many opportunities as possible to tell the interviewer what is wrong. The specific techniques discussed below can help you to do just that.

Interviewing Techniques

Opening the interview. Once you have introduced yourself and agreed upon the purpose of the meeting, ask a general question that allows your client to begin wherever he or she chooses. You might begin with, "What brings you to see me today?" or "Can you tell me what has been troubling you?"

If a client seems very anxious at the start of your interview and has difficulty responding to an open-ended question, you might ask some specific neutral questions concerning age, marital status, and living situation, to allow the client some time to get more comfortable.

Allow the interview to flow freely. Let clients describe the events of their lives in any order they choose. Your comments and questions should flow naturally from what the client says. Rather than jump from one topic to another, stay with the client—encourage him or her to elaborate on thoughts and feelings. Later in the interview, you can guide the client to fill in any gaps in the story without abruptly changing the subject. For example, if a client has spent the first half of the interview reviewing recent events, you might turn the conversation to the client's past with, "You mentioned your family, could you tell me more about your background?" If you keep in mind an outline of what needs to be covered, you can later rearrange what the client has said in an orderly form for your written report.

The inexperienced interviewer is often tempted to ask a prepared list of questions and follow a prescribed order in gathering information. However, this will simply restrict the client's options to tell you what is wrong, and this approach will give the impression that you are not really listening.

Provide structure for clients who have trouble ordering their thoughts. Some people—such as those suffering from severe anxiety or psychosis—may be confused by open-ended questions and may respond to them by rambling incoherently. In such cases, you must

Table 1–1. Some interviewing principles.

Allow the interview to flow freely rather than jumping from one topic to another.
Provide structure for clients who have trouble ordering their thoughts.
Phrase your questions to invite the client to talk.
Avoid leading questions.
Help clients to elaborate on thoughts and feelings.
Avoid jargon.
Use the client's words whenever possible.
Avoid asking questions that begin with "why?"
Take note of the client's strengths.

---

more actively structure the interview, both so that you can gather information about the client and so that the client does not become increasingly anxious and disorganized. A general question like, "Tell me about your background" is not likely to evoke a cogent response from such a client. Instead, you must show the client precisely where you want the interview to go, with specific questions such as, "What was your father's occupation?" and "How old were you when he died?" You may shift back and forth from a more-structured to a less-structured interviewing style as the interview proceeds; your goal is to tailor the specificity of your questions to your client's needs.

Phrase your questions to invite the client to talk. How you phrase questions will have an enormous impact on the information you gather. *Open questions* allow the client to elaborate; *closed questions,* which require short answers (often "yes" or "no"), leave little room for detail. Some examples:

Closed: Have you felt depressed for a long time?
Open: Can you tell me how you feel when you are depressed?

Closed: Are you from a large family?
Open: Tell me about your family.

Open questions help people reveal relationships between their symptoms and events in their lives. Closed questions keep the client quiet and make *you* do all the work. Using closed questions leaves you with the impossible task of knowing which out of possibly hundreds of closed questions will get to the root of the client's problems. And unless you prepare these questions ahead of the interview, you'll be compelled to concentrate so hard on thinking them up as you go that you will lose touch with what the client is saying.

Avoid leading questions. Like closed questions, leading questions are conversation-stoppers. They imply that you already know how the client feels. In the case of a man whose brother had just died, a typical leading question would be, "Did you feel sad when your brother died?"

This question sends a clear message that you expect the client to feel sad. In fact, the client may have hated his brother, and must then confront the choice of challenging your expectation or concealing his real feelings. The obvious nonleading question in this instance would be, "How did you feel when your brother died?"

In short, don't assume that clients will react to events as you do. Leave them ample opportunity to explain how they really feel.

Help clients to elaborate. When clients seem to run out of steam or come to a stopping point, a nod may suffice to show them that you are eager to hear more. Or you may offer an encouraging comment like, "Tell me more about that," "Please go on," "Oh?" or "And?"

You may also echo a key word or phrase from the client's statement. For example, if the client said, "My wife thinks I'm impossible to live with," you could say, "Impossible to live with?"

You may want to help the client focus on feelings. For example, you could ask, "How did you feel about that?" or "How did you feel when that happened?"

And to get the client to be more specific when he or she is speaking in generalities, you could ask, "Can you give me a specific example?" or "What do you mean when you say 'crazy'?"

Reflect your clients' feelings back to them. This technique involves echoing the *tone* the client has conveyed. This helps in two ways. First, when you show clients that you are trying to understand how they feel, you communicate your concern and thereby encourage them to open up. Second, reflecting clients' feelings in this way serves to test your own perceptions—that is, to confirm or deny that you have understood. Here are some examples:

Client: I can't seem to accomplish anything. Nothing has worked out for me in my life. Why should I expect the future to be different?
Interviewer: You seem pretty discouraged.

Client:　　It just isn't fair. My husband walked out and left me flat. He had no right.
Interviewer: You sound pretty angry with him.

When you do correctly verbalize clients' feelings, they will confirm it by elaborating further. You may help them in this way to see their feelings more clearly. But if you have not understood your clients, they will then have a chance to correct you.

Remember: reflecting the client's tone does not involve *sympathy.* Avoid making statements like, "Your story makes me feel terrible," or "That's absolutely awful!" Your goal is *empathy,* which means understanding how the other person feels, and not necessarily sharing those feelings.

Paraphrase the client's thoughts. This technique is similar to reflecting the client's feelings, but focuses on ideas more than emotions. Like reflecting feelings, paraphrasing the client's thoughts lets the client know that you are listening and trying to understand. It provides a check on your perceptions, and helps the client clarify his or her comments. Examples of paraphrasing include the following:

Client:　　That medicine I'm taking is no good.
Interviewer: You mean, when you took it you did not feel better?

Client:　　I come in here and talk to you, but what good is it doing me?
Interviewer: You're wondering whether our talks have helped you.

Another useful technique is *summarization*—recapitulating and condensing what the client has said. Summarization encompasses both thoughts and feelings. It is similar to reflecting feelings and paraphrasing, but summarizing allows you to cover more material or a longer time span. The following are a few instances in which summarizing may help clarify what the client has said:

• When the client's discussion has been long-winded, rambling, or confusing.
• When the client appears to have talked about everything important on a specific subject.
• When you want to ensure that you and the client have a mutual understanding of what has been discussed so far, so that you may move on to other matters.

- When you want to highlight certain ideas or events that you believe to be particularly important.

Here are some examples of summarization:

Interviewer: So for the past three months you have been hearing your dead mother's voice tell you that you should kill yourself. Since this began, you have been unable to go to work and have refused to leave your bedroom.

Interviewer: So you have felt depressed ever since your brother became ill, and for the past several days you have had trouble falling asleep and have not felt like eating.

Additional Tips on Interviewing

Avoid jargon. Our daily language has become increasingly "psychologized" in recent years, but psychological jargon usually confuses rather than clarifies. Also, your use of jargon may make the client feel dehumanized. Clients themselves sometimes use jargon to avoid genuine feelings. For example, the client who "explains" his recent suicide attempt as "a temporary decompensation due to a reactive depression" has told you absolutely nothing about what prompted him to try to kill himself, or how he feels about it. Therefore, take care not to use jargon, and when clients (or colleagues) use it, be sure to ask them what they mean. Inexperienced interviewers are often reluctant to ask clients to explain such terms as "depression" or "psychosis." However, if you ask for such explanations, you will be surprised at the many meanings offered. In addition, you will begin to understand more about your client's particular language.

Be careful, too, about assigning a diagnostic label to the client's problem during the interview. Such labels are rarely of any use to the client at this point and may be frightening or confusing.

Use the client's words as frequently as possible, rather than your own. This is particularly important, for example, in dealing with sexual matters, in which the different ways people use to describe their experiences are practically infinite. If a client says that he or she is "gay," use the client's term during the interview rather than a word like "homosexual," which may have different connotations for the client. Of course, if a client should use a self-denigrating term, like "queer," you might want to note the client's word choice and substitute a more neutral choice of words in your own speech. The principle of using the client's terminology applies to virtually all subjects, but particularly to matters about which the client is likely to be sensitive.

Avoid asking questions that begin with "why." Clients do not usually know "why," and asking implies that you expect them to produce facile explanations. With your help, clients will discover more about the roots of their problems as they reflect upon their lives during the interview and in subsequent sessions. When you are tempted to ask "why," rephrase your question so that it elicits a detailed response, such as, "What happened?" "How did that come about?" or "What thoughts do you have about that?"

Thoughts versus feelings. In the interview, most people will use a mixture of ideas and emotions to paint a picture of their lives. However, some people keep a tight rein on their emotions and will dwell exclusively on ideas and explanations—that is, they will intellectualize to protect themselves from uncomfortable feelings. With such people, it is very helpful to emphasize emotion in your interview by asking how they *feel*. Conversely, other people deal with problems and anxiety almost exclusively in emotional terms, such as, "Oh, I get so upset I just can't think straight." For them, it helps to emphasize their capacity to think by asking questions like, "What do you think about that?"

Often, the client's immediate response to a difficult or anxiety-provoking question is, "I don't know." Rather than immediately asking another question, you may get more information if you just sit quietly after an "I don't know" response, or ask the client, "What comes to mind?" and see what happens.

Sensitive subjects should be approached tactfully but not avoided. After initially refusing, the client may discuss difficult or embarrassing material if you rephrase your question or return to the topic at a later time.

Take note of the client's strengths. People seek mental health care because they have problems, and these often obscure positive personality traits and accomplishments. If you listen for strengths and show interest in them, you will convey to your clients a sense that you want to get a balanced view of their situation. If clients do not offer any examples of how they feel good about themselves, you might ask, "What are you proud of?" or "What do you like about yourself?" The reply will give you important information about self-esteem.

Humor. Humor can be a wonderful tool in building an alliance with your client. Be careful, though, for it can backfire. Clients may use humor defensively to avoid unpleasant feelings or to keep you amused. Your own use of humor may be misunderstood as ridicule. The key is to stay in tune with how your client is feeling—and when you're not sure of those feelings, ask.

Keep track of where the interview is going. While it is important to allow clients to tell their stories as they choose, the time in which you must complete the evaluation is usually limited. Thus, you should not hesitate to guide clients to more relevant matters if they ramble or repeat themselves. Keep track of time, so that you have a chance at the end of the interview to ask about topics that may have been ignored or that need to be explored further.

YOUR REACTIONS TO THE CLIENT

In the clinical interview, you are your own best and most important diagnostic instrument. Thus, your emotional reactions to the client constitute invaluable data. Your reactions not only tell you how the client makes others feel, but they may tell you how the client feels behind all of his or her defenses (for example, the helplessness you feel in talking with a woman who intends to commit suicide may reflect her sense of helplessness in the face of intolerable emotional pain). If the client awakens in you strong feelings of anger, depression, sexual arousal, or anxiety that you do not acknowledge, you may be rendered incapable of effective listening and may miss key aspects of the client's problem.

Anxiety is probably the most common obstacle to effective listening. It is only natural to be somewhat anxious as a beginning interviewer. But sometimes particular clients (such as threatening ones) or particular topics (such as suicide) arouse so much anxiety that the interviewer screens out anxiety-provoking information. For example, when a depressed client speaks casually of having a loaded gun in the house, the interviewer may become so frightened that he or she does not hear what has been said, or minimizes the seriousness of the situation. The anxious interviewer may even unwittingly change the subject and leave the client's suicidal thoughts unexplored. If you allow yourself to be aware of your anxiety and examine its source, you will be much less likely to retreat from difficult subjects during the interview. (For more detailed discussion of anxiety in dealing with violent clients, see Chapter 14.)

Identifying with the client is another common occurrence among inexperienced interviewers, and this can hinder an accurate assessment of the client's problems. You may mistakenly assume that you share certain feelings or experiences with your client. This assumption could distort the facts and hamper your work, as in the following case example:

> A young man seeks a psychological evaluation at his college health service, complaining that he can never complete his term papers on time, and that he is in jeopardy of flunking out of college. The psychologist, an intern, comments to the client that she, too, had difficulty completing assignments on time during college and graduate school. She assumes that she and her client are alike in this respect; that his symptom, like hers, is confined to his schoolwork, that he will "grow out of it," and that his fears of academic failure are exaggerated. The intern reassures him that the problem is not serious and sends him home.

In this case, the intern has failed to learn that her client procrastinates in every area of his life: He is routinely late for appointments, never pays bills on time, and always keeps his dates waiting (apologizing profusely for his lateness when he finally arrives). His problem is much more pervasive than hers, and causes him to be much more dysfunctional.

In addition, the intern does not recognize that their respective symptoms have very different roots. The intern struggles with her concerns about surpassing her mother in terms of professional education and advancement, and her trouble meeting deadlines in her work reflects a conflict between her wish to excel and her fear of losing her mother's love if she does. The undergraduate, by contrast, is caught in a more global struggle to exert control over all aspects of his life, and he stubbornly refuses to submit to what he sees as other people's demands. Because she has mistakenly equated her client's situation with her own, the intern does not get an accurate picture of this man's problem, and she intervenes in a way that is not likely to be helpful.

When you start to feel that you and your client are in some way alike, tread carefully. Make sure you differentiate what you know about yourself from what you know about your client. As a general rule, avoid talking about your own life. Doing so usually diverts the focus from the client's problems.

Avoid premature reassurance. You may be tempted to allay the client's fears with such assurances as, "Everything will be fine" or "There is nothing seriously wrong with you." However, reassurance is only genuine when 1) you have explored the precise nature and extent of the client's fears, and 2) you are certain of what you are telling the client. Premature reassurance can actually heighten the client's anxiety, by giving the impression that you have jumped to a conclusion without doing a thorough evaluation, or that you are just saying what you think the client wants to hear. It also leaves the client alone with his or her fears about what is "really" wrong. Instead of minimizing these fears, try to find out more about them. When, for example, the client expresses fears of being incurable, you might explore this area with an open-ended question: "What do you mean by incurable?" Or you might say, "You seem quite worried about this. Tell me more about it."

Address what is going on in the room. If the client speaks incoherently, for example, or is actively hallucinating in your office, it will most likely be a relief to both of you if you acknowledge the client's distress and try to clarify what you do not understand. Even the most disorganized clients often know when they are not making sense. If you are confused, say so.

Set limits on inappropriate behavior. Although understanding is your goal in the interview, there are times when you must simply put a stop to what the client is doing. This includes threats and menacing behavior, refusal to leave the office, and disruptive behavior in the office or waiting area. When, for example, a manic individual wants to remove his clothing, or an angry client threatens to throw an ashtray through your office window, you must put a stop to such behavior before you can go on with the interview. You might acknowledge the client's distress with a comment like, "You seem to be having difficulty controlling yourself. We'll have to stop our meeting until you are able to sit quietly again." As discussed in more detail in Chapter 14 (Violence), you should never continue an interview when you feel that you or the client may be physically harmed. If a client's behavior becomes unmanageable, do not hesitate to stop what you are doing and summon help.

CLOSING THE INTERVIEW

As the interview comes to a close, leave a few minutes for any comments or questions that the client has yet to voice. Often, clients will save critical information or profound concerns for the end of the session.

You might signal the close of the interview with a question such as, "In the minutes remaining, is there anything you'd like to add?" or "Is there anything else you think I should know?"

Also, ask your client if he or she has any questions for you. People are understandably anxious about their problems, and may ask you such questions as "What do you think is wrong?" or "So tell me, can you help me?"

Obviously, there are no pat answers to such questions, in part because the feelings and fears that prompt them are unique to each client. Your job is to provide as straightforward a reply as possible. And don't be afraid to admit that you do not yet know the answer, and that it may take more time to fully understand your client's problems. In the long run, a relationship built on honesty will be much more beneficial than one based on false reassurance.

This chapter has focused on the fundamentals of conducting a clinical interview. Chapter 2 will give you an overview of the psychodynamic principles of mental functioning and normal human development. You will need this psychological framework in order to make sense of what your clients tell you about their lives.

REFERENCES

MacKinnon RA, Michaels R: The Psychiatric Interview in Clinical Practice. Philadelphia, WB Saunders, 1971

Nicholi AM Jr (ed): The Harvard Guide to Modern Psychiatry. Cambridge, Mass, Harvard University Press, 1978, pp 3-40 (Chapter 1 contains a general discussion of interviewing technique and the doctor-patient relationship.)

Sullivan HS: The Psychiatric Interview. New York, WW Norton, 1954

Chapter 2

Psychodynamics: Some Basic Concepts

Psychodynamics refers to the study of mental forces and how they motivate behavior. For thousands of years, human beings have struggled to elucidate and schematize the nature of mental life, and a great many models of the mind have been put forward.

Modern psychodynamic theory is founded on the work of Sigmund Freud (1856–1939). His ideas about mental structure and functioning have been widely applied clinically to help understand and relieve many of the symptoms of the mentally ill.

Freud has been a controversial figure in Western culture for nearly a century, and his ideas continue to be closely scrutinized and hotly debated among thinkers in virtually all areas of the social and biological sciences. But Freud's work did not arise out of a vacuum, and was in many respects evolutionary rather than revolutionary. Specifically, Freud incorporated the concepts of many important eighteenth and nineteenth century theorists into his schemata of mental life. There is much that remains controversial in Freud's work, and—as he himself was quick to point out—much that is in need of revision. Nevertheless, Freud's ideas have profoundly influenced our way of thinking about the human mind and human behavior. His concepts have permeated virtually every aspect of our culture including the arts, politics, philosophy, and education.

This chapter does not attempt to teach Freudian psychology, but only to define some of the "household words" in the language of psychodynamics that you are bound to encounter in your clinical work. To the student who has had no prior clinical experience in mental health, psychodynamic theories will likely seem confusing and even nonsensical. Phrases like "the unconscious mind" and "oedipal rivalries" may seem, to the uninitiated, abstract and removed from real experience. But psychodynamic concepts are best learned not from books, but by talking with clients, watching others perform interviews, and discussing your clinical experiences with colleagues and supervisors. Once you have developed a curiosity about the forces that cause your clients emotional distress, you will be much more likely to find the psychodynamic theories of Freud and others to be intelligible, helpful, and even exciting.

MAPS OF THE MIND

Freud put forth two major models for understanding mental life: the topographic model and the tripartite model. Modern psychodynamic theory rests on both of these.

The Topographic Model: Conscious/Preconscious/Unconscious

The discovery of the unconscious may well be Freud's most important contribution to modern thought. The idea that each of us has an ongoing mental life that operates *without our awareness* is an astounding concept. Freud first presented this idea in 1900, in *The Interpretation of Dreams*, in order to explain such phenomena as the forgetting of dreams and our ability in dreams to recall hitherto forgotten events from early life.

His topographic model divides the mind into three "agencies," based on the extent to which the thoughts, feelings, and perceptions in each agency are accessible to our awareness. These agencies of the mind are not tangible—they do not occupy physical space in the brain—but are simply metaphors; that is, they are theoretical constructs that help us organize our clinical observations.

The *conscious* includes all thoughts and feelings we are aware of, including sensory input from the environment as well as input from "within"—i.e., from the preconscious.

The *preconscious* contains all those ideas, feelings, and memories available to us when we choose to focus attention on them. For example, most of us do not maintain the threat of nuclear war in the forefront of consciousness, but the thought is available when we choose to focus on it. A primary function of the preconscious is to censor—to police our psyche and to prevent unconscious thoughts that might generate anxiety from reaching consciousness. The censor operates either by completely blocking access of unconscious material to consciousness, or by disguising unconscious material so that the conscious mind cannot recognize it.

For example, a young girl's unconscious sexual longing for her father would arouse considerable anxiety if she became aware of it, so her censor represses her incestuous impulses. The censor may block these sexual feelings entirely, or disguise them as their opposite—i.e., as hatred. In the latter case, the girl would be using the defense of *reaction formation* (see below), and would be aware only of an aversion for her father. Her sexual yearnings would remain buried in the unconscious.

The *unconscious* contains ideas, impulses, feelings, and fantasies that lie out of reach of the conscious mind and cannot be made conscious by focusing one's attention. This material has been banished from awareness—i.e., it has been repressed because it is in some way unacceptable, as in the example noted above. Unconscious material may reach consciousness when the censor is relaxed, as in dreams, or when it is overpowered and neurotic symptoms result. (For example, if the young girl's repressed incestuous impulses toward her father intensified, she might develop a conscious reaction against these impulses that took the form of a snake phobia.)

Along with these three aspects of the mind, Freud's topographic model includes two types of thought processes—primary process and secondary process.

Secondary Process
Secondary process is the mode of thinking with which we are most familiar. Our conscious and preconscious mental activities are carried out in secondary process thought, which makes sense to us and to the people with whom we communicate. It is logical, it is not filled with gross inconsistencies, and it is relatively well organized. Secondary process thought is governed by the *reality principle*—i.e., it respects the constraints of the real world. Thus, for example, the rules of secondary process dictate that today cannot be yesterday or tomorrow, and one cannot be in two places at once. These are, of course, statements of the obvious, and secondary process seems obvious because it appears to most of us that this is the only type of thinking

we do. But there is another type—primary process—that is strikingly different.

Primary Process

Primary process is unorganized mental activity that seems foreign to us because it operates primarily in the unconscious. Primary process thinking does not respect logic, contains no sense of time, allows for blatant contradictions and inconsistencies, and aims at immediate gratification without regard for the demands of the real world. Dreams are the best examples of primary process thinking. (For example, in a dream you may be five years old but also a college student, the year may be 1993, and your professor may look exactly like your mother.) The rules of logic do not apply in primary process thinking, but certain other mechanisms operate to make primary process seem bizarre to our conscious minds. The most important of these mechanisms are listed below:

Symbolism: An object or idea comes to signify something else—based on a resemblance between the original and its substitute (e.g., a banana may symbolize a penis).

Condensation: Several concepts or objects become fused in a single symbol (e.g., one's father, boss, and minister may become the same person in a dream).

Displacement: Emotions, ideas, or wishes are transferred from their original substitute (e.g., anger might be displaced from a parent to a teacher).

Dreams exhibit all of these characteristics, and this is why a dream often seems like nonsense after you wake up. Also, in your clinical work you will likely be able to detect primary process in the speech of severely psychotic people, whose ability to censor unconscious material is impaired.

Primary process is a normal part of conscious mental activity in children below the age of five. For example, young children commonly use *magical thinking,* i.e., they equate thinking with doing, and believe that their wishes actually define what is real. Hence, a child may believe that wishing someone dead will make it happen. As children grow, they become increasingly aware of the relationship between fantasy and reality and cease to use magical thinking. Other primary process modes of thought (such as denial) also gradually disappear under the pressures of the child's expanding knowledge of the real world.

The Tripartite Model: Id/Ego/Superego

Freud's topographic model categorized mental *content* according to whether or not it was available to consciousness, but this scheme did not account for the different types of mental *functions* that he encountered in his work with patients. Dividing the mind according to functions and forces, he devised the tripartite model of id, ego, and superego. Like the divisions of the topographic model, the id, ego, and superego are not concrete entities but metaphors that clinicians have found useful in differentiating one type of mental function from another.

Id

The *id* is the name given to our most basic biological drives and our most primitive impulses. The guiding force of the id is the *pleasure principle*—i.e., the tendency to demand immediate satisfaction of desires, seek immediate pleasure, and avoid pain. The id encompasses states of pain and rage; cravings of sexual longing, hunger, and thirst; and the drive for self-preservation.

Id impulses and instincts are for the most part unconscious. The aspects of instinctual drives that do reach our awareness have usually been censored—i.e., "laundered" to look more respectable to our conscious adult selves.

Ego

In everyday language, the word *ego* has come to refer to self-love or self-esteem. The psychological usage of the term, though, is quite different from this. The ego is the part of the personality that mediates between inner strivings and the realities of the world. It comprises all of those faculties of thought, feeling, perception, and action we use to harmonize the urges of the id with the requirements of the external environment and the inhibitions and aspirations of the superego (see below).

The ego strives to maintain mastery over the drives of the id, and it is the ego that delays gratification and substitutes more acceptable pleasures for less acceptable ones. The ego contains the compromising, evaluating, puzzle-solving, and defense-creating aspects of the personality. Ego functions are largely, but not entirely, conscious.

The ego develops as the growing infant interacts with the environment—especially with parents and other caregivers. Ego development includes the acquisition of defensive maneuvers for self-protection, as well as intellectual functions like comprehension, judgment, and language. The mature individual with a healthy ego is someone who is flexible in handling various life stresses, rather than one who must repeatedly resort to inflexible, maladaptive behaviors under pressure.

Superego

The superego, like the ego and the id, is a metaphor. The fictional character who most closely personifies the superego is Jiminy Cricket, who sat on Pinocchio's shoulder and acted as his guardian of moral standards and promoter of personal ideals. Freud conceived of the self-critical faculties of the mind as constituting a separate psychic agency that observes and evaluates our thoughts, feelings, and actions, comparing actual ego functioning with ideal standards. The superego consists of what we commonly call the "conscience," as well as the standards known as the *ego ideal.*

Each of us develops an image of the person he or she would like to become. This "ideal image" is derived from the standards of behavior that we perceive in parents, teachers, and other important people in our childhood. The ego ideal is highly individual. It provides our inspiration to achieve and directs our strivings for gratification.

Children also adopt many of the prohibitions and obligations of parents and other important figures, by accepting parental dictates as demands of absolute obedience. This process by which parental standards and morality are incorporated into one's personality is a central part of superego formation and is thought to begin around the age of four to six years, and continue throughout life. As the child's social sphere expands, parental morality no longer seems absolute, while the standards of peer groups, teachers, and other admired figures take on new importance. Many, though not all, aspects of superego are conscious.

People who develop harsh and strict superegos are their own cruelest taskmasters. They are often rigid, inhibited, anxious, and very unhappy. Those with more tolerant superegos can be flexible and accept their limitations without giving in to impulses that violate their own or society's fundamental moral ideals.

The id, ego, and superego exist in a constantly changing relationship. A disturbance in the checks and balances of these three agencies often results in mental discomfort, unacceptable behavior, or both. The id and superego largely remain out of our awareness until they cause trouble—e.g., when an unacceptable instinctual impulse becomes conscious and arouses anxiety, or when criticism by the superego prompts feelings of guilt. The well-adjusted individual makes compromises intuitively that resolve conflicts among id, ego, and superego.

PSYCHOSEXUAL DEVELOPMENT

Freud postulated the existence of two basic human drives: libidinal instincts and aggressive instincts. *Libido* refers to sexual energy, though the term is also used more broadly to refer to all strivings for pleasurable experience. He put forth the idea that the child's strivings for pleasure are organized and modified in a series of developmental stages. In each stage, the child has particular needs to be met and problems to be solved.

According to Freud, the way we negotiate each of these stages is crucial, for "unfinished business" from any one stage is carried with us as development proceeds, and can become a source of psychopathology in adult life. The stages of psychosexual development are briefly outlined in Table 2-1 and described below. The timetable for these stages is only a crude approximation, since each child develops at his or her unique pace.

Oral Stage (Birth to 18 Months)

The newborn infant needs total care, and so must immediately begin to form relationships with other human beings. The mouth is the part of the body through which pleasure is secured and hunger satisfied. The mouth thus becomes the focus for a variety of the infant's sensations, interests, and activities. Because of its pleasure-giving potential at this stage, the mouth is spoken of as an *erogenous zone*. The infant's primary relationship is, in most cases, with the mother, although "good mothering" at this stage may actually come from any caregiver(s), male or female, whose attention to the infant is warm and consistent. Such caring lays the foundation for a sense of security and basic trust in others that the infant will carry into later life, while a lack of caring may establish a deeply rooted sense of mistrust and insecurity.

The infant must learn to tolerate frustration when his or her urgent demands are not instantly met. Contact with the mother cannot ever be as immediately or constantly gratifying as the infant would wish, and the child must cry in order to make certain needs known. This frustration, if not unduly prolonged, prompts the infant to develop healthy self-soothing techniques and defense mechanisms that protect against overwhelming excitement and rage. It also helps

Table 2–1. The stages of psychosexual development.

Stage	Age	Description
Oral	0 to 18 months	The mouth is the focus for sensations and activities. "Good mothering" now lays the foundation for a sense of security and basic trust in others.
Anal	1½ to 2½ years	The child finds pleasure in experiencing control over bodily needs. This period ideally fosters self-control, independence, the ability to give, and personal pride.
Phallic	2½ to 4 years	The focus of attention shifts to the genitals. The child begins to explore the world more autonomously and learns to take pride in his or her abilities. This stage is crucial in developing a stable sense of self-worth.
Oedipal	4 to 6 years	The child longs for a special relationship with the parent of the opposite sex and has feelings of jealousy and hostility for the parent of the same sex. Resolution requires development of a special relationship with the same-sex parent.
Latency	6 to 12 years	The child masters physical, intellectual, and social skills; identifies with those of the same sex; and learns mastery of impulses.
Adolescence	Teen years	Physical maturation heightens interest in sexual activities. The adolescent is preoccupied with personal identity and how others perceive him or her. The adolescent ideally assumes more responsibilities for self-control and self-direction.

the infant differentiate between self and others, as it becomes clear that mother is a separate being who is not always present when the infant wants her.

We often label adult emotional states *infantile* if they are reminiscent of behavior at the oral stage of development, i.e., states characterized by urgent demands, extreme dependence, lack of responsibility for or consideration of others, and a very low tolerance for frustration. People with such characteristics are said to have *oral personalities*, and they are commonly preoccupied with fantasies and needs that focus on the mouth.

Anal Stage (1½ to 2½ Years Old)

As the infant's nervous system matures, it becomes possible to recognize and control the need to eliminate. This is a pleasurable experience for the child, both because of a growing awareness of the sensations involved in the excretory functions, and because of the new experience of control over bodily needs. During toilet training, the child and the parent interact around the child's control of bowel and bladder function, and this interaction is thought to influence later personality traits.

The child must make compromises between primitive wishes to do whatever he or she pleases, and the rewards obtained by conforming to the demands of important caregivers. Ideally, this period fosters the beginnings of self-control, independence, the ability to give, and a sense of personal pride. However, if toilet training is harsh and the parents are punitive, the child may develop strong attitudes of shame and disgust, and be both fearful of and enraged at controlling caregivers. In later life, these unresolved problems of self-control may manifest themselves as rigid behavior patterns. The four classic traits of the *anal character* are aptly described by the following mnemonic:

Parsimony,
Orderliness,
Obstinacy, and
Punctuality.

Obviously, toilet training is only one of the areas of childhood experience in which issues of self-control and societal expectation emerge. It has become a symbol in our culture for a developmental step that all children must take in the process of becoming social beings.

Phallic Stage (2½ to 4 Years Old)

The focus of the child's attention gradually shifts from the mouth to the anus to the genitals. At this stage, the penis or clitoris is a "new" discovery and a source of pleasure. The differences between the sexes become more discernible to children at this age, promoting the beginnings of identification as male or female. In addition, the child's increasing motor and intellectual capacities make it possible to explore, to be curious, and to take initiative and pride in solving simple problems. Ideally, parents greet such initiatives with pleasure, which mirrors the child's own sense of accomplishment, while setting realistic limits on the child's sense of his or her unlimited power (e.g., not letting the toddler run into the street). This stage is thought to be crucial in developing a stable sense of self-worth—i.e., that one is an attractive and lovable human being.

Psychoanalytic theorists trace many of the origins of narcissistic personality disturbance to problems in the phallic stage of development. They posit that children whose self-esteem does not consolidate during this stage develop into adults who are plagued by persistent feelings of inferiority, extreme sensitivity to perceived slights or insults, and constant excessive reliance on the responses of others as measures of their worth.

Oedipal Stage (4 to 6 Years Old)

Oedipus, you will recall, was the tragic hero of Sophocles' drama about a man who unwittingly murdered his father and married his mother. According to Freud, this Greek classic has remained compelling to audiences for centuries because it recaptures a fantasy that children experience and subsequently repress.

The *Oedipus complex* refers to the child's increasing longings for a special relationship with the parent of the opposite sex. Along with these longings go feelings of jealousy and rivalrous hostility toward the "competition"—i.e., the parent of the same sex. Thus, little boys feel as if they are competing with father for mother's love, and little girls see mother as a rival for father's affections.

Children at this stage both hope and fear that their murderous and incestuous wishes will come true. Because they cannot yet differentiate clearly between fact and fantasy, children develop the concern that their wishes will hurt their rival, and that the rival will retaliate. This is the fear that psychoanalytic theorists refer to as *castration anxiety.*

How does the child resolve this romantic dilemma? The normal resolution to the Oedipus complex involves recognizing that this incestuous pursuit is futile, and giving it up in favor of a special relationship with the same-sex parent. The child identifies with the rival and adopts many of the same-sex parent's goals, standards, and behaviors. Instead of wanting to marry mother, the little boy settles for growing up to be like father and marrying a woman who is like mother. For little girls, the process is similar, but at present there is great controversy among psychological theorists about how little girls deal with the Oedipus complex.

Resolving the Oedipus complex requires that the child, to some extent, begin to identify with the parent of the *opposite* sex. Thus, the little girl who cannot "have" Daddy can be partly satisfied by becoming like Daddy in some respects—e.g., by adopting certain of her father's interests or attitudes. Children normally emerge from the oedipal stage having identifications with both parents.

People who develop neurotic symptoms are thought to have been unable to successfully resolve the Oedipus complex. Thus, you will often hear the term "oedipal" used synonymously with "neurotic." By contrast, the term *pre-oedipal* (or *pre-genital*) is reserved for more severe illnesses like personality disorders and psychoses, implying that these more severe disturbances originate in the oral, anal, or phallic stages of development.

Latency Stage (6 to 12 Years Old)

The term *latency* refers to Freud's observation that sexual curiosity seemed to become dormant or latent during this period, to reemerge in adolescence with renewed force. However, the term is something of a misnomer in that sexual interests do not disappear during this phase, but remain present throughout childhood.

Latency is a time for mastering a host of physical, intellectual, and social skills. The child's world enlarges beyond the nuclear family to include school and other activities outside the home. This affords the opportunity to identify with new role models—e.g., teachers, peers—and to modify or solidify behavior patterns learned in the family. In this period, the child normally identifies strongly with those of the same sex. The emphasis is on learning social skills and mastering one's own impulses—hence the latency-age child's fascination with games that have elaborate rules and rituals (e.g., hopscotch, "tag"). The child learns about the pleasures and pains inherent in dealing with peers. Failure to conform to peer-group standards can result in ostracism and a sense of inferiority, but successful mastery of age-appropriate skills can foster a sense of pride and social acceptance.

Adolescence

The onset of puberty, with the rapid maturation of the genitals, stimulates a heightened interest in sexual activities. However, the adolescent's drive toward maturation is not confined to sexuality. Adolescents become preoccupied with personal identity and how they are perceived by others—hence the adolescent's concern that he or she dress, speak, and act "cool."

Standing on the threshold of independence from parents, adolescents identify strongly with groups of peers as a means of separating themselves from their families. They try out emancipatory behaviors (e.g., smoking, drinking, staying out late with friends), often rejecting many of the values and demands of their parents in favor of peer group mores. Courtship and first sexual activities normally occur during this phase. Ideally, the adolescent becomes freed from parental controls, while assuming more responsibility for self-control and self-direction. Adolescence lays the groundwork for mature sexual relationships based on mutual respect.

Development does not end with adolescence, of course, but continues throughout life. The preceding discussion is a very crude sketch of Freudian developmental theory. The process by which human beings mature is infinitely complex, and our understanding of it is far from complete.

MECHANISMS OF DEFENSE

Each of us uses a variety of techniques to relieve tension and shield ourselves from painful experiences. However, not all of our self-protective maneuvers are carried out consciously. Those techniques that we employ unconsciously to alleviate anxiety and eliminate conflict are termed *defense mechanisms*. The defenses listed in Table 2-2 and described below are among those most commonly encountered in clinical practice. The first 12 defense mechanisms are "immature" in that they may work to protect the person who uses them from distress, but they do so at a significant cost (e.g., by grossly distorting reality). The "mature" defenses do not require such distortions.

Repression, the fundamental mechanism of defense that underlies all others, is akin to forgetting. It involves forcing thoughts, memories, and feelings into the unconscious and actively keeping them out of awareness. Repression is responsible for lapses of memory (e.g.,

Table 2–2. Some common defense mechanisms.

Immature	Mature
Repression	Altruism
Denial	Humor
Retroflexion	Suppression
Acting out	Anticipation
Projection	Sublimation
Splitting	
Reaction formation	
Conversion	
Dissociation	
Displacement	
Intellectualization	
Isolation of affect	

forgetting the hour of a dreaded examination) or seemingly inexplicable naiveté. The apparent ignorance which results from repression is often accompanied by symbolic behavior that suggests that the repressed material is not really forgotten (e.g., the woman who is unaware of her sexual attraction to her therapist, but who dresses seductively for her appointments). Repression prevents us from recognizing our own thoughts and feelings, while *denial* prevents the recognition of external reality.

Denial involves disbelieving a fact of external reality in order to avoid pain or anxiety. Denial often results in grossly distorted thinking and behavior, as in the case of the man who refuses to accept the death of his wife and goes on "communicating" with her as though she were still alive. People commonly use denial to avoid recognizing the presence of serious physical illness, and may delay consulting a physician about ominous symptoms until it is too late (e.g., the woman who denies the growing lump in her breast for many months). Denial is not conscious—i.e., it involves more than simply pretending that something is not so. Unacceptable facts are banished from awareness entirely, and the individual has no access to them.

Retroflexion (turning against the self) is an unacceptable impulse or feeling (usually hostile) made acceptable by deflecting it from its original object back upon the self. This is most commonly seen among people who are labeled "depressive" or "masochistic" (e.g., the woman who berates herself for being a bad wife after she is abandoned by a physically abusive husband). *Hypochondriasis* is related to retroflexion, and involves transforming a reproach toward others into somatic complaints. It allows the individual to bemoan his or her condition in lieu of complaining about others.

Acting out is a term used too often and too loosely to describe any client's behavior that mental health professionals do not approve of. When used correctly, the term *acting out* refers specifically to the process of acting on an unconscious wish or impulse in order to avoid being aware of the emotion that accompanies it. In other words, action is used in the service of remaining unaware of intolerable feelings— e.g., a man who behaves with uncharacteristic promiscuity and who has no awareness of sexual longings for his therapist.

Projection is a process by which motives and feelings unacceptable to the self are unconsciously attributed to others instead. For example, a man who struggles to fend off his own unconscious homosexual impulses may complain, "Every man on the street makes homosexual advances toward me." Projection is used both by people whose thinking is grossly out of touch with reality (as in the example above), and by healthier individuals as well. Racial and other forms of prejudice are based on the use of projection.

Splitting involves dissociating positive and negative aspects of oneself and others, and compartmentalizing them into "all good" or "all bad" images. People who use splitting see themselves and others in black-and-white terms, dividing the world into "good guys" and "bad guys." This relieves the anxiety that comes with recognizing ambivalence—e.g., that one can be mad at someone one loves.

Reaction formation occurs when unacceptable unconscious impulses are disavowed and *opposite* conscious attitudes and behaviors are adopted. For example, a man whose strong sexual urges are severely repressed may lead a campaign for censorship of "salacious" literature in school libraries; a woman who unconsciously despises her children may smother them with undue affection.

Conversion takes the unconscious conflicts that would otherwise give rise to anxiety and instead gives them symbolic external expression through some bodily symptom—such as hysterical blindness or paralysis (e.g., a woman whose arm suddenly becomes paralyzed due to her unacceptable impulse to stab her unfaithful husband). Conversion is a major defense used in hysterical neurosis.

Dissociation involves a temporary but drastic modification of one's character or of one's sense of personal identity to avoid emotional distress. Examples of dissociation include such states as sleepwalking, amnesia, and multiple personality. Even acting in the theater may involve dissociation, as when it allows the actor a "safe" way to express instinctual wishes that would be unacceptable in real life.

Displacement redirects feelings from an original object to a more acceptable or less dangerous substitute. This defense is commonly found in everyday life—i.e., as when a man who is angry at his boss takes it out on his family.

Intellectualization involves thinking about instinctual wishes in affectively bland terms in order to avoid experiencing strong emotions.

Isolation of affect involves separating an idea from the feelings associated with it and generally banishing these feelings from consciousness. This defense is closely related to intellectualization. It is characteristic of people with obsessive-compulsive personality styles. People use isolation to protect themselves from emotions they find threatening or unacceptable—e.g., sexual or angry feelings. Thus, a man who is enraged at his wife may be totally unable to feel his anger, but finds himself preoccupied with emotionless, matter-of-fact thoughts about hurting her. While extensive reliance on isolation can hamper one's ability to form satisfying relationships and to experience life fully, isolation can be useful in certain situations. For example, health care professionals who routinely deal with people who are in pain usually need to isolate thoughts from feelings to prevent being overwhelmed and rendered incapable of performing their jobs.

All of us, when under stress, occasionally fall back on some of the defenses listed above. However, healthier individuals do not rely heavily on any of these, but instead allay anxiety and diminish intrapsychic conflict by using the following, more adaptive defenses.

Altruism involves constructive and instinctually gratifying service to others, including philanthropy and other activities from which one derives vicarious or more direct pleasure. Unlike reaction formation, altruism is gratifying to the person who uses the defense.

Humor facilitates our ability to express feelings and focus on anxiety-provoking thoughts without causing distress to ourselves or others. Forbidden wishes can be expressed in comic fashion and not acted upon.

Suppression involves a conscious decision to postpone paying attention to an unpleasant subject. This is in contrast to repression, which operates unconsciously and is therefore beyond conscious control. Suppression includes minimizing misfortunes, "keeping a stiff upper lip," and postponing *but not avoiding* difficult experiences. (Consider Scarlet O'Hara's famous line in *Gone with the Wind,* "I'll think about that tomorrow.")

Anticipation involves planning for future discomfort in a realistic fashion to effectively decrease anxiety, e.g., by carefully planning for an impending separation from a loved one.

Sublimation supports much of civilization. It consists in diverting unacceptable instinctual drives (e.g., sexual and aggressive impulses) into personally and socially acceptable channels. One common example is competitive sports, in which aggression is "tamed" and channeled, but not inhibited. Many artistic endeavors are thought to result from sublimated libidinal energies.

PSYCHODYNAMICS IN CLINICAL PRACTICE

What relevance do these maps of the mind, developmental stages, and mechanisms of defense have to your clinical work? After all, no one has ever seen an ego, or measured the size of an Oedipus complex. Yet despite their intangibility, psychodynamic concepts can be invaluable tools in helping you make sense out of symptoms and behaviors that might otherwise seem nonsensical. Indeed, Freud was among the first to advocate the idea that psychological symptoms (such as obsessions and phobias) have meaning, and that they represent the human mind's complex and often ingenious efforts at easing intrapsychic distress.

You will not often hear your clients talk directly about these concepts—about their defenses or their developmental problems—but you will hear "derivatives" of them. For example, a client is not likely to tell you about (or even to recall) his difficulties with a rigid and punitive parent around the issue of toilet training at age two. But you may see him replay this traumatic situation by struggling with a series of "unreasonable" bosses over his working conditions, or by struggling with you over whether or not he will pay his bill.

As you hear more about a client's life, you will discover recurring themes—like strains of music that thread through a symphony—and you can usually relate these themes to problems the client experienced at particular stages of development. In attempting to master issues not resolved in childhood, people continually recreate infantile problems in many areas of their adult lives. Much of psychotherapy, particularly in treating neuroses and personality disorders, consists of helping people to discover these "leftover" problems, along with the defenses used to keep from recognizing them.

Of course, Freud did not have the last word on concepts about mental functioning. Great advances continue to be made in our understanding of the human psyche. Ego psychology, object relations theory, and self-psychology are among the most important post-Freudian schools of thought that you are likely to encounter as you learn more about psychodynamic concepts. And as your understanding of psychodynamics deepens, your skill as a clinician will increase, regardless of the field of medicine you choose.

Psychodynamic concepts can be of great help to you in organizing the many details of a client's life story. Even in a single interview, you can learn enough to relate many of the recurrent problems in clients' adult lives to their childhood experiences, and begin to outline some of the defenses and psychological conflicts that cause or exacerbate their current distress. The next chapter discusses the process of taking a history, a process that will be greatly enhanced by your familiarity with the basic ideas about mental functioning discussed above.

REFERENCES

American Psychiatric Association: A Psychiatric Glossary, 5th ed. Washington, DC, American Psychiatric Association, 1980

Freud A: The Ego and the Mechanisms of Defense, rev. ed. New York, International Universities Press, 1966

Gedo JE, Goldberg A: Models of the Mind: A Psychoanalytic Theory. Chicago, University of Chicago Press, 1973 (An excellent review of psychoanalytic theories of mental structure and function, beginning with Freud.)

Kolb LC: Personality development, in Modern Clinical Psychiatry, 10th ed. Philadelphia, WB Saunders, 1983, pp 58-79 (An overview of human development, written from a psychoanalytic perspective.)

Nemiah JC: Foundations of Psychopathology. New York, Oxford University Press, 1961 (A general introduction to psychodynamic concepts, with lively case examples.)

Vaillant GE: Theoretical hierarchy of adaptive ego mechanisms. Arch Gen Psychiatry 24:107-118, 1971

CHAPTER 3

The Case History

This chapter deals with two separate but related tasks: taking a history, and reporting it to someone else. They are related, in that the information you gather in your interviews with the client provides the material for the case report. But that is the extent of their resemblance.

You can almost never adhere strictly to an outline in taking a mental health history. People do not talk about themselves in outline form, nor would you be an effective interviewer if you tried to force them to do so. You must keep an outline in your own mind, so that you will know which topics you want to cover in the course of your evaluation. But never use it as a checklist—this will only alienate your clients and limit the amount of information you can gather.

The outline of the case history presented in this chapter includes both a list of subjects to be covered in a mental health evaluation and some examples of interview questions that may help you explore these topics.

When reporting a mental health history, the history must be organized and presented in a way that gives readers (or listeners) a coherent picture of your client's current condition. Given that virtually any detail of the client's life may be relevant to his or her emotional state, you are likely to feel overwhelmed by the task of fitting all the information you have collected into a single presentation. It is therefore essential that you 1) pare down the history to include only those details you believe will help others understand your client's problems, and 2) adhere to an outline when you present a case verbally or in writing.

The case history is organized much like a standard medical history, as the outline in this chapter shows. In addition to familiarizing yourself with this outline, look at Appendix A, which contains a sample case report. This will give you a general idea of how a written evaluation is prepared. However, many mental health facilities have their own specific formats for these reports, and you should be sure that your evaluation summaries are consistent with the record-keeping system of the particular institution in which you work.

The initial evaluation summary is often the portion of the client's record that is most widely read—e.g., by new staff members coming to a ward or an outpatient clinic. The write-up therefore will be essential in communicating your client's situation to others. It should be clear, concise, and accurate. Beware of too much detail—after all, no one reads a 50-page treatise.

The outline included here is too detailed for most evaluations. You should take care to elaborate on aspects of the history that are germane to your client's current problems, but do not hesitate to cover less relevant categories in a cursory fashion. For example, if your client has a "negative" family history for mental illness, you need only write, "The client denies any history of mental illness or substance abuse in family members."

At a minimum, every area of the case history must be mentioned in every summary that you prepare. When in doubt about what to include in a case report, discuss your write-up with a supervisor—for both your own and the client's benefit.

OUTLINE FOR THE CASE HISTORY

The preparation of a case history should follow a standard outline (Table 3-1). The evaluation begins with a rough sketch of the client's situation. Identifying data such as age, sex, and occupation; the source of the client's referral to you; and the client's chief complaint orient your audience quickly to who the client is and why he or she has come to see you. Because these statements set the stage for the rest of the case report, they come first.

With this brief introduction, you have prepared your audience to learn about the client in depth. You begin with a description of the present problem, starting with its onset and proceeding chronologically to the date of your interview. You then place the client's current

Table 3–1. Organization of the case history.

Identifying data	Medical history
Referral source	Drug and alcohol history
Chief complaint	Mental status examination
History of the present problem	Formulation
Past history	Diagnostic impression
Family psychiatric history	Treatment plan

difficulties in the context of his or her childhood development and important formative experiences. (The description of the present problem and past history are usually the most detailed sections of the case report.) Information about the client's physical health, drug and alcohol use, and mental illness in family members completes the history.

The mental status examination—discussed in Chapter 4—is not actually part of the history. Rather, it is your description of the client as he or she appears and behaves in the interview. It is the mental health counterpart of a physical examination.

With all of this information in mind, your audience is then prepared to understand your assessment of the client's problems (the formulation of the case), your diagnostic impression, and your plan of treatment. By presenting the report in this order, you permit others to follow the thought processes that brought you to your conclusions about the case. Without such an outline, your report can easily become a barrage of disorganized detail in which you and your audience get lost.

Obtaining Identifying Data

Identifying data include:

- Name
- Age
- Marital status
- Sex
- Occupation
- Number of children
- Place of residence
- Number of previous admissions to psychiatric hospitals (if an inpatient).

This information alone can tell you much about the client's situation. For example, "This is the sixth psychiatric hospitalization for Mrs. Petrocelli, a 38-year-old divorced homemaker and mother of six who lives with her children in a Brooklyn apartment." Also detail the client's ethnic and religious background if this is particularly relevant to his or her current situation.

Referral Source

Find out how your client came to you, and you may learn something of his or her expectations. For example: "My brother says this is the best clinic in the state."

Chief Complaint

Ask the question "What brings you to see me?" to elicit the client's chief complaint. *In the client's own words,* record a one-sentence description of what is wrong.

History of the Present Problem

Where does the present problem begin? In many cases, the client will tell you, for example, "My wife died six months ago and I've been depressed ever since."

Determining when the client's current difficulties truly began is often difficult and requires some judgment about what may have precipitated his or her emotional distress. You may, for example, choose to date the onset of the present problem from the time a prominent symptom appeared (e.g., a first suicide attempt), from the date of a first psychiatric hospitalization, or from the time of a major personal loss (e.g., abandonment by a spouse). Whatever you decide, though, make sure to arrange the events of the history of the present problem in *chronological* order—that is, bring the reader (or listener) from the onset of the problem right up to the time the client came for help.

Explore in detail the client's chief complaint and other problems that hamper his or her life at present (Table 3-2). Note when these problems began, as well as how persistent they have been. Describe any prominent psychological symptoms (e.g., hallucinations, memory loss, panic attacks), and any mood changes reported by the client. Be particularly thorough in documenting previous suicidal or homicidal thoughts or acts. Pay attention to any physical symptoms that have been present during the illness. Determine the degree to which

Table 3–2. Exploration of current problems in the client's life.

Onset of problems (time, setting)
Duration and course (chronic vs. episodic)
Psychological symptoms
    Symptoms of psychosis
    Cognitive problems
    Mood changes (irritability, depression, elation)
Somatic symptoms
    Medical conditions
    Vegetative signs (loss of appetite, weight loss, insomnia, decreased energy, agitation or retardation of thought and action, decreased sexual energy and interest, mood worsens in morning and improves during day)
    Neurological symptoms
    Somatic complaints without physical basis
Severity of problems—degree of impairment in functioning
Possible precipitants

---

these problems have impaired the client's relationships with others and his or her ability to function at work. Also, note any circumstances in the client's life that may have precipitated the present crisis.

Map the Current Problems in the Client's Life

Onset of problems (time, setting). The time and setting of onset may not be clear (e.g., "I've been depressed all my life"), but this should be noted.

Duration of problems. Has the problem been present continuously or has it recurred intermittently?

Psychological symptoms. Describe in detail any disturbances of thought or perception that are central to the client's present problem. While such symptoms are reported in the mental status examination when the client actually exhibits them during the interview, they are included in the history of the present problem when they are part of the client's history (for example, "The client reports that for the last six months he has heard his dead father's voice commanding him to kill himself"). Note the following:

- Symptoms of psychosis, such as hallucinations, delusions, disassociative states, or ideas of reference.

- Cognitive problems, such as impaired memory or concentration.
- Mood changes, such as

Irritability: Rage, violent thoughts or acts. Techniques for exploring homicidal thoughts and fantasies are outlined in Chapter 14.

Depression: Guilt, hopelessness. Recent suicidal thoughts and acts should be reported in the history of the present problem. Techniques for exploring suicidal feelings are outlined in Chapter 13.

Elation: Outline extent of hyperactivity (for the symptoms of mania and hypomania, see Chapter 6).

Somatic symptoms. These include medical conditions that seem to be an integral part of the present problem. Describe the course of illness and any treatment (past and present). Note the following:

- Vegetative signs, such as anorexia (loss of appetite), weight loss, insomnia, energy, agitation or retardation, and decreased sexual energy and interest (see the section on Depression in Chapter 6).
- Neurologic symptoms, such as seizures or a recent head trauma.
- Somatic complaints with no known physical basis.

Severity of problems. To what extent have current problems interfered with the client's ability to work and to participate in relationships? Some clients are totally incapacitated by mental illness, while others function very well at daily tasks despite emotional distress.

Possible precipitants. Pay close attention to what was going on in the client's life at the time symptoms developed, and pay close attention to changes in important relationships (friends, lovers, family), job or financial situation, school performance, or physical health.

Always Try to Answer the Question "Why Now?"
What prompted the client to seek help this week rather than last week, this month rather than next month? Many times, the problem has been present for quite a while, but some key event in the client's life has upset an equilibrium and made life less tolerable.

For example, a woman comes to you seeking help for agoraphobia (a fear of being alone or on her own in public places), from which she has suffered for the past 12 years. During this time, she has been afraid to go out of the house unless accompanied by her husband, and cannot stay alone in the house unless she can speak to him by telephone at regular intervals while he is at work. Why does she seek help now, after 12 years? On close scrutiny, you discover that her husband is about to be promoted to a job that will require him to travel for several days each month, and the client is enraged that he is "abandoning" her.

Does the Client Know Anyone Who Has Had Similar Problems?

For example, you may discover that your 30-year-old depressed client has a mother who also became depressed at age 30. Identification of this kind often exists just outside the client's awareness. Yet it may be very important in determining the types of symptoms the client develops as well as when during the client's life these symptoms first take hold.

How Has the Client Dealt with These Problems to Date?

First, detail any efforts clients have made to cope on their own or get help from others. Then, mention the client's previous history of mental health care, if any. This includes psychotherapy, medications, hospitalization, along with the client's response to these treatments. How the client felt about previous therapists may give you clues to the kind of relationship he or she is likely to form with a therapist in the future.

PAST HISTORY

The past history summarizes the client's life, in chronological order, from infancy until the present problem began. Deciding which details of a client's past are pertinent to his or her current distress is not always easy. But two aspects of your client's early life are almost always relevant and deserve particular attention.

Relationships with Parents, Siblings, and Other Important People During Childhood

As is discussed in Chapter 15, our childhood relationships exert a powerful influence on how we deal with people as adults. In the case of the agoraphobic woman described above, you might discover that she had an intense attachment to her mother, that she felt herself to be like her mother in every way, and that she and mother were "inseparable pals" throughout her childhood.

Major Milestones in Growing Up

How we react as children to times of stress or separation from parents—starting school, at onset of puberty, leaving home—often carries over into our behavior under similar circumstances as adults. For example, it would not be surprising to discover that the agoraphobic woman was terrified of going to kindergarten and missed many days of school during the months it took her to overcome her fear. Nor would it be surprising to learn that at age 18 she turned down a scholarship to a college in another city, and did not leave her parents' home until she married at age 26.

Past history places the client's current problems in a broader context, helping you to see patterns of behavior that have persisted throughout the client's life. Thus, although most people seek mental health care because they are concerned about the present, it is worth your while to spend some time learning about the past in the course of your evaluation.

The points to be explored in a client's history are outlined in Table 3-3 and described more fully below. Bear in mind that there is more detail here than will be applicable to any one client's situation.

Table 3–3. Outline of the past history.

Family constellation (father, mother, siblings, others living at home)—
    important family relationships, major separations or losses

Infancy
    Birth order
    Birth history
    Developmental milestones

Childhood
    Health—hospitalizations
    Preschool years
    Starting school—academic performance
    Friendships

Adolescence
    Onset of puberty
    Early sexual experiences
    Peer relationships
    Experimentation with drugs, alcohol

Adulthood
    Education
    Military experience
    Employment
    Social life/friendship
    Romantic relationships
    Sexual history
    Marriage
    Children

Family Constellation

List age and occupation of the client's father, mother, siblings, and others living at home—relatives, babysitters, other caretakers. Describe their personalities and relationship with the client. Include disruptions in this relationship due to illness, death, or separation. Questions that may be helpful in eliciting this information include the following:

- Tell me about your family.
- Who took care of you when you were small?
- Who were you closest to in your family?
- Who do you feel you are most like among those in your family?

Infancy

The client's place in the family. A client's birth order can provide valuable clues about his or her family role (e.g., the "baby" or the "little mother"). Also inquire about how much attention clients received from parents and others (e.g., a mother with four children all under age six will obviously have less time and energy to devote to individual children than a mother of two). The birth of younger siblings is usually a major event in a child's life.

The client's birth history. Was the pregnancy planned or unplanned? Note any complications of pregnancy or delivery.

Developmental milestones. Did the client have difficulty in learning to walk or talk? Was the client considered by parents to be a "bright" or "slow" child? The client will not remember the early months of life, but what one has been told about birth and infancy becomes an important part of one's self-concept (e.g., "You were always a fussy, unhappy baby," or "You were smarter than every other kid in the neighborhood").

Childhood

Note any major family event—e.g., illness, death, divorce, separations, moves.

Preschool years. Note activities, caregivers, playmates. Helpful questions include "How far back can you remember?" and "What do you recall about your life before you started school?"

Health. Any hospitalizations? Note prolonged separation from family as a result of these.

Starting school. Inquire about the client's relationships to teachers and peers, school performance, extracurricular activities, what the client hoped to be when he or she grew up, whether the client had to change schools owing to moves or disciplinary problems. Typical questions include the following:

- What do you remember about starting school?
- What were you like in elementary school?

Adolescence

Ask about the onset of puberty in the client's life and accompanying emotional reactions to physical changes. Note where the client acquired initial information about sex. Detail information about early sexual experiences (heterosexual and homosexual), peer relationships, quality of friendships, and experimentation with drugs and alcohol. Questions might include the following:

- Tell me about junior high school/high school.
- From whom did you learn about sex?
- Did you have any romantic relationships as a teenager?
- Did you have any close friendships?

Adulthood

Information relevant to the present problem should be included in the history of the present problem.

Education. Note the level achieved and aspirations for further education, in the past or the present.

Military experience. Every client of appropriate age should be asked about military experience. Veterans of the Vietnam War may be prone to special problems stemming from wartime experiences.

Employment. Stability, satisfaction, relationships with peers and authorities, and job performance are all factors that should be included.

Social life and friendships. Describe leisure activities and re-
ligious/moral values.

Romantic relationships. Characterize lovers, stability of relationships. People commonly choose lovers based on their earliest important relationships—i.e., they seek lovers who remind them in some
ways of parents or other caregivers.

Sexual history. Note degree of intimacy and satisfaction, sexual
orientation, sexual dysfunction. Many people with mental disorders
are troubled by sexual dysfunction, and a simple question may open
up an entire area of emotional distress—e.g., "Is there anything about
your sex life or sexual feelings that is troubling you now?"

Marriage. Describe relationship with spouse, satisfaction in marriage, separations, divorce.

Children. List their ages and describe the client's relationship
with each. Also describe disruptions in these relationships due to
illness, death, separation. Note any miscarriages or abortions, since
these often have a major impact on family life.

FAMILY HISTORY OF MENTAL ILLNESS

This is a critical part of every evaluation. Ask about any relatives of the
client (including grandparents, aunts, uncles, cousins) who have had
emotional problems, who have seen a mental health professional,
who have been hospitalized for mental illness, or who have had
problems with drug or alcohol abuse. Pursue any "yes" responses to
these questions by inquiring about the following:

- Symptoms of the illness,
- Course of the illness (chronic versus episodic),
- Types of treatment (medication, psychotherapy, "shock treatment,"
  hospitalizations), and
- Responses to various treatments.

Relatives are either biologic ("blood relatives") or nonbiologic
(related to the client by marriage). Biologic relatives may suffer from
disorders that are thought to be genetically transmitted (e.g., major
affective disorders), which would increase the chances that your client

might suffer from the illness as well. The occurrence of emotional disorders in nonbiologic relatives is also important, because what has happened to family members is likely to influence your client's ideas regarding mental illness (e.g., "I'm afraid I'll be locked up in an asylum like my stepfather was").

MEDICAL HISTORY

Major medical problems should be explored in detail. Note major medical conditions, current treatment for them, disabilities, and any other medical facts pertaining to the client's psychological state. Pay particular attention to a history of neurologic disorders, especially seizures or head trauma. Be sure to list all current medications—including over-the-counter drugs—since these can profoundly affect your client's emotional state. Obtain relevant medical records from doctors and other health care facilities. Clients who have physical complaints but have not obtained a recent physical examination should be advised to do so, and inpatients should undergo physical examination upon admission.

DRUG AND ALCOHOL HISTORY

Note types of drugs and alcohol used. Also detail how frequently and in what amounts these are taken as well as symptoms of withdrawal and other complications (e.g., hepatitis resulting from the use of dirty needles). If drug use is a major problem, include it in the history of the present problem. When inquiring about drugs, use terms the client is likely to be familiar with (e.g., "angel dust" instead of PCP); see the table of commonly abused drugs in Appendix B. Also, inquire about so-called "social use" of drugs like alcohol, marijuana, and cocaine. Clients who heavily abuse these substances may rationalize their behavior as "just being sociable" (see Chapter 12).

MENTAL STATUS EXAMINATION

For a detailed discussion of the mental status examination, see Chapter 4. The results of the mental status examination can usually be summarized in a short paragraph. Each aspect of the mental status examination (appearance and behavior, speech, emotions, thought, etc.) must be mentioned. Where no abnormalities are present, you may simply say so without elaborating.

CASE FORMULATION

The case formulation is the clinician's attempt to integrate all the data collected during the evaluation and to arrive at a tentative understanding of the factors contributing to the client's problems. Basically, your formulation assesses the biological and social forces that have fostered the development of the client's personality style and current illness. This assessment is based on what you have learned from the client's history and mental status exam. In short, your formulation summarizes the case for the reader. It does not include a diagnosis, but rather it musters evidence in support of your diagnostic impression.

Composing a case formulation need not be an intimidating task; two or three well-organized paragraphs will usually suffice. The outline below may help you organize your formulation.

Introduction

In one or two sentences, describe your client, the presenting problem, and your understanding of why the client seeks help at this particular time. Summarize the client's symptoms and the extent to which they cause distress to the client and/or others. Also note how the symptoms impair the client's ability to function in his or her usual daily tasks and in ongoing relationships.

Biological Factors

Discuss any organic problems present (e.g., seizure disorder, endocrine abnormality) and how these might contribute to the client's problem. Include drug or alcohol abuse. Also note any predisposition to illness caused by organic factors (e.g., a history of minimal brain dysfunction in childhood) or family history that might suggest a genetic contribution to the problem. If no biologic factors have been noted, state this explicitly.

Psychological Factors

Psychodynamics. Note the client's major conflicts, defense mechanisms, and personality strengths and weaknesses. Also, describe the type and quality of relationships your client is capable of forming with men *and* women (see Chapter 2).

Social situation. Comment on your client's current life situation, including his or her important relationships and occupational status, as well as changes in these.

Mental status. Note any important findings from your own mental status examination of the client (e.g., delusional thinking, paucity of expressed emotion).

Hypotheses About Causes

Try to link the biologic and social factors in a coherent statement about how the client's illness came about. Obviously, this statement will be somewhat speculative, but it may provide you with hypotheses that you can test as treatment proceeds. Note any patterns you see in the course of the illness—recurrent decompensations, a slow but constant deterioration, or specific somatic or environmental precipitants (e.g., a client who becomes psychotic every time his wife gives birth to another child).

DIAGNOSTIC IMPRESSION

You will be called upon to make a tentative diagnosis based on your formulations. Keep in mind that accurate diagnosis is difficult and often requires observation of the client over time. Thus, your initial impression may change as you get to know your client better and watch how he or she responds to treatment.

The *Diagnostic and Statistical Manual of Mental Disorders,* Third Edition (*DSM-III*) should be available in the health care facility where you are working. You can compare your client's signs and symptoms with the various sets of diagnostic criteria in *DSM-III* to see which syndromes most closely fit your client's condition. Once you have done this, you will probably want to discuss your diagnostic impression with a supervisor.

DSM-III organizes diagnosis along a series of five axes (the use of this multiaxial system is explained on pages 23-32 of *DSM-III*):

Axis I: Clinical syndromes. This includes all mental disorders except personality disorders and developmental disorders.

Axis II: Personality disorders and specific developmental disorders. The separation of personality disorders from other disorders is clinically useful, because many clients will have a personality disorder underlying another clinical syndrome. In such cases, clients will be assigned both Axis I and Axis II diagnoses (e.g., manic-depressive illness on Axis I, and compulsive personality disorder on Axis II).

Axis III: Physical disorders and conditions. This category is self-explanatory. Your primary concern in arriving at a diagnostic impression should be with Axis I and Axis II, for all clients with mental disorders will have diagnoses in either Axis I or Axis II, or in both. Clients may have more than one diagnosis in any of the first three axes, but where no diagnosis is made (e.g., when no physical or personality disorder is present) it is sufficient to write "no diagnosis" beside the appropriate axis number.

Axis IV: Severity of psychosocial stressors. This axis allows for the identification of specific stresses that seem to have precipitated or exacerbated the client's current condition. Considered here are interpersonal, family, occupational, financial, legal, developmental, and physical factors.

Axis V: Highest level of adaptive functioning in the past year. This category allows you to judge how well your client has been able to function at work, in social relations, and during leisure time in the previous year. This information is likely to have some prognostic significance, since clients usually return to their previous levels of functioning after an episode of illness. (For example, a man who is now floridly manic but worked effectively as a corporate executive between manic episodes in the past year is likely to return to this high level of job performance when the current crisis passes.)

You will want to consult *DSM-III* to see how to evaluate your clients' situations with respect to psychosocial stressors (Axis IV) and highest level of functioning (Axis V). In many health care facilities, the use of Axis IV and Axis V is optional.

An example showing how to use the multiaxial system for diagnosis is included in Appendix A. Further examples can be found in *DSM-III*, on pages 30 and 31.

Along with your diagnoses, you may want to include one or more diagnoses that have not been ruled out—i.e., diagnoses you feel have not been excluded and that still warrant serious consideration. However, avoid entering unsubstantiated diagnoses into a client's permanent record, since government agencies and insurance companies may have access to such documents and could be misled by inappropriate diagnostic labels.

TREATMENT PLAN

The treatment plan is your recommendation regarding how the client's problems can best be alleviated. It may include any of the many therapies listed in Chapters 15 and 16. Often, more than one treatment will be recommended. Of course, a treatment plan that involves drug therapy should be planned in conjunction with the physician who will prescribe the medications. For example, the treatment plan for a depressed client seen as an outpatient might read as follows: "Trial of tricyclic antidepressants, supportive psychotherapy once weekly, and one or more meetings with the client and her husband to assess marital difficulties."

The treatment plan is based on many factors, the most important of which is your assessment of what is wrong. In addition to diagnosis, however, you must consider the following.

What Is Your Client's Most Pressing Problem?

Obviously, you must attend to emergencies first. For example, a severely depressed young man may be an excellent candidate for treatment with antidepressant medication, but his clear suicidal intentions make it impossible to begin any drug treatment until he can be prevented from harming himself. Thus, hospitalization would be the most important recommendation at this time.

How Receptive Is Your Client to Various Forms of Treatment?

You might, for example, decide that a woman with anorexia nervosa needs a behavior modification program to help alter her eating patterns, and twice-weekly psychotherapy to work on the severe personality disorder that underlies the eating problem. However, the client denies that she has any emotional difficulties and vehemently rejects the idea of psychotherapy, despite your emphatic recommendation. She does, however, accept a referral to a behavior therapist, and you list insight-oriented psychotherapy as a possible future treatment in your plan.

What Services Are Available to the Client?

To some extent, you must gear your treatment plan to the resources available in your area. Suppose, for example, you are working in a busy urban mental health clinic and a young man comes to you in acute distress over a failed romance. Although it is apparent that he has persistent difficulties with women and could benefit from long-term insight-oriented psychotherapy, you know that there are no staff members available at this time to provide long-term treatment. However, the clinic can offer short-term psychotherapy that provides the client with support and helps him weather the current crisis. He may choose to seek long-term therapy at some future time.

What Are the Client's Financial Resources?

Ideally, money would never need to be considered in deciding on a treatment plan. But in fact, mental health care is costly, and clients often need treatment over a period of months or years. Thus, it is imperative that you help clients plan for ongoing care that is financially feasible. For example, the parents of a young man with schizophrenia may be willing to exhaust their entire savings to pay for initial care in a private hospital rather than send him to a state-run facility. However, this would not be in the client's best interest, since he will almost certainly need long-term follow-up care as an outpatient and will require financial assistance from his family for a long time to get the treatment he needs.

In devising a treatment strategy, do not hesitate to recommend further evaluative procedures when you feel that important questions about the client's condition remain unanswered. This includes consultations by other professionals (e.g., a consultation by a neurologist for a suspected seizure disorder), psychological testing (e.g., an intelligence test to rule out mental retardation), and meetings with rehabilitation specialists (e.g., to assess a client's ability to work).

The next chapter covers a particular part of the mental health evaluation, the mental status examination. The chapter is designed not only to familiarize you with the structure of this examination, but also to define for you many of the most important terms used to describe the symptoms of mental illness.

REFERENCES

American Psychiatric Association: Diagnostic and Statistical Manual of Mental Disorders, 3rd ed. Washington, DC, American Psychiatric Association, 1980, pp 23-34

Cameron PM, Kline S, Korenblum M, et al: A method of reporting formulation. Canadian Psychiatric Association Journal 23:43-50, 1978

MacKinnon RA, Michaels R: The Psychiatric Interview in Clinical Practice. Philadelphia, WB Saunders, 1971

Nicholi M Jr (ed.): History and mental status, in The Harvard Guide to Modern Psychiatry. Cambridge, Mass, Harvard University Press, 1978, pp 3-40

CHAPTER 4

The Mental Status Examination

The *mental status examination* (MSE) is an assessment of the client's current state of mind. Like a physical examination, the MSE evaluates the client's functioning in the here and now; like physical findings, the client's mental status may change over time.

The term "mental status examination" is used to refer both to 1) the process of gathering information about the client's state of mind during an interview and 2) the section of the case report reserved for this information. The MSE is recorded separately from the history in evaluation summaries and progress notes, as a way of distinguishing what you observe about the client from what the client tells you about himself or herself.

The outline of the MSE presented in this chapter is very detailed (see summary in Table 4-1). This may give you the impression that a mental status examination takes four or five hours to complete. Do not be misled. In most cases, you will not need to devote more than a few minutes of an evaluation interview to a formal exam, because most of the necessary information about mental status will come not from asking specific questions but from your observations of the client's appearance, behavior, and manner of speaking in the course of routine conversation.

Table 4–1. Summary outline of the mental status examination.

Appearance and behavior
  Dress and grooming
  Posture and gait
  Physical characteristics
  Facial expression
  Eye contact
  Motor activity
  Specific mannerisms
Speech
  Rate
  Pitch, volume, clarity
  Abnormalities
Emotions
  Mood
  Affect (variability, intensity, lability, appropriateness)
Thought
  Process (flow of ideas, quality of associations)
  Content
    Distortions (delusions, ideas of reference, depersonalization)
    Preoccupations (obsessions, phobias, somatic concerns)
    Suicidal or homicidal ideation
Perception
  Illusions
  Hallucinations
Sensorium and intellectual functions
  Consciousness
  Orientation
  Concentration
  Memory (immediate, recent, and remote)
  Fund of knowledge
  Abstraction
  Judgment
  Insight
Attitude toward the interviewer

When Do You Do a Mental Status Exam?

Actually, you assess a client's mental status every time you meet, but in most cases, you do this informally. A detailed and careful MSE is usually part of an initial evaluation. This serves as a baseline examination with which to compare your impressions of the client on subsequent meetings. For example, you may notice that a client who has just been admitted to the hospital has trouble concentrating on your interview with her, because she hears her grandmother's voice telling her to jump out of your office window. As part of your MSE, you test her other intellectual functions and discover that she also has difficulty remembering recent events (e.g., what she ate for breakfast). In your follow-up interviews, you need not go through an entire formal MSE again, but can simply test those areas where you noted abnormalities on admission, such as perception, concentration, and recent memory. In this case, as treatment alleviates auditory hallucinations, the client may recover both her ability to concentrate and her ability to remember recent events.

Do you do a formal mental status exam with every new client? Clinicians disagree on this issue. Some insist that you can gather all the information you need about a client's mental state from informal conversation alone. They argue that asking structured questions (e.g., asking the client to interpret proverbs or do simple arithmetic) alienates you from the client and destroys any rapport that has developed between you in the course of the interview. Other clinicians warn that abnormalities of mental functioning can be masked by the client and go unnoticed in an unstructured interview, and that formal questioning is the only way to elicit them.

There is no clear way to resolve this debate. With each client you see, you must use your judgment about the extent to which formal testing of mental functions is necessary to answer your questions about the client's condition. Certainly, it is incumbent upon you to learn how to do a complete mental status examination as part of your training in mental health.

Often, clients will tell you about abnormalities of mental functioning that are symptoms of their presenting problem and that you need to explore in a formal MSE. For example, if an elderly client tells you that he has trouble remembering to turn off the stove at home, you will want to do a careful evaluation of his memory, along with other intellectual functions. Clients will usually give you clues to important abnormalities, either in what they tell you (e.g., "I keep hearing voices") or in how they tell it to you (e.g., continually losing the train of thought in midsentence). If you pay attention to these clues and explore in depth anything that seems unusual, you are likely to pick up any important abnormalities in the client's mental state.

Determining the Presence of Psychosis

One of the most important questions you will need to explore in the MSE is whether the client is currently psychotic. But first you must understand what we mean when we use the term "psychotic."

Surprisingly, there is some debate among clinicians on this point. Many textbooks define *psychosis* as a major mental disorder in which thinking, emotions, communication, and behavior are so severely impaired that they significantly interfere with the individual's capacity to meet the ordinary demands of daily life. This definition emphasizes loss of functioning.

However, many people who are severely impaired in their daily lives (e.g., those with severe personality disorders) would not be considered psychotic. And some people who harbor carefully concealed delusions (e.g., that their thoughts are being monitored by foreign spies) may nevertheless function well at jobs and even manage to maintain a family life.

There is no single definition that will satisfy all clinicians. For practical purposes, psychosis may be defined as an inability to distinguish between what is real and what is not, even when evidence of reality is clearly available. We speak of the psychotic individual as having impaired *reality testing*—i.e., being unable to test subjective ideas and experiences against objective facts of the external world.

The loss of the ability to test reality is an essential aspect of psychosis. Those whose misperceptions of reality can be corrected by evidence are not said to be psychotic.

A hallmark of psychosis is confusion between what comes from one's own mind and what emanates from the outside world. The psychotic person loses a sense of boundaries between inside and outside. Some common psychotic beliefs are that one can control others' thoughts, that external forces have put thoughts into one's own head, or that other people can read one's thoughts—all involve the notion of a "permeable" mind. Hallucinations, which are by definition psychotic, are internal stimuli (e.g., hearing voices) that are falsely believed to be of external origin.

In the narrow definition given above, psychosis involves false ideas or perceptions about oneself and the world that cannot be altered even when evidence of their falsehood is presented. In reality, there is no precise boundary between psychotic and nonpsychotic thinking, for false ideas and perceptions are held by people with varying degrees of tenacity. You must watch and listen carefully for evidence of psychosis, since it can be well masked in an interview. The most common psychotic symptoms you will see involve disorders of thought content (e.g., delusions) or disorders of perception (e.g., hallucinations); these are described in some detail below. Bizarre forms of speaking and behaving are also commonly associated with psychosis.

Psychosis is not, in and of itself, an illness. It is a symptom of a wide variety of illnesses, ranging from drug overdoses to manic-depressive illness. Some disorders involve psychotic symptoms by definition (e.g., schizophrenia), while others may or may not include psychotic symptoms (e.g., depression). An individual may be psychotic for a period of minutes, or for many years. Psychotic symptoms often wax and wane in their severity, but they may remain unchanged over long periods of time. Thus, each time you interview a client you must reassess whether psychosis is present.

Using the Mental Status Exam

Although specific mental illnesses are associated with particular abnormal findings in the MSE, beware of jumping to diagnostic conclusions based on the MSE alone. Each symptom in this outline can occur in any of several disorders. A given symptom provides only a small portion of the evidence required to make a diagnosis. The client's history and course over time will provide critical data. If you rely only on the MSE, you will often be fooled.

Avoid using this outline for the MSE as a checklist; the exam should vary according to each client's needs. Let the client's history and your own judgment guide you to explore in detail only those areas of mental functioning about which you have specific questions.

In many cases, you will have more than one meeting with the client you are evaluating, so you need not gather all the necessary information at one sitting. After a first meeting with a new client, you may find it helpful to seek the advice of a supervisor in deciding which aspects of the MSE to explore in follow-up interviews. Do not, however, neglect to ask about suicidal and homicidal ideation in the first interview with *every* new client you see. Dangerousness to self or others is a mental health emergency, and its assessment must not be postponed or overlooked.

APPEARANCE AND BEHAVIOR

The client provides a wealth of information without saying a word. Take care not to overlook the many things you can learn through nonverbal communication.

Dress and Grooming

Grooming is an important indicator of a client's ability to care for himself or herself; manner of dress often provides valuable clues to a client's self-image. Dress may be seductive or slovenly or overly fastidious. Depression or psychosis may prevent normally well-groomed individuals from attending to personal hygiene, and they may become disheveled and disorganized. Any change in appearance should be explored with the client and family, documenting when the change occurred and under what circumstances.

Posture and Gait

Rigid posture and gait may indicate clients' anxiety. Physical handicaps are almost always of great emotional significance to the client and should be noted.

Physical Characteristics

Note the client's apparent versus chronological age (young-looking, old-looking), physical health (vigorous, frail), and weight (obese, emaciated).

Facial Expression

The client's facial expression often mirrors his or her mental state (e.g., sad, suspicious, angry, silly, bland, mobile).

Eye Contact

Note whether the client makes frequent eye contact with you, avoids a direct gaze, stares into space, or glances furtively about the room. Eye contact often decreases with increasing anxiety or paranoia. Clients with psychosis or dementia, who cannot concentrate on the interview, may not focus on you visually.

Motor Activity

Observe the client's physical activity during the interview. Constant restlessness and pacing may signal anxiety, agitated depression, or mania. Slow movements and little reactivity are signs of the psychomotor retardation common in depression, drug reactions (e.g., extrapyramidal side effects), and *catatonia*, a state in which the client becomes immobile, with muscular rigidity or inflexibility. Catatonia may be accompanied by stupor or excitement, or by a refusal to cooperate with others (negativism).

Specific Mannerisms

Repetitive gestures such as tics or grimacing should be noted. Also, pay attention to agitated behaviors (e.g., hand-wringing, hair-pulling) that may accompany anxiety or depression. People who are taking antipsychotic medications should be observed for involuntary movements of the tongue and mouth or the extremities (these are suggestive of tardive dyskinesia), and for the general motor restlessness that is characteristic of akathisia (for an explanation of these side effects, see Chapter 16).

SPEECH

This category of the MSE is reserved for observations about the way the client speaks. By contrast, your observations about what the client says are included under Thought (below).

Rate

- *Pressured speech* is very rapid, frenzied speech that may exceed the speaker's physical powers of articulation and/or the listener's ability to comprehend. It is often present in the manic phase of manic-depressive illness.
- *Rapid speech* is found in a variety of other conditions, most commonly in acute anxiety states.
- *Slowed speech* is common among depressed people who have generalized psychomotor retardation.
- *Mutism* (i.e., absence of speech) occurs in some severely psychotic people.

Pitch, Volume, and Clarity

Speech may, for example, be described as high-pitched, infantile, loud, whispered, mumbled, or garbled.

Abnormalities

- *Stuttering:* Note the extent to which this interferes with conversation; circumstances that alleviate or exacerbate stuttering.
- *Speech impediment:* Note the nature of the impediment, and extent to which it interferes with communication.
- *Aphasia:* the loss of facility in language comprehension or production at the level previously possessed. It is commonly found in people who have brain damage (e.g., secondary to strokes). *Amnesia* (or *anomic*) *aphasia* is the loss of the ability to name objects. *Broca's aphasia* is a syndrome characterized by the loss of the ability to produce spoken and (usually) written language, although the individual retains the ability to understand language. *Wernicke's*

aphasia is a syndrome that involves the loss of the ability to comprehend language, coupled with the production of inappropriate language (e.g., nonsensical speech).

EMOTIONS

The client's emotional state consists of both mood and affect. *Mood* is a pervasive and sustained emotion experienced by the client. *Affect* refers to the outward manifestation of mood, i.e., the way the client shows feelings. Mood and affect are not always the same, and the range of emotions clients report and display is vast—e.g., depression, despair, hopelessness, anger, irritability, tenseness, anxiety, panic, terror, elation, emptiness, guilt, self-loathing.

Mood

Clients often volunteer information about how they feel during an interview, but it may be helpful to ask about mood (e.g., "How would you describe your general mood recently?"). If it is possible, use the client's own words to report the quality and intensity of mood, and note whether the client reports a change in mood in the course of the interview.

Affect

Predominant affect. In the course of the interview, note the client's predominant expression of emotion, e.g., depression, elation.

Variability. Normally, emotional tone varies in the course of conversation, from animated to subdued, from sad to happy, etc. Disturbances of affect often destroy this variability, so a depressed client may not brighten up even when discussing pleasant subjects, and a manic client may be incapable of maintaining a calm and sober attitude in the interview.

Intensity. Emotional reactivity may be increased or decreased. Increased reactivity is common among histrionic individuals, who show intense disproportionate emotional responses (e.g., rage if you arrive two minutes late). Decreased reactivity is also common: *blunted affect* refers to a generalized decrease in affective intensity, while *flat affect* describes a more extreme situation—the virtual absence of any evidence of emotion. Blunted and flat affect are classically seen in schizophrenia. Blunted affect is also a symptom of Parkinson's disease; among clients in mental health care settings, it is more commonly a side effect of antipsychotic (neuroleptic) medication (see Chapter 16).

Lability. Watch for rapidly shifting and unstable emotional reactions, particularly among clients who suffer from affective (depressive) disorders. Depressed people are often unable to control sudden tearful outbursts, while manic individuals experience uncontrollable bouts of rage or laughter.

Appropriateness. You must judge whether the client's affective responses are appropriate to his or her thought content and to the interview situation. For example, the client who speaks with apparent indifference about a recent death in the family or abandonment by a spouse may unconsciously be trying to avoid experiencing emotional pain.

THOUGHT

You evaluate thought processes and thought content based on what the client says. *Thought process* refers to the way the client puts ideas together—to the associations between ideas and to the form and flow of thoughts in conversation. *Thought content* refers to ideas the client communicates. A *thought disorder* is a disturbance of content or process, or of both. A *formal thought disorder* specifically denotes abnormal thought process.

Thought Process

Rate and flow of ideas. Clients frequently use the term *racing thoughts* to describe being flooded with ideas and unable to keep up with them. This condition is often seen in anxiety states, as well as in psychosis (e.g., mania, schizophrenia). If you suspect this condition, you might ask, "Do your thoughts ever go so fast you cannot keep up with them?"

In the case of *retarded or slowed thoughts,* people experience their thinking as slowed down, and may consider their minds empty of thoughts. This condition is seen in depressed people.

Circumstantiality involves thinking that is delayed and indirect in reaching a goal or getting to the point. This style is common in obsessional people and in schizophrenics.

Blocking is a sudden obstruction or interruption in the spontaneous flow of thought, perceived by the client as an absence or deprivation of thought. It is seen in schizophrenia and in severe anxiety states.

Perseveration is the tendency to emit the same verbal response again and again to varied stimuli. This may range from constant repetition of one word to an inability to shift the focus of conversation away from one particular topic (e.g., "night and day, night and day, night and day. . .").

Associations. Associations are the relationships between ideas. Normally, these relationships are intelligible to the listener; i.e., one idea seems to follow from another. Disturbances in the associative process may be quite subtle and, when one idea does not appear to follow from another, you may erroneously assume that your attention lapsed from what the client was saying. When something does not appear to make sense, *always* ask for clarification.

Loose associations involve the shifting of ideas from one subject to another in an oblique or unrelated manner; the speaker is generally unaware of the disturbance. An example of a loose association is, "I'm tired; all people have toes." Loose associations are commonly seen in psychotic states.

Flight of ideas is skipping verbally from one idea to another. Speech is fragmented and associations are determined by chance or by temporal factors. This is commonly seen in clients who are manic.

Tangentiality is a style of speech in which the individual replies to questions in an oblique or irrelevant way (e.g., when asked about his mother's illness, a client embarks on a lengthy discussion of the various "get well" cards his mother has received).

Clanging involves using the sound of a word, rather than its meaning, to give direction to the flow of ideas (e.g., "I'm sad, mad, bad.") It is sometimes present in mania.

Punning is used in a similar way, substituting for logic as a means of associating one idea with another; it is seen in mania (e.g., "What's the weather like? Is the sun out? He's out in the yard playing with his new football.").

Other Abnormalities of Thought Process. These may include the following:

- *Neologisms* are new words or condensations of several words that are not readily understood by others. This disturbance is seen in schizophrenia and organic brain syndromes (e.g., a paranoid man used "plickening" to mean "the plot thickens").

- *Word salad* is a jumble of words and phrases that lacks any comprehensive meaning or logical coherency. It is characteristic of schizophrenia.
- *Echolalia* is a parrot-like repetition of another's speech.

Thought Content

Clients' ideas about themselves and the world are frequently at the core of their presenting problems. Careful exploration of unusual or pervasive thoughts will often assist you in making a diagnosis.

Here are two helpful rules to keep in mind when assessing thought content:

1. *Always* ask for clarification when you do not understand something the client has said.
2. Begin with general questions and move on to specifics.

Some open-ended questions for assessing abnormal thought content include, "Have you had any unusual or troublesome experiences?" "Have you had any strange or disturbing thoughts?" "Have you had thoughts you feel other people would not understand?" If you get positive answers to any of these general questions, explore unusual thoughts in more detail, using the categories below.

Delusions

A *delusion* is a false belief firmly held despite incontrovertible and obvious proof or evidence to the contrary. Further, the belief is not one ordinarily accepted by other members of the person's culture or subculture. Delusions are hallmarks of psychotic illness, although they do not occur in all psychotic individuals. These beliefs may affect all areas of a person's thought and functioning, or they may be "encapsulated" and confined to one particular topic. Examples of delusions are illustrated in Table 4-2.

Delusions of grandeur. Exaggerated ideas of one's importance or identity (e.g., "I am the Messiah"). You may discover these with such questions as, "Do you feel you have special knowledge or powers?"

Delusions of persecution. Ideas that one has been singled out for harassment (e.g., "The FBI is out to get me."). Interview questions might include, "Do you think anyone wants to hurt you or has spread lies about you?"

Table 4–2. Types of delusions.

Delusions of grandeur
   "I am the Messiah."
Delusions of persecution
   "The FBI is out to get me."
Delusions of control
   "A computer puts these angry thoughts in my head."
Somatic delusions
   "I don't care what the doctors say; I know that I have cancer."
Thought broadcasting
   "People always know what I'm thinking."
Ideas of reference
   "The President sends me special messages during his television press
     conferences."

Delusions of control. The idea that one's feelings, thoughts, or actions are imposed by some external source (e.g., "A computer puts these angry thoughts in my head.") or, conversely, that one can control others' feelings, thoughts, or actions. To elicit such thoughts, you might ask, "Have you felt that your thoughts were influenced or controlled by some outside force?" or "Do you feel that you can control the thoughts of others?"

Somatic delusions. False beliefs about body image or body function (e.g., "I don't care what the doctors say; I know that I have cancer"). You might explore somatic delusions with a general question: "Has anything unusual happened to your body?"

Thought broadcasting. The notion that other people can read one's thoughts. Your question could be, "Do you feel that others can hear your thoughts or read your mind?"

Ideas of Reference
Ideas of reference involve incorrectly interpreting casual incidents and external events as having direct personal reference. These ideas often reach delusional proportions; that is, the person believes them despite evidence that they are false (e.g., "That newspaper headline was a secret signal to me from the President that he needs my help in Washington"). You may elicit such ideas with a question like, "Do you feel you receive special messages that others do not (on television, over the radio, etc.)?"

Depersonalization

Depersonalization is a sense of unreality or strangeness concerning the environment, the self, or both. *Derealization* refers to feeling detached from one's environment. A client may describe feeling "like I have stepped outside of myself and watch myself doing things," or say, "I feel as if everything is unreal and those around me are actors in a play." Depersonalization and derealization are common in anxiety states as well as in borderline personality disorder.

Preoccupations

An *obsession* is a persistent, unwanted idea that cannot be eliminated by logic or reasoning. The obsessive thought is usually consciously distasteful to the person but is often unconsciously desired (e.g., "I'm afraid my father will by hit be a truck."). Obsessive thoughts often occur along with *compulsions*, which are persistent unwanted urges to perform acts that are contrary to one's ordinary wishes (e.g., compulsive hand-washing).

A *phobia* is an obsessive, persistent, unrealistic fear of an object or situation. Some common phobias are *acrophobia* (fear of heights), *agoraphobia* (fear of leaving a familiar home setting, fear of open spaces), *claustrophobia* (fear of closed spaces), *mysophobia* (fear of dirt and germs), and *xenophobia* (fear of strangers). For a detailed discussion of phobias, see Chapter 8.

Morbid preoccupations (e.g., with guilt or death) are often found in depressed people. When these concerns with personal guilt and worthlessness are frankly out of touch with reality, they are said to be of delusional proportions.

Suicidal and Homicidal Ideation

Assessment of suicidal and homicidal thoughts are part of *every* MSE. Actively raise these issues in the first interview with *every* new client. This includes assessing thoughts, plans, potential for action, deterrents to action, and the client's feelings about these suicidal and/ or homicidal ideas. If you have reason to suspect that a client may become suicidal or homicidal, you must constantly reassess and monitor these aspects of the client's mental status. For a more complete discussion of homicidal and suicidal clients, see Chapters 13 and 14.

PERCEPTION

Human beings are continually barraged by a wide range of stimuli from the five senses. Perceptual disorders involve misinterpreting sensory input (an *illusion*) or perceiving sensory input in the absence of any actual external stimulus (a *hallucination*). Thus, hearing one's name in a train whistle is an illusion, while hearing one's name called in a silent room is a hallucination.

Illusions

Illusions may be of pathological or nonpathological origin. Seeing a face in a cloud and hearing voices in the rustle of leaves are common experiences but, in the face of reasonable evidence, the normal person recognizes these as misinterpretations. However, illusions also occur in toxic states (e.g., drug intoxication), in acute anxiety states, and in schizophrenia.

Hallucinations

Hallucinations are perceptions the client believes to be real despite evidence to the contrary—i.e., the client perceives something that does not exist. Hallucinations are invariably symptoms of psychosis and may be seen in all types of psychotic illness. They may also be induced by such factors as drugs, alcohol, and stress. They may involve any of the five senses.

Helpful general questions for eliciting reports of hallucinations include, "Do you ever hear voices or see things other people do not hear or see?" and "Does your mind ever play tricks on you?"

Auditory hallucinations are the most common in psychiatric illness, particularly in schizophrenia. It is useful to document what the client hears and to ask the identity of the speakers (e.g., "I hear my mother's voice telling me to kill myself.").

Visual hallucinations are less common than auditory ones but are often found in toxic (i.e., substance-induced) psychoses, and less often in schizophrenia and mania (e.g., "I see a devil with red eyes staring at me.").

Olfactory hallucinations (smell) are encountered in schizophrenia and in lesions (i.e., abnormalities) of the temporal lobe of the brain.

Gustatory hallucinations (taste) are rare and are usually associated with olfactory hallucinations.

Tactile hallucinations (touch) occur mainly in toxic states (e.g., in the toxic state resulting from liver failure) and drug withdrawal syndromes. For example, the sensation that insects are crawling under the skin occurs in delirium tremens (DTs) and in cocaine toxicity.

In evaluating hallucinatory experiences, it is important to note the *circumstances* in which hallucinations occur, with an eye to the possible precipitating factors (e.g., "What was going on when you heard these voices?"), and the *content* of the hallucinations (e.g., threatening, benign, grandiose, accusatory, religious, sexual). Content often provides important clues to the client's fears and wishes, and may identify general areas of intrapsychic conflict. Your questions might include "Whose face did you see in the dark?" or "Whose voice was it, and what did they say?"

Always try to ascertain whether the client's consciousness is clear or clouded at the time the hallucinations occur. If consciousness is clouded, look to drugs and organic processes (physical illnesses) as likely causes. A careful history of drug and alcohol use is critical to understanding hallucinations diagnostically.

Be sure to differentiate pathologic hallucinations from *hypnagogic* hallucinations, which are false sensory perceptions healthy people experience midway between being awake and falling asleep.

Finally, be alert to unreported hallucinatory experiences during the interview, e.g., when the client does not attend well to you and instead appears to be paying attention and even responding to internal stimuli.

SENSORIUM AND INTELLECTUAL FUNCTIONS

Mental illness commonly involves disturbances in cognitive functioning. A person who is overwhelmed with emotional difficulties (as in depression) or flooded with internal stimuli (as in psychosis) is often unable to focus energy and attention on ordinary intellectual tasks. *Dementia* is a mental disorder in which the primary symptom is a loss of intellectual function.

This area of the MSE is the main one in which specific tests can be of use in the clinical interview (see Table 4-3). However, only test particular intellectual functions if the client's history or behavior in the interview gives you reason to suspect derangement. Further evaluation can be accomplished by observing the client over time or by obtaining psychological testing.

Consciousness

The presence or absence of a clear state of consciousness is a crucial factor in diagnosis. Clouded or fluctuating levels of consciousness suggest an organic etiology (drug or metabolic toxicity, organic brain syndromes). Record whether the client is *hyperalert, alert, drowsy, confused, stuporous,* or *unconscious.* Note whether alertness is steady or varies during the interview.

Table 4–3. Tests of cognitive functioning.

Function	Test
Orientation	
Time	"What is today's date?"
Place	"What is the name of this place?"
Person	"What is your full name?"
Concentration	Serial 7's (or 3's)—ask the client to subtract 7's (or 3's) in succession, starting from 100. Counting backward from 20.
Memory	
Immediate	Digit span—ask the client to repeat a series of random numbers, first forward and then backward.
Recent	Ask the client to remember three unrelated objects and recall them after 15 minutes.
Remote	Ask about names and dates from the client's earlier life; ask the client to name the U.S. Presidents beginning with the current one and going backwards.
Fund of knowledge	"Who is the Vice-President of the United States?" "What are the colors of the American flag?" "How far is it from New York to Los Angeles?" "What is a thermometer?"
Abstractions	Proverbs—ask the client to interpret a proverb (e.g., "A stitch in time saves nine"). Similarities—ask the client what two things have in common (e.g., table and chair).
Judgment	Ask what the client would do in a social situation that requires judgment (e.g., on smelling smoke in a crowded theater).

Orientation

Awareness of *time, place,* and *person* is a basic cognitive capacity that remains intact even in many severely disturbed mental states. Disturbances in orientation are common in delirium, dementia, and drug-induced psychosis, but are less commonly found in people with acute affective illnesses and schizophrenic disorders. You can test for orientation with a few simple questions:

Time. Ask for the time of day (approximate), day of the week, season, year (ask, for example, "What is today's date?").

Place. Determine the client's awareness of the present location: the building (hospital, office), street, town (ask, for example, "What is the name of this place?").

Person. Test the client's identification of self and examiner (ask, for example, "What is your full name?" " What is my name?")

Concentration

Concentration is the ability to focus and maintain one's attention on a desired set of stimuli. A number of disorders can disturb this capacity, but it is most common in depression, anxiety, and psychosis. Gross disturbances in concentration will affect the client's ability to pay attention and answer your questions during the interview. If you suspect abnormalities, the following tests are useful:

Serial 7s (or 3s). Ask the client to subtract 7s (or 3s) in succession, starting from 100. Most people will be able to perform five or more operations without difficulty, but those who have difficulty concentrating will rapidly lose track of their calculations.

Counting backwards. Particularly if the client's mathematical ability may be insufficient to perform the task of serial 7s, ask the client to count backward from 20. Again, those with concentration difficulties are likely to drift away from the task before completing it.

Memory

Memory function is generally divided into three categories: *immediate, recent,* and *remote.* Much can be learned about memory as the client tells his or her story during the interview. Test specific memory functions only when you have reason to suspect memory deficits on the basis of the client's history and clinical condition.

Immediate memory. Use *digit span* to test immediate recall; that is, ask the client to repeat a series of random numbers (e.g., 2—6—8—9—3—1—5) immediately after you, first forward, and then backward. Normal persons can repeat an average of seven digits forward (± 2) and five digits backward. However, when concentration is impaired (e.g., in depression), the client may be unable to attend to the task and will *appear* to have a memory deficit when none exists.

Recent memory. Ask clients how they spent the last 24 hours and what they ate for breakfast, lunch, and dinner. Or ask them to remember three unrelated objects (e.g., lamp, umbrella, telephone) and then recall these objects in 15 minutes.

Remote memory. Ask the client important names and dates from his or her earlier life (e.g., birth, marriage, school, jobs), or ask about less personal past events (e.g., "Name as many Presidents as you can, starting with the current one and going backward").

If memory impairment is observed, note the client's reaction to the deficit and any efforts to cope with it. These efforts may include *denial*—acting as if the deficit did not exist; *confabulation*—inventing stories about situations or events that are not remembered; and *circumstantiality*—"beating around the bush" in an effort to mask the memory deficit. Clients who recognize that they have memory impairment may react to your questions with anxiety, depression, or hostility.

Memory deficits may be confined to particular time spans. In *amnesia*, a specific area of experience becomes inaccessible to conscious recall. *Anterograde amnesia* is memory loss for events that occurred after a significant point in time, while *retrograde amnesia* is memory loss for events that occurred before a significant point in time.

The number of disorders that can impair memory is great, but common causes include the following:

- *Organic lesions* as a result of tumors, strokes, or abuse of alcohol (Korsakoff's syndrome frequently involves short-term memory loss). Both presenile and senile dementia also involve recent memory loss, initially without impairment of remote memory.
- *Trauma:* Post-traumatic amnesia (e.g., after a severe concussion) is common and is usually predominantly anterograde with a mild retrograde component.
- *Psychological disorders:* Depression, anxiety, and psychosis impair immediate and recent memory, along with concentration, by distracting the client and making it difficult for him or her to focus on the environment.

Fund of Knowledge

A person's accumulation of knowledge is lifelong and varies with educational and cultural background. However, a person with chronic psychological disturbances may have difficulty in obtaining and processing information for long periods, and will therefore have a poor fund of knowledge. This can usually be judged during the interview. Specific test questions include:

- Who is the President of the United States?
- Who is the Vice President?
- What are the colors of the American flag?
- How far is it from New York to Los Angeles?
- Name three countries in the Middle East.
- What is a thermometer?

Abstraction

For adults, normal thought process involves the ability to shift from the specific to the general and to grasp the whole, as well as the particulars, of a given situation. The mind continually categorizes, relying on symbolic thinking to organize details. *Concrete thinking* involves difficulty in shifting from the specific to the abstract. This disorder is prevalent in the various forms of psychosis, particularly in schizophrenia. Concrete thinking can be masked in conversation, so if you suspect psychosis, use the following specific tests to assess the client's powers of abstraction.

Proverbs. Ask the client to interpret a proverb, couching it in terms of "How would you explain to someone the meaning of (proverb)?" Use such proverbs as "A stitch in time saves nine," "A rolling stone gathers no moss," and "People who live in glass houses shouldn't throw stones." Obviously, there are no "right answers" in interpreting proverbs. However, people whose thinking is overly concrete will be unable to infer general meaning from the particulars. For example, a concrete interpretation of the "glass houses" proverb might be "If you throw rocks at others, they'll throw rocks back and break your glass house."

Similarities. Our ability to see relationships among seemingly different things is based on a capacity for abstract thinking. You can test this capacity by asking about similarities—"What do these things have in common?" (for example, apple and orange; table and chair; baseball and tomato). A person whose thinking is very concrete will have difficulty seeing any relationships or similarities between these objects.

Judgment

As you listen to the client's history, you should learn a great deal about his or her ability to make and carry out plans and to discriminate accurately and behave appropriately in social situations. People who have poor impulse control or who have been inadequately socialized will often demonstrate faulty judgment. Drug abuse, brain damage, psychosis, depression, and anxiety are among the many causes of impaired judgment.

Formal questions to assess judgment include, "What would you do if you smelled smoke in a crowded theater?" (e.g., get up and leave, tell the usher, run, scream "Fire!") or "What would you do if you found a stamped, addressed letter on the ground?" (e.g., mail it, open and read it).

Insight

Insight refers to clients' awareness and understanding of their illness. People vary enormously in how accurately they perceive themselves and their problems.

Some helpful questions in evaluating insight include "What are your reasons for seeking help?" "Do you feel that you have emotional problems right now?" "Do you feel that you need help in understanding and learning to cope with these problems?"

ATTITUDE TOWARD THE INTERVIEWER

Attitude is the client's response to you, the interviewer. Mental disorders commonly involve disturbed interpersonal relationships. During a clinical interview, the client may display such problems by acting them out with you—e.g., by adopting an attitude of hostility or seductiveness that is inappropriate to the interview situation. Clients often adopt surface attitudes in an effort to compensate for deeper problems, e.g., a frightened man may adopt a hostile and aggressive manner in an effort to hide his fear. Attitudes provide valuable clues to how people defend themselves against unpleasant feelings.

Although it is not sufficient for diagnosis, the client's attitude can lend support to tentative diagnostic formulations. Paranoid individuals are characteristically suspicious, evasive, and arrogant, while manic people are frequently impatient and uncooperative. Schizophrenics manifest reserved, remote, and seemingly unfeeling attitudes; depressed people are often apathetic, hopeless, and helpless. People with organic brain syndromes (e.g., dementia) classically demonstrate distractibility and apparent indifference to their condition. The following considerations are important in documenting attitude:

- In what ways does the client engage or distance you?
- Does the client become more or less comfortable as the interview proceeds?
- Does the client show an ability to form an alliance and work with you?

REPORTING THE MENTAL STATUS EXAMINATION

When you report the MSE to others orally or in writing, follow the outline in Table 4-1. Each major category of the MSE (appearance and behavior, speech, emotions, etc.) should be mentioned in its proper order, and when there are no abnormalities you may be brief (e.g., "Speech was clear and normal in rate").

Although you may use many of the terms defined in this chapter, beware of relying heavily on jargon, for it does not convey an adequate picture of a person's mental state. Particularly when you document abnormal findings, use specific examples and quotes from the interview to illustrate your points. For example, it is not enough to report "auditory hallucinations"; instead, note that "The client reported hearing his mother's voice calling his name during the interview."

Report the MSE with enough detail that a reader or listener who does not know the client can get a clear understanding of the client's state of mind at the time of the interview. The two examples presented below are designed to show you how two very different clients might be described.

CASE EXAMPLES

The following examples will give you some perspective on what is involved in recording an MSE. It need not be a long and overly detailed endeavor. The MSE report can usually be written in one paragraph, but this will depend on the requirements of the mental health care facility in which you are working. Be sure to report the findings of the MSE in the order given in this chapter.

Example 1

Mr. A is a well-functioning man who presented to an outpatient clinic with mild anxiety and marital difficulties. His MSE is provided below:

Mr. A presented as a tall, slender, well-dressed, and meticulously groomed man who looked his stated age of 35. He sat stiffly during the meeting, with a worried facial expression, and made intermittent eye contact with the interviewer. Speech was clear and normal in rate but at times halting, mood was moderately depressed and anxious, and affect varied appropriately with the content of the interview. No abnormalities of thought or perception were noted, and the client denied any current suicidal or homicidal ideation. Intellectual functioning was grossly intact with apparent above-average intelligence, good judgment, and moderate insight into the nature of his difficulties. Mr. A related to the interviewer in a formal and deferential manner throughout the meeting.

Example 2

Mrs. B is a chronic schizophrenic woman who is being readmitted to a psychiatric hospital for an acute exacerbation of her psychosis and suicidal impulses. Her MSE is provided below:

Mrs. B is an obese, disheveled-looking woman who presented with poor personal hygiene and looked older than her stated age of 46. She sat hunched over in her chair during the interview, with a fixed and bland facial expression, staring at the clock on the wall. She occasionally grimaced and made continuous rapid darting movements with her tongue. Speech was slow and halting, and at times quite loud. She reported "feeling like I'm dead," and her affect was flat and did not vary during the interview. Abnormalities of thought process included occasional episodes of racing thoughts during the interview, loose associations, and tangential replies to questions. The client also used neologisms infrequently (e.g., "glidders," "crickly"). She insisted that the CIA was trying to poison her, and she reported believing that CIA agents could hear her thoughts. She denied homicidal ideation, but reported urges to harm herself using knives "because I would enjoy seeing the blood run out my veins." She reported seeing men in military uniforms with rifles standing in each corner of the interview room waiting to take her prisoner, but denied any auditory hallucinations. She was oriented to time, place, and person, and her intelligence appeared to be average. There were marked cognitive impairments, notably in concentration (she could only repeat 3 of 7 digits and could not count backwards from 20 beyond 15). Recent memory function was difficult to assess due to her distractibility. Remote memory (date of birth, marital history) was grossly intact. Thinking was markedly concrete on proverb interpretation ("People who have large windows might get them broken with rocks"), judgment was poor, and she had little insight into the nature of her illness. She related to the interviewer in an aloof manner.

REFERENCES

American Psychiatric Association: A Psychiatric Glossary, 5th ed. Washington, DC, American Psychiatric Association, 1980

Donnelly J, Rosenbert M, Fleeson W: The evolution of the mental status—past and future. Am J Psychiatry 125:997-1002, 1970

Nicholi AM Jr (ed): History and mental status, in The Harvard Guide to Modern Psychiatry. Cambridge, Mass, Harvard University Press, 1978, pp 25-40

Part II

INTRODUCTION

The third edition of the *Diagnostic and Statistical Manual of Mental Disorders* (*DSM-III*) lists more than a hundred mental disorders. Obviously, you cannot be introduced to all of them at once, nor would such an introduction be of much use to you as an introduction to the field. You will get a better understanding of mental illness if you familiarize yourself with the more common disorders first, and expand your knowledge to more esoteric subjects as your clinical experience deepens.

This section includes the syndromes you are most likely to encounter as you work in outpatient and inpatient mental health facilities. Chapter 5 focuses on schizophrenia, an illness that accounts for a substantial proportion of those who are chronically mentally ill. Chapter 6 deals with affective disturbances (depression and mania) and Chapter 7 with personality disorders, two categories that encompass much of the psychopathology you will see in your clinical work.

The discussion of personality disorders in Chapter 7 is designed to introduce you to various character styles, as well as to the personality disorders themselves. Since features of human personality such as obsessive-compulsive traits are common to normal people and neurotics, as well as those with personality disorders, an understanding of personality types is relevant to every client you see, not just those who fit the *DSM-III* criteria for personality disorders.

A variety of disorders are grouped in Chapter 8. Anxiety disorders are ubiquitous in our society, and both agoraphobia and panic attacks have been the focus of much research and public attention in recent years. Similarly, eating disorders have lately been recognized as being more prevalent in the general population than was previously believed. The personal and social costs of somatoform disorders are very great, for these emotional illnesses manifest themselves in physical symptoms for which no organic cause can be found, often after expensive and exhausting medical work-ups.

Chapter 9 deals with two disorders characterized by global intellectual impairment—dementia and delirium. Dementia, a significant cause of morbidity and mortality in the elderly, is discussed at length. Delirium is discussed only briefly in this chapter, since it commonly stems from underlying somatic illness that is treated by medical and surgical personnel.

Finally, Chapter 10 offers an introduction to the special problems of children and families. Because the manifestations of many mental disorders in children differ significantly from those of adults, it is important to become familiar with the basics of child psychopathology and treatment. Family work has always been closely associated with child psychiatry, and more recently it has become a more autonomous clinical specialty. An understanding of the rudiments of family dynamics is essential to the clinical care of adults as well as children.

The literature on each of the disorders discussed in the following chapters is vast. These chapters are meant to serve merely as starting points from which you can go on to do further reading.

CHAPTER 5

Schizophrenia

More than a century ago, the French psychiatrist Benedict-Augustin Morel watched a 14-year-old boy deteriorate rapidly because of a severe mental illness. The boy had been a good student, but in a matter of months he seemed to have become "demented"—his thoughts were confused and his behavior disorganized. Morel called this devastating illness *demence précoce* (precocious dementia). The term came to be widely used to describe a syndrome we now know as *schizophrenia*.

Schizophrenia has been described as the "cancer" of mental illness—in fact, the two diseases are similar in many ways. We do not know what causes schizophrenia, nor do we know how to prevent it; our efforts at managing the illness once it occurs have met with limited success. The emotional and financial cost of schizophrenia to those who suffer from the illness and to their families is often astronomical. The pessimism with which many lay people and mental health professionals approach the schizophrenic individual resembles the aversion often shown to cancer victims.

What is schizophrenia? It is a syndrome that involves a highly altered sense of inner and outer reality to which the afflicted person responds in ways that impair his or her life. This altered sense of reality—the psychotic core of the illness—shows itself in disturbances of perception, thinking, emotion, speech, and physical activity. The term literally means "splitting of the mind," and lay people often misuse the word to describe someone with a "split" or multiple personality. But schizophrenia refers instead to incongruity between different mental functions, e.g., between thought content and feeling, or between feeling and motor activity. The schizophrenic may, for example, talk of sad or terrifying events while laughing or showing no emotion whatsoever.

Schizophrenia is a syndrome that probably consists of multiple disorders with varying causes, courses, and treatment outcomes. The diagnostic label covers many different clinical pictures, and symptoms vary so greatly from one individual to another that it is impossible to present a classic picture of the disorder. The diagnosis may, for example, apply equally well to the hypervigilant scientist who suspects others of plotting against him, to the homemaker who believes she is controlled by her dead mother's voice, and to the withdrawn and apathetic teenager who broods incessantly on the reality of existence. Symptoms also vary within the same individual over time, so that a schizophrenic person who is psychotic and totally unable to function one week may next week be capable of good reality testing and able to perform adequately on the job.

DIAGNOSIS

Schizophrenia must be diagnosed entirely on the basis of the client's history and clinical observations, for there are no independent laboratory tests to verify the presence or absence of the disorder. Since the diagnosis has important implications for prognosis and treatment, mental health professionals have struggled for more than a century to arrive at precise criteria for identifying schizophrenic individuals. The latest effort—by the authors of the third edition of the *Diagnostic and Statistical Manual of Mental Disorders* (*DSM-III*)—is summarized in Table 5-1.

Since these criteria emphasize chronicity, you must get a history of psychotic symptoms over at least six months, or observe the person for some time, before the diagnosis can be certain.

CHARACTERISTIC SYMPTOMS

What are the "characteristic" symptoms that must be present for at least six months in order to diagnose schizophrenia? The most common ones are described below. Clients may have only one symptom, or they may exhibit many simultaneously. *It is very important that the client give clear signs of chronically disordered thinking.*

Table 5–1. Diagnostic criteria for schizophrenia.

Characteristic psychotic symptoms—most importantly, hallucinations or delusions
The presence of these symptoms continuously for more than six months
Loss of functioning in at least two areas of life (e.g., work, school, social relationships, self-care)
Onset before age 45
Chronic course
Symptoms are not due to an affective illness, organic brain syndrome, or mental retardation

Hallucinations

Auditory hallucinations are most common. They may consist of sounds, identifiable voices, or even continuous dialogues among several voices. These can be particularly dangerous to the client, or to others, if hallucinated commands are obeyed. Visual, tactile, and olfactory hallucinations occur less often in schizophrenia (they are more commonly associated with organic causes of psychosis).

Also seen in schizophrenia are *coenesthetic hallucinations*—perceptions of altered states in body organs, such as "My stomach is rotting" or "My head is growing larger."

Delusions

Falsely held beliefs that cannot be corrected by presenting the person with the facts are particularly common in schizophrenia. Often these involve erroneous notions about the permeability or transparency of the mind, e.g., that one's thoughts are being controlled by an outside force, that thoughts are being inserted or withdrawn by an outside force, or that thoughts are being broadcast to others. Also common are ideas of reference and delusions of persecution (for discussion of these terms see Chapter 4).

Emotional Disturbance

Blunted or flattened emotional tone is the classic affective symptom of schizophrenia. People who exhibit flat effect can remain so expressionless that they appear to be wearing masks. Other emotional disturbances may accompany this disease, in particular, affect that is inappropriate to thought content (e.g., laughing about a friend's death).

Volitional Disturbance

The person's will and ability to carry out plans may be paralyzed by negativism, or by an irrational fear of his or her own destructive powers (e.g., a client may believe that he has the power to single-handedly destroy the universe—and be terrified lest he do so).

Disturbed Speech

Common disturbances of speech include loose associations, incoherence, concreteness, "private" language understood only by the client, making up new words, and echoing the speech of others.

Disturbed Motor Activity

Activity may be markedly decreased, as in catatonia, or increased, as in excited states. Schizophrenics may exhibit robot-like behavior, bizarre repetitive mannerisms, or echopraxia (mimicking others).

CLINICAL PICTURE

By themselves, these symptoms and diagnostic criteria cannot give you a feel for what people with schizophrenia are like. Although the clinical picture may vary greatly from one person to another, certain characteristics are common to most people who have the disease.

A person typically develops schizophrenia in adolescence or early adulthood—e.g., a student whose grades begin to decline for no apparent reason and who begins to spend more time lying in bed "daydreaming." Or the person may be a homemaker who stops spending time with friends, instead spending time apparently lost in thought, and stops paying attention to her appearance. The incipient schizophrenic often begins to communicate in ways that seem odd or nonsensical, e.g., discussing some special personal meaning in a newspaper headline, or using words in eccentric ways. Performance at daily tasks declines as the person withdraws into his or her own world. The schizophrenic may initially show considerable anxiety and hypersensitivity to perceptual and interpersonal stimuli, but increasing absorption in an inner world makes it more and more difficult for him or her to pay attention to what is going on in the environment. This *prodromal phase* may last for days or months. However, some people do not develop schizophrenia in this way but suddenly experience a psychotic "break." Thus, the active phase may be the first sign of illness.

Whether or not there is a prodrome to the illness, all schizo-phrenics have what is called an *active phase,* in which their psychosis is most evident and they appear most severely disturbed. It is in this phase that someone is likely to be convinced that he is Jesus Christ, or to believe that the KGB has poisoned his drinking water, or to insist that his intestines are riddled with cancer, despite doctors' assurances to the contrary. In this phase, a client may believe that her thoughts are controlled by an office computer at her husband's office, or that her five-year-old son is trying to murder her, or that she receives messages from her dead mother over a radio station. A schizophrenic individual may hear voices commanding him to collect garbage in his bedroom, or to lead his family in jumping out a fifth-story window. Or he may see snipers shooting at him whenever he attempts to leave his house. Such delusions and hallucinations sound bizarre to us, but they are quite real to schizophrenics and may prompt them to act in strange and dangerous ways. To complicate matters, schizophrenics may be so withdrawn and guarded that they are unable to describe their psychotic symptoms to you. Or they may describe them without any show of feeling and thus give the false impression that they are not in any real distress.

The active phase of schizophrenia may last indefinitely or only a few weeks. When this phase subsides (with or without treatment), the schizophrenic person does not return to his or her baseline level of functioning but is left with chronic symptoms that constitute the *residual phase.* In many ways this phase is like the prodromal phase, in that the individual is usually not floridly psychotic or agitated, but is still obviously impaired. If hallucinations or delusions persist in this phase, they are usually less emotionally charged than before. Flat-tened affect is common, as is poor performance at work, at school, and at household tasks. In fact, impairment of functioning varies, so that some chronic schizophrenics who are in the residual phase of their illness are able to work (albeit with reduced effectiveness), while others are unable to function at all or even to care for themselves.

Some require chronic care in psychiatric hospitals, but most are able to live either on their own or in community-based programs such as halfway houses (see the discussion of Treatment below). Speech and thought commonly remain odd or eccentric, and schizophrenics in the residual phase usually continue to behave in peculiar ways (e.g., talking to themselves in public) and remain socially withdrawn.

The most important feature of the residual phase is that the person remains impaired. A return to normal premorbid functioning is the exception rather than the rule. Thus, if you encounter a "schizo-phrenic" client who gets back to baseline functioning after a psychotic

Table 5–2. Factors that help predict the clinical course of schizophrenia.

Poor prognosis	Good prognosis
Premorbidly withdrawn and isolative	Good premorbid social functioning
Premorbid personality disorder	No premorbid personality disorder
No identifiable precipitating events	Precipitating events
Insidious onset	Abrupt onset
Early onset (childhood, adolescence)	Mid-life onset
Little confusion in clinical picture	Confusion prominent in clinical picture
No family history of affective illness	Family history of affective illness

episode, you should question your diagnosis and consider other possibilities (e.g., an affective disorder or drug-induced psychosis).

Once a first psychotic episode occurs, the schizophrenic person's clinical course is quite variable. A small number of people recover with little or no residual deficit, but the more common course is one of exacerbations and remissions of the illness throughout life. Some schizophrenics have increasing residual impairment after each acute exacerbation of their psychosis, while others appear to stabilize at one suboptimal level of functioning.

How do you predict which schizophrenics will have a deteriorating course and which will stabilize or get better? To date, we cannot make such predictions with much reliability. Some factors that have been correlated with specific outcomes among schizophrenics are shown in Table 5-2.

A COMMON AND DANGEROUS COMPLICATION

Suicide and *suicide attempts* are common among schizophrenics. Suicide is frequently attempted during the onset of a first psychotic episode, when schizophrenics feel that something terrible is happening that they do not understand and that is beyond their control. Schizophrenics also try to kill themselves during the periods of depression that occur in the course of the illness. Floridly psychotic individuals are at particular risk for suicide, since hallucinations or delusions may dictate self-destructive acts and they may obey these internal commands quite impulsively. Roughly 20 percent of schizophrenics attempt suicide over the course of their illness, and 2 to 3 percent of schizophrenics actually kill themselves.

Homicide is much rarer, although catatonic and paranoid people are more prone to violence than those in other categories.

SUBTYPES OF SCHIZOPHRENIA

It has long been apparent that schizophrenia as a diagnostic umbrella covers a variety of clinical conditions, and many schemes of sub-categories have been proposed that attempt to separate schizo-phrenics according to symptoms, clinical course, and outcome. The subtypes of schizophrenia listed in *DSM-III* are of limited value in this respect, and many schizophrenics do not fit neatly into any one diagnostic subcategory. Nevertheless, since you will hear these sub-types used in clinical work, they are described briefly below.

Disorganized type. The disorganized type includes the primary symptoms of incoherent speech and blunted or inappropriate affect, with extreme social impairment but without well-developed delu-sional systems. These people often have a history of poor premorbid functioning, experience an early and insidious onset of the illness, and follow a chronic course without significant remission.

Catatonic type. The catatonic type refers to a clinical picture dominated by psychomotor disturbance. This may take the form of catatonic stupor or rigidity, catatonic excitement, catatonic posturing, or negativism (see Chapter 4). For reasons that are unclear, this type is now relatively rare in Europe and North America.

Paranoid type. The paranoid type is quite common and involves the presence of grandiose, jealous, or persecutory delusions or hallu-cinations with persecutory or grandiose content. Unlike disorganized or catatonic schizophrenics, paranoid schizophrenics sometimes show very little impairment in functioning (e.g., a paranoid security expert may function adequately on the job). Gross disorganization of behavior is rare among paranoid schizophrenics—they often speak clearly, and some can behave quite appropriately in social situations that do not arouse their paranoid fears. The onset of this type tends to occur later in life than the other subtypes, and symptoms remain more stable over time.

Undifferentiated type. The undifferentiated type is simply a cate-gory for schizophrenics whose prominent psychotic symptoms do not fall within any of the main categories listed above.

Subtypes are probably most useful as a kind of shorthand for describing a specific clinical picture of schizophrenia. Do not worry much about classifying an individual by subtype; it is not usually of major importance to the client's care. What *is* important, however, is that you take utmost care in differentiating schizophrenia from other diagnoses.

DIFFERENTIAL DIAGNOSIS

Accuracy in diagnosing schizophrenia is of critical importance, but it is the ideal rather than the reality in modern practice. Many disorders mimic schizophrenia, and schizophrenia varies so greatly in its clinical presentation that it is often mistaken for other syndromes. Because "schizophrenia" implies chronicity and intractability, the diagnostic label can have devastating effects on clients and families when applied incorrectly. On the other hand, correct diagnosis may provide some measure of relief to people who are struggling to understand their illness and to families attempting to plan for future care and proper treatment.

The process of differential diagnosis is often difficult, because there are several disorders that are commonly confused with schizophrenia and that must be ruled out before the diagnosis can be made with confidence.

Mood Disorders (Affective Illness)

Mania and psychotic depression often present with hallucinations, delusions, and bizarre behavior; they are easily confused with schizophrenia. You should suspect a mood disorder

- When the client develops prominent affective symptoms of depression or mania *before or along with* the onset of psychosis (schizophrenics often show affective symptoms, but these occur *after* psychosis has developed, often in reaction to it).
- When the client has a *complete* remission and functions normally between psychotic episodes.
- When the client has a biological relative who has a history of a remitting psychotic illness, since this is more suggestive of a mood disorder.

For a detailed discussion of mood disorders, see Chapter 6.

Schizoaffective Disorder

This diagnosis is made when both chronic psychosis and mood disturbance are prominent and you are unable to distinguish between schizophrenia and a mood disorder.

Organic Mental Disorders

Organically based psychosis may look exactly like schizophrenia with respect to delusions, hallucinations, incoherence, and bizarre affect and behavior. The cause may be drugs (particularly amphetamines or phencyclidine), metabolic disease (e.g., liver failure), a neurologic condition, or infection. If disorientation, confusion, and impaired memory are prominent, it is a good rule of thumb to suspect underlying medical illness or drug toxicity. In evaluating acute psychosis, a thorough history, physical examination, and laboratory screening are essential to rule out medical illness (see Chapters 9 and 12).

Personality Disorders

Transient psychotic symptoms may occur in people with personality disorders—particularly in schizotypal, borderline, and schizoid individuals who become psychotic under stress. However, these people will recompensate completely within hours or days. It is the brevity of the psychosis and the fact that the psychotic symptoms are felt to be "alien" that distinguish such people from schizophrenics. Paranoid personality disorder involves pervasive suspicion and mistrust that impairs relationships with others, but it does *not* include delusions or other chronic symptoms of psychosis (see Chapter 7).

Paranoid Disorders

Paranoia is the dominant symptom in this condition. Psychosis may take the form of well-systematized delusional beliefs, but disordered thinking is not prominent, as it is in paranoid schizophrenia.

Brief Reactive Psychosis

This condition, which occurs in individuals under severe stress, may look exactly like schizophrenia. It is here that observing the client over time is crucial, since reactive psychoses clear rapidly (days to weeks) without residual impairment. Reactive psychosis is frequently seen in adolescents.

EPIDEMIOLOGY

Schizophrenia is ubiquitous. It is found in every culture and in every part of the world with roughly the same frequency. It affects men and women equally, and most people develop the illness in their late teens or early twenties. It is estimated that between 100,000 and 150,000 new cases of the disease are diagnosed annually in the United States. Between 500,000 and 1 million cases now exist in this country.

Schizophrenia is more prevalent among lower socioeconomic groups within urban populations—perhaps because of the downward mobility forced on people by the debilitating effects of the illness, and possibly because the stresses of lower-class life (e.g., poverty, crime) serve as precipitants in those who are susceptible.

WHAT CAUSES SCHIZOPHRENIA?

The cause of schizophrenia, like the cause of cancer, has eluded researchers for years, and few people retain much hope that any single etiologic factor underlies this disorder. Research has been plagued by many difficulties, not the least of which has been the lack of an objective and universally accepted definition of the illness itself. Investigators have looked for a clear relationship between schizo- phrenia and gross pathologic changes in the brain, early childhood development, metabolic disorders, neurochemical abnormalities, and endocrine dysfunction—thus far, without success.

The Dopamine Hypothesis

To date, the most widely discussed notion of a biologic cause of schizophrenia has been the dopamine hypothesis. It is based on the idea that the mechanism of action of antipsychotic medications can shed light on the pathophysiology of the schizophrenic disorders they treat.

Antipsychotic drugs have been shown to block postsynaptic dopamine receptor sites in the brain. This has led investigators to speculate that schizophrenia might involve excessive levels of activity of dopamine as a neurotransmitter. This hypothesis would explain the therapeutic effects of antipsychotic drugs in schizophrenia, but it presents several problems:

- Evidence of increased dopamine activity in the brains of schizo- phrenics has *not* been found.

- Although the dopamine-blocking effects of these medications appear to coincide with their antipsychotic effects, it has *not* been shown that dopamine blockade is the mechanism by which psychosis is ameliorated.
- These drugs are not specifically antischizophrenic, but have antipsychotic effects in other illness, like mania and psychotic depression.

Thus, the dopamine hypothesis remains unproven, and research into the biology of schizophrenia continues.

Heredity Versus Environment

To what extent is schizophrenia rooted in human genes? To what extent is it caused by the environment? Recent research has yielded important findings, as discussed below.

Genetics. The case for a genetic basis in schizophrenic disorders has been supported by a variety of studies, including *adoption studies,* which reveal a significant concentration of schizophrenia in the biologic relatives of schizophrenics reared in different environments, and *twin studies,* which show consistently higher concordance for schizophrenia among identical twins (~40 percent) than among fraternal twins (~20 percent). In other words, when one twin is schizophrenic, the other is much more likely to be schizophrenic if the twins have identical genetic make-up.

Such studies lend support to the hypothesis that genetic factors play an important causal role in schizophrenia, but probably a role that varies from person to person. It is still unclear whether such genetic predisposition is specific to schizophrenics or occurs broadly within the general population.

Environment. Genetics alone cannot explain why some individuals become schizophrenic while others do not. This is most clearly seen in pairs of monozygotic twins when only one of the twins is schizophrenic.

In looking for environmental causes, researchers have explored the hypothesis that people with one certain personality type (e.g., schizoid personality) are more vulnerable to schizophrenia than others, but in fact many different personality types are found among people who later develop schizophrenia. Investigators looking at family interactions have found evidence that the families of schizophrenics show more communication deviance (i.e., illogical, inconsistent, and/or tangential communications) and lower general competence than families that have no schizophrenia. However, this evidence of preexisting family pathology only establishes a casual (rather than causal) relationship between pathology in family functioning and schizophrenia.

Contrary to earlier hypotheses that certain types of families *cause* schizophrenia, there is increasing evidence that the families of schizophrenics are quite diverse. You must be sensitive to such diversity, helping families to modify behavior patterns that aggravate the schizophrenic's psychotic symptoms, but also helping to alleviate the misplaced burden of guilt many families bear when they feel they are entirely responsible for one member's illness.

Although the appropriate genes may be a necessary precondition for schizophrenia, genetic factors alone do not account for the development of the illness. Thus, the nature-versus-nurture debate is only useful in sorting out the relative contributions of heredity and environment in individual cases. It seems safe to posit an interactive relationship between genes and the environment. It may be that a *vulnerability* to schizophrenia is transmitted genetically but that the development of the illness itself depends on the presence of environmental factors that have yet to be elucidated.

TREATMENT

The treatment of schizophrenia can be an arduous process for clients, families, and clinicians alike. No cure exists for this tenacious disease, so therapeutic efforts are aimed at management of symptoms and at social and psychological rehabilitation. Like cancer, schizophrenia has invited the discovery of "miracle cures," none of which has proved effective. The major treatment modalities we currently use—medications, psychosocial therapies, and hospitalization (see Table 5-3)—are all of limited efficacy and all have the potential to be harmful as well as helpful. Nevertheless, carefully designed treatment programs can help many schizophrenics to regain lost functioning and a greater sense of psychological well-being. Long-term support is necessary for most schizophrenics, to maximize both their ability to function and their quality of life.

Psychosocial Treatments

Hospitalization. Until the middle of this century, the treatment of choice for schizophrenia was long-term custodial care. Many schizophrenics remained in psychiatric hospitals most of their lives. Today, long-term inpatient treatment still occurs, but it has been largely

Table 5–3. Major modalities used in treating schizophrenia.

Psychosocial treatment
  Hospitalization
  Psychotherapy
  Rehabilitation—social, vocational
  Aftercare—day treatment, halfway houses
  Education about the illness for clients and families

Somatic therapies
  Antipsychotic medications
  Lithium
  ECT
  Antidepressants

eliminated by programs of *deinstitutionalization*. These programs are based on the idea that hospital stays should be short and used for crisis intervention, to stabilize schizophrenic individuals so they can return to life in their communities. Obviously, this is less costly than long-term hospitalization.

Advocates of this policy also argue that emphasis on returning to the community promotes greater personal autonomy and higher-level functioning than a lengthy stay, during which people become accustomed to being cared for by others. Advocates of long-term hospitalization argue that lasting psychological change takes time and is more likely to occur in the protective and structured setting of an inpatient unit. At present, deinstitutionalization is the prevailing policy in mental health care; the number of schizophrenic inpatients in the United States has decreased by more than half in the last 20 years.

When should a schizophrenic client be hospitalized?

- *At the onset of a first psychotic episode.* To facilitate a thorough diagnostic work-up, to keep the client safe, and to initiate medication and psychotherapy while the client is under close observation. These treatments can then be continued in an aftercare program when the client is discharged.
- *When the client poses a danger to self or to others.* Suicidal and homicidal threats or gestures are especially serious among psychotic people, who may lack the judgment and impulse control to keep from acting on hallucinated commands or delusional beliefs.
- *When the client is unable to care for himself or herself.* People who cease to be able to protect, clothe, and feed themselves need support until their functioning returns. Some schizophrenics have been ill

for so long that they have *never* learned to care for themselves. These people can benefit from the intensive social skills programs that are offered in many long-term treatment facilities.

● *When the client has lost important social supports.* Clients who function well with a network of supportive people and activities (family, friends, therapists, jobs) may decompensate when this network is disrupted. Changes in home life, work, or treatment may precipitate loss of functioning and even psychosis, warranting hospital admission and crisis intervention.

Note that the return of psychotic symptoms is not, in and of itself, an indication for hospitalization of schizophrenic clients. When community support exists and clients are not dangerous to themselves or others, crisis intervention with medication and/or intensified psychological treatment can be attempted on an outpatient basis.

Management of hospitalized schizophrenics. During acute episodes of psychosis, the schizophrenic's behavior may be difficult to manage. Many agitated, suicidal, and violent people require locked inpatient units. Verbal limits may be sufficient to control behavior, and threatening individuals often calm down when confronted with the fact that their behavior is frightening to others. Seclusion rooms (quiet, sparsely furnished areas) are helpful in decreasing the noise and activity around an overstimulated psychotic person who may be flooded with hallucinations and racing thoughts. When verbal limits, reassurance, and seclusion do not suffice to calm the person and control dangerous behavior, physical restraint and/or chemical restraint may be necessary (see Chapter 14).

As the acute symptoms subside, the schizophrenic can be integrated into the inpatient community. Ideally, the inpatient unit should have structured activities and group meetings in which people can improve their social skills, modify inappropriate behaviors, and support one another in coping with the stresses of their illnesses. This *milieu therapy* provides the backdrop for the action of medications and the individual and family therapies discussed below. A major focus of hospital admission should be careful planning of comprehensive treatment that can continue when the individual leaves the hospital.

The goals of hospitalization usually include resolution of a suicidal or homicidal crisis, improved hygiene and behavior to allow the person to return to life in the community, improved judgment and reality testing, stable remission of symptoms, the ability to care for oneself (with or without support) outside of the hospital, and the ability to comply with an outpatient treatment program. When these goals are achieved, when the client has arranged a stable living situation, and when adequate outpatient treatment has been provided for, the client is usually ready for discharge. Outpatient treatment may include medication, individual and/or group therapy, day treatment, and job rehabilitation.

Repeated hospital admissions are the norm in schizophrenia. Nearly 70 percent of all admissions of schizophrenics are readmissions. Frequently, a life crisis will prompt the client to become disorganized, discontinue medication and other treatment, and decompensate to the point that hospitalization is required.

Psychotherapy. There is widespread disagreement about the type of psychotherapy that is helpful to schizophrenics. *Supportive individual psychotherapy* is nonintensive "here and now" treatment in which the therapist actively assists the client in understanding and coping with the reality of his or her illness and life circumstances. By contrast, *exploratory psychotherapy* is more intensive and focuses on the therapist-client relationship as a "laboratory" in which clients can gain insight into their psychological make-up and achieve lasting intrapsychic change. Since schizophrenics are usually severely handicapped in their ability to be close to others, the first goal of most therapies is to establish a stable, trusting relationship between therapist and client. Insight-oriented work often emphasizes the importance of helping the schizophrenic to label feelings and connect them to life experiences and to explore feelings that may be so stressful for the client that he or she lapses into disorganized ways of thinking.

Group therapy has been used with some success in helping clients understand and change their inappropriate ways of dealing with others. As mentioned above, *family therapy* can identify and help to change family patterns of behavior that exacerbate the client's illness. Family treatment can also be of great help in educating relatives about the illness and what they can expect in dealing with a schizophrenic family member.

The range of approaches to psychotherapy with schizophrenic clients is enormous, and no single approach has been shown to be superior to the others. The diversity of therapies thought to be effective in schizophrenia reflects the tremendous diversity of needs and personalities among schizophrenic individuals themselves.

Rehabilitation. Clients uniformly lose functioning in some areas of their lives as a result of schizophrenia, and must overcome intrapsychic and environmental obstacles to leading a productive life in the community again. All too often, the very process of hospitalization prompts clients to allow others to take over their lives for them—one of the unfortunate side effects of chronic institutionalization. Schizophrenics therefore need help in learning or relearning skills for life in the community. Successful rehabilitation can be a tremendous boost to clients' self-esteem as they come to feel more competent at taking care of themselves. Such rehabilitation efforts usually include job training and practice in cooking and other household tasks. Ideally, rehabilitation begins when the schizophrenic is in the hospital and continues after discharge.

Aftercare. The extent to which schizophrenic people can care for themselves on their own, outside a hospital setting, varies enormously. Some are able to live independently, while others need total care on a 24-hour basis. People who can live outside a hospital but require supervision in their daily activities (e.g., handling money, buying food) often do well in *halfway houses* or *cooperative apartments,* in which residents are supported by mental health professionals who either live in these facilities or staff them on a regular basis. However, such living arrangements are costly, and many schizophrenics are cared for in private homes by family members or friends.

Along with support in a living situation, schizophrenics who cannot work full-time or cannot work at all need structured daytime activities. For such people, *day treatment programs* are helpful. These programs are set up so that clients may spend all or part of the day in group activities and meetings designed to increase social and other skills, while providing close supervision of medication regimens for those who have difficulty with compliance. Day treatment programs are usually affiliated with hospitals or community mental health centers.

Somatic Therapies

Antipsychotic medications. Antipsychotic medications are the mainstay of somatic treatment in schizophrenia. They have revolutionized the management of the disease, both because of their acute sedative effects and because of their long-term antipsychotic effects. They do not cure the disease, but they have been shown to reduce confusion, anxiety, delusions, hallucinations, social isolation, and other symptoms of schizophrenia. The principles of treatment are discussed in detail in Chapter 16.

Antipsychotic medications are sedating; they may help calm agitated and acutely psychotic people within hours after treatment is begun. However, the maximum antipsychotic effect of these medications may not be reached for six weeks. Once the acute psychotic symptoms of schizophrenia have been controlled (usually in four to 12 weeks), the dosage can be reduced to a maintenance level of 20-50 percent of the amount needed in the acute crisis. The prescribing physician must carefully monitor the tapering of the dosage over several weeks so that it can be increased again at the first sign of a return of symptoms. Clients who cannot comply with an outpatient regimen of oral medication may be maintained on intramuscular injections of fluphenazine decanoate (Prolixin) every 10 to 14 days. Schizophrenics who are not maintained on antipsychotic medication after an acute psychotic episode have a relapse rate significantly greater than that of those who continue to take their medication once a crisis has passed. Thus, long-term maintenance therapy with antipsychotic medication is indicated for a great many people diagnosed as schizophrenic.

However, people must not be kept on antipsychotics indefinitely without reevaluation of their need for medication. Clients who have a complete remission that lasts six months or more, and those who are stabilized on low maintenance doses of antipsychotics, deserve a trial off all medications for two reasons:

- To determine whether a first psychotic episode was a reactive psychosis rather than the onset of a schizophrenic disorder (particularly important in young people, many of whom recompensate quickly after a first psychotic break), and
- To reduce the risk of tardive dyskinesia in people for whom maintenance medication is no longer essential (see Chapter 16).

Lithium. Lithium therapy has been found to be useful in a minority of people diagnosed as schizophrenic. It is not clear whether this is because lithium-responsive "schizophrenics" have been misdiagnosed and are really manic-depressive, or because there are some true schizophrenics who happen to respond to lithium. Particularly when the differential diagnosis between schizophrenia and mood disorder is difficult to make, a trial of lithium may be both diagnostic and therapeutic. Certainly lithium therapy should be considered whenever affective symptoms are a prominent part of a psychotic illness (see Chapter 16).

Electroconvulsive therapy (ECT). ECT has been found useful in alleviating the symptoms of catatonic stupor and catatonic excitement. However, its efficacy in relieving other symptoms of schizophrenia has not been clearly demonstrated (see Chapter 16).

Antidepressants. Despite the "flat, affectless" stereotype, people with schizophrenic disorders do sometimes become depressed. They are particularly vulnerable to depression after an acute psychotic episode has cleared and they must come to terms with what has happened to them. However, if a schizophrenic appears apathetic, inactive, and in low spirits, you must rule out the possibility that he or she has been overtranquilized and is suffering parkinsonian side effects, rather than depression. (This can be done by testing the person's response to an antiparkinsonian drug or to lowering the dosage of the antipsychotic drug.) For people who seem genuinely depressed rather than overmedicated, it is often useful to add a tricyclic antidepressant to the medication regimen (see Chapter 16). Observe such people closely, because tricyclics can precipitate psychosis.

Controversy in the Treatment of Schizophrenia

The introduction of antipsychotic medications has had a powerful effect on the management of schizophrenia. Some psychopharmacologists argue that the only mode of treatment that has proven to be effective is medication, and that psychotherapeutic intervention in schizophrenia is of little use.

On the other hand, advocates of psychotherapy in schizophrenia argue that medication alone is not sufficient, that the effectiveness of medication depends on the psychosocial context in which it is given, and that medication only reduces psychotic symptoms but does not affect the client's social or personality development.

In fact, there can be no single correct treatment, since "schizophrenia" almost certainly consists of multiple disorders. The range of treatments and combinations of treatments used effectively reflects the variability inherent in the disease itself. What is useful to some schizophrenic individuals may be useless or even harmful to others. *Most effective treatment regimens combine somatic and psychosocial therapies.*

Despite our best therapeutic efforts, schizophrenics still occupy nearly half the psychiatric hospital beds in this country. And despite the effectiveness of new antipsychotic medications, the disease continues to leave a significant percentage of schizophrenics with real deficits, while the prevalence of schizophrenia in the United States remains unchanged.

REFERENCES

American Psychiatric Association: Diagnostic and Statistical Manual of Mental Disorders, 3rd ed. Washington, DC, American Psychiatric Association, 1980, pp 181-194

Baldessarini RJ: Schizophrenia. N Engl J Med 297:988-995, 1977

Cancro R: Advances in the diagnosis and treatment of schizophrenic disorders, in American Handbook of Psychiatry, vol. 7, 2nd rev ed. Edited by Arieti S. New York, Basic Books, 1981, pp 285-296

Green H: I Never Promised You a Rose Garden. New York, New American Library, 1977 (A moving fictionalized account of a young woman's experience of her illness and improvement during intensive psychotherapy.)

Gunderson JG: Major clinical controversies, in Psychotherapy of Schizophrenia. Edited by Gunderson JG, Mosher LR. New York, Jason Aronson, 1975, pp 3-22

Kety SS: Genetic aspects of schizophrenia. Psychiatr Ann 6:6-15, 1976

MacKinnon RA, Michaels R: The Psychiatric Interview in Clinical Practice. Philadelphia, WB Saunders, 1971, pp 230-258

Matthysse S, Lipinski J: Biochemical aspects of schizophrenia. Ann Rev Med 26:551-565, 1975

Pope G Jr, Lipinski JF Jr: Diagnosis in schizophrenia and manic-depressive illness. Arch Gen Psychiatry 35:811-828, 1978

Shader RI, Jackson AH: Approaches to schizophrenia, in Manual of Psychiatric Therapeutics. Edited by Shader RI. Boston, Little, Brown, 1975, pp 63-100

CHAPTER 6

Mood Disorders

The *mood disorders* (also called *affective disorders*) encompass a spectrum of emotions ranging from deep depression to unbounded elation and mania. An elated or depressed mood dominates the clinical picture, but mood is by no means the only problem for the client with a mood disorder. Physical symptoms, self-destructive behavior, loss of social functioning, and impaired reality testing frequently go hand in hand with depression and mania, posing difficult and sometimes life-threatening problems for clients and their families.

We are all subject to mood changes in our daily lives. Feelings of sadness and disappointment are a normal part of human existence; fortunately, so are feelings of happiness and elation. How, then, do we distinguish "normal" moods from "abnormal" ones? On what basis are mood states labeled abnormal? Here are some questions to use in attempting to identify pathological mood changes:

- *How intense is the mood, and how long does it last?* Pathological mood states are unduly prolonged and severe.
- *Do physical symptoms accompany the mood change?* Impaired body functioning is common, including disturbances of sleep, appetite, and sexual activity.
- *Does the mood disrupt normal daily activities?* Impaired performance often occurs in the usual social roles, e.g., home life, work, school, hobbies.

101

- *Is the client's ability to recognize reality impaired?* For example, is the mood change accompanied by hallucinations, delusions, or confusion?
- *Does the mood put the client or others in danger?* The danger may be direct, i.e., suicidal or homicidal intent; or indirect, as a result of impaired judgment.

As in so many other illnesses, the causes of affective disorders remain a mystery and are the subject of intense research and heated debate. Diagnosis rests almost entirely on the client's history, symptoms, and behavior. However, since depression and elation can present themselves in many ways, diagnosis is not always easy. For years, clinicians have debated how best to fit the mood disorders into diagnostic categories, using different hypotheses about causation and various groupings of symptoms. The most basic and least controversial classification of affective disorders is the bipolar-unipolar dichotomy (Table 6-1).

Bipolar affective disorders are conditions in which both depression and elation are present at different times in the course of the illness or, more rarely, disorders in which there are only episodes of elation. This category includes *manic-depressive illness* and a milder form of bipolar illness, *cyclothymic disorder.*

Unipolar affective disorders involve episodes of depression, but no episodes of elation. Depression may be chronic or episodic, may occur only once or recur again and again. This category includes *major depressive disorder* and the milder and more chronic *dysthymic disorder.*

The distinction between unipolar and bipolar illness has been made not only on the basis of symptoms, but also on the basis of different genetic and familial patterns, different responses to intervention with medication, and different physical and biochemical characteristics.

Table 6–1. Major forms of affective illness.

Type	Key to diagnosis

Bipolar
  Manic-depressive illness
  Cyclothymic disorder
	History of episodes of elation, with or without a history of depression

Unipolar
  Major depressive disorder
  Dysthymic disorder
	History of depression without any history of elation

UNIPOLAR DISORDERS

Depression is the most common of mental illnesses. All of us have friends, acquaintances, or relatives who have at some time been clinically depressed. In fact, at least one out of 10 adults experiences one or more episodes of depression during his or her lifetime. Researchers estimate the lifetime risk to be as high as 30 percent.

Some depressed people obtain professional help, but many others do not. Probably only 10 to 25 percent of those with depressive disorders seek treatment. It is essential that all human service professionals recognize the signs and symptoms of these ubiquitous disorders.

The clinical picture of depression varies tremendously. One client may present with tearfulness and self-reproaches, another with low back pain and chronic fatigue, and a third may be terrified that his spouse is trying to kill him. Yet all three of these clients may have depressive disorders and may even respond to the same treatment modalities. No single symptom is present in all depressive syndromes. Feeling sad or "down in the dumps" is the most common experience of depressed people, but even a depressed mood is not universal. There are clients who report no mood disturbances but have the classic physical signs of depression and respond beautifully to treatment with antidepressant medication.

Symptoms

Given the variety of forms that depression assumes, the list of symptoms is long. Some of the most common symptoms of the depressive disorders are listed in Table 6-2 and described below, grouped according to the mental and physical functions they impair. A client may be troubled by one or by many of these afflictions at any given time.

Affective Symptoms
Depressed mood. More than 90 percent of depressed people experience prolonged moods of sadness or discouragement, or a sense of "not caring anymore." A depressed mood usually colors the client's entire mental life; it is pervasive and dominant. A small percentage of depressed people do not experience a depressed mood but manifest other symptoms. One clue to the diagnosis in such cases is that the client's situation often saddens the interviewer, even though the client does not report sadness. Depressed children often do not complain of dysphoria but constantly wear sad facial expressions.

Table 6–2. The symptoms of depression.

Affective	Motivational
Depressed mood	Loss of interest in usual
Anhedonia	activities
Anxiety	Feelings of hopelessness and
	helplessness
	Suicidal thoughts or acts
Vegetative	Cognitive
Sleep disturbance	Sense of guilt, worthlessness,
Appetite disturbance	and low self-esteem
Loss of energy	Difficulty in concentrating
Decreased libido	Psychosis
Psychomotor retardation	
Psychomotor agitation	Psychosomatic
	Bodily complaints

Anhedonia. The inability to derive pleasure from previously pleasurable activities is an almost universal symptom of depression. Activities that may cease to be enjoyable include eating, sex, hobbies, sports, social events, and family functions.

Anxiety. Most depressed clients experience anxiety—i.e., inner distress with dread, fear, or anticipation of danger—along with such autonomic nervous system dysfunctions as sweating, palpitations, rapid pulse, or "butterflies in the stomach." Because anxiety and depression often go hand in hand, it may be difficult to distinguish clients who are depressed from those who have primary anxiety disorders (see Chapter 8).

Vegetative Symptoms

These refer to specific physical problems that often accompany a depressed mood. The presence or absence of vegetative symptoms is of primary importance in predicting response to somatic therapies for depression. You should therefore inquire about vegetative symptoms whenever the diagnosis of depression is a possibility.

Sleep disturbance. The majority of depressed clients experience some form of insomnia. This may involve difficulty falling asleep (*early insomnia*); clients with this complaint often report "tossing and turning" while they ruminate on life events. Others complain of waking up during sleep—often from nightmares—and returning to sleep with difficulty (*middle insomnia*). Particularly common is early-morning awakening (*terminal insomnia*); clients wake up at 5:00 or 6:00 A.M. or earlier and cannot get back to sleep. Hypnotic medications (e.g., barbiturates, benzodiazepines) are often unsuccessful in prolonging sleep in depressed people, and antidepressants are generally more effective.

Although insomnia is the norm, some people (particularly children, young adults, and those with bipolar illness) experience *hypersomnia*, or sleeping too much.

Appetite disturbance. Many depressed people experience a loss of appetite (*anorexia*) with or without weight loss. In taking a client's history, you should always document the amount of any weight loss and the period over which it occurred. Weight loss may be small or quite large, even life-threatening. A minority of people—particularly young women and people with bipolar illness—will experience overeating (*hyperphagia*) and binge eating (*bulimia*) as a symptom of depression. In such cases, weight gain usually results.

Loss of energy (anergy). Depressed people commonly experience fatigue and loss of energy in the absence of exertion, and describe this as feeling "run down" or "like all the energy has been drained out of my body." They may believe they suffer from a vitamin deficiency, and some severely depressed people believe that their decreased energy is caused by cancer or tuberculosis. Some experience *diurnal variation* in mood and energy level—i.e., depression is worse in the morning and improves somewhat during the day.

Decreased libido. A loss of sexual interest and energy commonly plagues depressed people. It may cause an increase in marital tensions and a lowering of the client's already fragile self-esteem. In men, the most common presenting symptom is impotence. You must inquire specifically about sexual dysfunction when depression is suspected, because many people are too embarrassed to volunteer such information.

Psychomotor retardation. Many depressed people exhibit an actual retardation of thought, speech, and action. Sparse replies to questions, monotonous and slowed speech, fixed gaze, and slowed body movements are all part of this syndrome, which may be severe enough to resemble catatonia.

Psychomotor agitation. Some depressed people—particularly the elderly—experience agitation rather than retardation. This involves an unpleasant restlessness or tension, an inability to relax or to sit still. Such people appear "fidgety." Unlike elated individuals whose activity is purposeful, agitated people simply make tension-relieving efforts, such as hand-wringing, pacing, nail-biting, and hair-pulling.

Motivational Symptoms

Loss of interest in usual activities. Depressed people not only experience a loss of pleasure, but also a decrease in motivation, often in all areas of life. Work, home life, and other pursuits come to seem dull and uninteresting. Ability to perform one's usual tasks may decline.

Feelings of hopelessness and helplessness. People who are very depressed feel they cannot cope with even the smallest of tasks, including personal hygiene and grooming. Work, school, and household duties can suddenly appear unmanageable to the depressed person. The individual who sees nothing but misfortune in the future may lose all impetus to carry on. Getting out of bed in the morning may take hours.

Suicidal thoughts or acts. Suicide is the most serious complication of depressive disorders and, unfortunately, it is all too common. One percent of all depressed clients kill themselves within 12 months after the onset of a depressive episode. Among clients who suffer from recurrent depressions, 15 percent eventually commit suicide. Depressed clients are at the highest risk for suicide in the six- to nine-month period after they have achieved some symptomatic improvement. Why this seeming paradox? It may be because the client has regained enough energy and motivation to carry out a suicide plan, but has not regained enough of a positive outlook on life to be able to choose an alternative to self-destruction.

Cognitive Symptoms

Sense of guilt, worthlessness, and low self-esteem. People who are depressed often berate themselves for perceived shortcomings that they exaggerate but feel are obvious to others. Such people are unable to realistically evaluate their own performance at daily tasks. Their low self-esteem may vary from mild feelings of inadequacy to severely critical auditory hallucinations as described under the section on Psychosis below.

Difficulty in concentrating. Depressed people may be so completely preoccupied with inner thoughts that they have difficulty paying attention to their environment. They often complain of "poor memory" or of being unable to keep their minds on such pastimes as reading or watching television. Because demented people also have problems with memory and concentration, it is sometimes difficult to differentiate depression from dementia in the elderly (see Chapter 9).

Psychosis. Depression may be severe enough to include psychotic symptoms, most commonly hallucinations and delusions. The content of these hallucinations and delusions is usually consistent with the depression (*mood congruent*). For example, psychotically depressed people may suffer from the deluded belief that they are being persecuted because they are sinful or inadequate ("My husband is trying to kill me because I'm a bad wife"); hallucinations frequently take the form of voices that berate depressed people for their shortcomings.

Somatic Symptoms
Bodily complaints. Besides the classic vegetative symptoms of depression, a variety of somatic symptoms are part of the depressive syndrome. In fact, internists and general practitioners of medicine are barraged with such complaints; the most frequent are headaches, backaches, muscle cramps, nausea, vomiting, constipation, heartburn, shortness of breath, hyperventilation, and chest pain. Many depressed people undergo various examinations, x-rays, and laboratory tests; some even undergo surgery. Too frequently, the diagnosis of depression is only considered after numerous diagnostic studies have failed to reveal an organic basis for the illness and the physician concludes that it is "all in the patient's head." Careful inquiry will often uncover other symptoms besides "aches and pains" that point more clearly to the diagnosis of depression.

Classifying Depressive Disorders

The long list above makes it clear that there is tremendous variety in the symptoms of depression. The variations in types of depression become almost infinite when you consider precipitating factors, family histories, and clinical courses. Some people become depressed after obvious traumatic events; others seem to sink into depression for no apparent reason. Some clients have family trees laden with depressed relatives; others have no family history of mental illness. Some people experience discrete, limited episodes of depressive symptoms; others complain that they have been depressed all their lives.

How can we make sense out of this vast array of clinical presentations? Many classification systems have been proposed, most of them based on unproven theories about what causes depression. A newer system, based on symptoms and clinical course, is put forward in the *Diagnostic and Statistical Manual of Mental Disorders*, Third Edition (*DSM-III*).

DSM-III defines two basic depressive syndromes: *major depressive episode* and *dysthymic disorder*. In a major depressive episode, symptoms are severe and persistent, and the illness has a discrete, episodic quality. In dysthymic disorder, symptoms fluctuate and are less severe, psychosis is not present, and the illness is chronic and long-term. The diagnostic criteria are summarized below.

Major Depressive Episode
A major depressive episode is marked by the following:

1. A *dysphoric mood* that is prolonged and persistent.
2. At least four of the following symptoms present nearly every day for at least two weeks:

   • Increased or decreased appetite;
   • Insomnia or hypersomnia;
   • Psychomotor agitation or retardation;
   • Loss of interest or pleasure in usual activities;
   • Decreased sexual drive;
   • Loss of energy;
   • Feelings of worthlessness, self-reproach, or guilt;
   • Impaired ability to think clearly or concentrate;
   • Suicidal ideation.

3. No psychotic symptoms during periods of normal mood.
4. Depression is not due to another condition, such as bereavement or an underlying schizophrenic disorder.

Two subtypes of major depressive episode are singled out in *DSM-III* for special mention:

• *Depression with psychotic features*, which includes gross impairment in reality testing: usually delusions, hallucinations, or depressive stupor (the individual is mute and unresponsive), and
• *Depression with melancholia*, which involves a loss of pleasure in

usual activities, and at least three of the following six symptoms: a depressed mood, worsening of depression in the morning, early morning awakening, psychomotor retardation or agitation, anorexia with or without weight loss, and excessive or inappropriate guilt. The emphasis in this subtype is on vegetative signs and diurnal variation in mood—the classic picture of what is often called "involutional melancholia."

Dysthymic Disorder

Dysthymic disorder, also called *depressive neurosis,* has the following diagnostic criteria:

1. Mild depressive symptoms, present for at least two years, that are not severe or persistent enough to constitute a major depressive episode.
2. Depression may be episodic or constant, but a period of normal mood lasts no longer than a few months.
3. Prominent depressed mood or loss of interest in usual activities during depressed periods.
4. At least three of the following symptoms during periods of depression:

   - Insomnia or hypersomnia;
   - Low energy level;
   - Feelings of inadequacy or low self-esteem;
   - Decreased effectiveness at school, work, or home;
   - Decreased attention or ability to concentrate;
   - Social withdrawal;
   - Loss of interest in pleasurable activities;
   - Irritability or excessive anger;
   - Inability to respond with pleasure to praise or reward;
   - Less activity or talkativeness, feeling slowed down or restless;
   - Pessimistic attitude toward the future, brooding about the past, self-pity;
   - Tearfulness, crying;
   - Recurrent thoughts of death or suicide.

5. Psychosis is not present.
6. Another mental disorder may be present, e.g., a personality disorder or anxiety disorder.

Dysthymic disorder can be distinguished from major depressive disorder by the criteria listed in Table 6-3.

Table 6–3. Comparison of major depressive episode and dysthymic disorder.

Feature	Major depressive episode	Dysthymic disorder
Dysphoric mood	Yes	Yes
Severity of symptoms	Severe	Mild to moderate
Impaired functioning	Prominent	Less prominent
Psychosis	May be present	Not present
Persistence of symptoms	Present every day	Usually fluctuating
Duration of symptoms	Every day for two weeks	On and off for two years

Older Systems of Classification

The *DSM-III* diagnostic categories, now widely used, should replace older and less accurate systems. Some more traditional ways of classifying depression will be briefly described here, for they are still used by many clinicians, and you will continue to hear older diagnostic labels used in day-to-day clinical work.

Endogenous versus reactive depression. Endogenous versus reactive depression reflects a long-standing debate about the cause of depression.

Endogenous depression refers to a syndrome thought to come from inside—i.e., it results from internal biological factors and seems to have a life of its own, rather than being dependent on environmental influences. The hallmarks of endogenous depression are prominent physiological disturbances (sleep, appetite, energy); absence of environmental precipitants (deaths, personal losses); and stable premorbid personality patterns without self-pity, hypochondriasis, or self-dramatizing attitudes.

Reactive depression, by contrast, refers to a syndrome triggered by factors in the environment, rather than biological factors. Such depressions are characterized by obvious precipitating events and life stresses, the absence of significant vegetative disturbances, fluctuation of symptoms according to psychological and environmental factors, and unstable, "neurotic" premorbid personality patterns.

The value of the endogenous-reactive dichotomy lies in calling attention to the importance of the vegetative signs of sleep disturbance, weight loss, decreased energy, and psychomotor retardation or agitation. It also emphasizes the favorable response of these symptoms to antidepressants and electroconvulsive therapy (ECT). However, the problem with this dichotomy is that very few depressed people fall into one category or the other; most lie somewhere on a continuum between the endogenous and reactive extremes. For example, almost all depressed clients, if pressed, can cite some recent adverse events in their lives that might be termed precipitants. And many depressed people have both obvious life stresses and clear vegetative signs. To further complicate matters, the presence of precipitating life stresses does not rule out a favorable response to medication or ECT.

Psychotic versus neurotic depression. Psychotic versus neurotic depression refers both to the ability to test reality and to the severity of the depression.

Psychotic depression is used quite specifically to denote depression in which the person has lost the ability to test reality, and this is often manifested by delusions, hallucinations, or profound confusion. Roughly 10 percent of all depressed clients have psychotic symptoms. But the term has also been used more broadly to denote depression with severe impairment in social and personal functioning, inability to perform daily tasks, and withdrawal from others. Psychotic depressions are thought to be biologically based.

In *neurotic depression* reality testing remains intact and, more broadly, day-to-day functioning is not significantly impaired. The term implies social and psychological origins, rather than a biological cause.

This distinction is another dichotomy of limited usefulness. Applied to depression, the term psychotic is ambiguous, since it can refer either to specific psychotic symptoms or to the severity of the syndrome. Considering the wide spectrum of severity of depressive disorders, it is rather arbitrary to decide that one person has a depression of psychotic severity while another's is simply neurotic.

However, the presence or absence of specific psychotic symptoms is an essential piece of data in the evaluation of every depressed client. Besides having implications for long-term treatment (to be discussed later), the presence of psychotic symptoms should alert the clinician to an increased risk of suicide and prompt consideration of a hospital admission.

Agitated versus retarded depression. Agitated versus retarded depression divides depressive disorders according to the motor disturbances that occur as part of the illness.

Agitated depression refers, quite simply, to the clinical picture that includes psychomotor agitation—excessive, unproductive, and tension-relieving activity, like hand-wringing, hair-pulling, nail-biting, and pacing, along with such vocal expressions of psychic pain as sighing or moaning. Agitated depressions are much more common in older people (peaking in the fifties and sixties), and often include psychotic symptoms. ECT and antidepressants are helpful in the treatment of agitated depressions.

Retarded depression refers to a clinical picture that includes psychomotor retardation—slowed, unspontaneous thought and action. The presence of psychomotor retardation predicts a good response to antidepressants.

The agitated versus retarded dichotomy is of particularly limited usefulness because many depressed people show a mixture of agitated and retarded features. Also, many depressed people have normal rates of psychomotor activity and do not fall into either category.

Differential Diagnosis

In making the diagnosis of major depressive episode or dysthymic disorder, you must rule out conditions that mimic depression, and underlying illnesses that manifest themselves secondarily as depression.

Organic causes. These are too numerous to list in their entirety, but the more common ones are listed below.

- *Drugs:* Among the many drugs that can cause depression are reserpine, propranolol, steroids, methyldopa, oral contraceptives, alcohol, marijuana, and hallucinogens. Amphetamine withdrawal can also produce a depressive syndrome, as can withdrawal from benzodiazepines and barbiturates.
- *Infectious diseases:* Including pneumonia, hepatitis, and mononucleosis.
- *Tumors:* Tumors often first present as depression, particularly cancer of the head of the pancreas.
- *Endocrine disorders:* Especially those of the thyroid, adrenals, or pituitary.
- *Central nervous system disorders:* Including brain tumors and strokes.
- *Systemic diseases:* Including anemias and nutritional deficiencies.

The routine evaluation of people with depression should include the screening measures shown in Table 6-4, as well as the additional measures that are done if the client's history or clinical presentation suggest a particular underlying problem.

Table 6–4. The medical work-up of the depressed client.

Routine screening measures
  Medical history—including drug use
  Physical examination
  Complete blood count (CBC)
  Routine blood chemistries (SMA-12)
  Thyroid function tests
  Urinalysis

Additional screening measures
  Neurology consultation
  Chest X-ray
  Electrocardiogram (EKG)
  Computerized tomographic (CT) scan

Dementia. Because demented people experience memory loss and difficulty in concentrating, it can be difficult to distinguish between depression and dementia, particularly in the elderly (see Chapter 9).

Psychological reaction to a physical illness. People who suddenly find themselves bedridden or functionally impaired because of a medical condition often react by becoming depressed.

Schizophrenia. Differentiating between psychotic depression and schizophrenia may be difficult. In schizophrenia, depressive symptoms usually follow the onset of psychosis; in psychotic depression, the mood disturbance precedes or coincides with the onset of psychosis. A history of normal functioning between psychotic episodes suggests affective illness, as does a family history of affective illness. Also, remember that schizophrenics may have secondary depressive episodes, particularly on recovering from an acute psychotic break.

Schizoaffective disorder. This is often called a "wastebasket diagnosis," because the label is given to people whose symptoms and clinical course make it impossible to differentiate between depression and schizophrenia.

Bipolar disorders. Those who present initially with depression may later manifest elation or mania as well, taking them out of the unipolar category. At this time, we are unable to predict which people who present as unipolar depressives will go on to reveal a bipolar illness instead.

Uncomplicated bereavement. A full depressive syndrome is frequently a normal reaction to the death of a loved one. It may include sleep and appetite disturbance. Such a reaction rarely begins more than two or three months following a loss, and it does not result in marked or prolonged functional impairment. Remember that the duration of normal bereavement varies widely among different ethnic groups.

Personality disorders. Many people with personality disorders—particularly borderline, histrionic, dependent, and obsessive-compulsive disorders—have depressive symptoms as well. The depression is often chronic, has fluctuating symptoms, and usually meets the criteria for dysthymic disorder.

Chronic alcohol dependence. Alcohol addiction is often associated with depressive symptoms. It is thought that many alcoholics are actually depressed and "self-medicate" underlying depression by drinking, but chronic alcohol abuse can also be the sole cause of depressive symptoms.

Anxiety. Because a large percentage of depressed people also experience anxiety, the task of distinguishing between anxiety disorders and depressive disorders is not always easy. As more and more studies point out the efficacy of antidepressant medication in treating panic disorders, the overlap between depression and anxiety becomes even greater. Anxious clients tend to complain more of bodily symptoms than do depressed clients.

Normal mood fluctuations. Obviously, all of us have experienced depressed feelings at some time in our lives. However, normal mood fluctuations are not as prolonged or as severe as those in dysthymic disorder and major depressive episodes. Moreover, normal mood changes do not interfere significantly with day-to-day functioning.

Clinical Course

Major depressive disorder. Symptoms of a major depressive episode usually develop over a period of days to weeks, but they may develop quite suddenly—particularly after a severe life stress. The depressive episode is sometimes preceded by several months of milder symptoms, by anxiety, or by panic attacks.

Most acute depressive episodes are self-limiting and have a good prognosis even without specific therapy, but somatic therapies (such as antidepressants or ECT) decrease the intensity of the symptoms and hasten recovery. Before the advent of somatic therapies, most acute depressive episodes lasted six to eight months; with these therapies, such episodes now last only several weeks. More than half of those who have a first major depressive episode go on to have one or more recurrences in their lifetime; a minority of people recover completely after one episode.

Most people return to their previous levels of functioning between depressive episodes, but about 15 to 30 percent of those with major depressions never return to their premorbid state of mental health; they have residual symptoms and social impairment. Factors that seem to predispose certain depressed people to a chronic "downhill" course are advanced age, a family history of depression, long-standing personality problems, and lack of social supports.

People who have recurrent depressive episodes are more likely to go on to develop a manic or hypomanic episode (bipolar illness) than those who only experience a single depressive episode.

Dysthymic disorder. Unlike major depressive disorder, dysthymic disorder has no clear onset, but seems to the client as if it had always been there. A chronic, rather than episodic, course is the rule. Social and occupational impairment may be mild or even moderate, but this is due to the chronicity of the symptoms rather than to their severity. Hospitalization is rarely necessary unless the client seriously plans or attempts suicide.

Epidemiology

Depressive disorders are ubiquitous. The following figures give a sketch of their distribution in the general population.

Morbid risk. At least 10 percent of adults in the general population have one or more major depressive episodes at some time in their lives. Some estimates place an individual's lifetime risk of developing a major depressive or dysthymic disorder as high as 30 percent.

Age at onset. Dysthymic disorder usually begins early in adult life. Major depressive disorder may begin at any age, and the age at onset is fairly evenly distributed throughout adulthood. Contrary to popular belief, depression is no more common among the elderly than among younger adults.

Sex. Major depressive disorder is roughly twice as common in women as in men, and dysthymic disorder has been estimated to be four to five times more common in women than men. The reasons for these differences are not fully understood.

Socioeconomic status. No strong or constant trend has been demonstrated, but depression appears to be somewhat more common in the higher social strata.

Marital status. There is no appreciable difference among single, married, divorced, and widowed people in the incidence of major depressive disorder. Some reports have shown increased incidence of dysthymic disorder among separated and divorced persons, but this trend is not striking.

Family history. There is a clear tendency for major depressive disorder to run in families. Familial patterns in dysthymic disorder have not been established.

Etiology

No single causal factor has been identified as the basis of depression. Indeed, the depressive syndromes are so varied in their course and symptomatology that discovery of a single cause of all depressive disorders is highly unlikely. Research points to many factors that seem to contribute to the development of depressive illness.

Genetics. Studies of the incidence of depressive illness in twins, families, and the general population strongly suggest a genetic basis for at least some depressive disorders. Evidence includes the fact that relatives of people with unipolar depressive illness have a higher frequency of depression than the general population. The prevalence of unipolar depression is greatest among first-degree relatives of unipolar depressives. Also, monozygotic twins have a greater concordance rate for depression than do dizygotic twins (i.e., if one twin suffers from depression, it is more likely that the other twin will also suffer from depression if he or she is identical rather than fraternal).

Neurochemical abnormalities. Much attention has been focused on chemicals that transmit nerve impulses from one neuron to another in the brain, particularly norepinephrine and serotonin.

Norepinephrine is found in both the central and peripheral nervous systems. Evidence suggests that in some forms of depression there is a central nervous system (CNS) deficiency of norepinephrine. Abnormally low levels of norepinephrine in the CNS correlate with low levels of its metabolite, 3-methoxy-4-hydroxyphenylglycol (MHPG), in the urine. And certain tricyclic antidepressants (e.g., imipramine, desipramine) block the reuptake of norepinephrine in presynaptic neurons, increasing the amount of norepinephrine that remains active as a transmitter, and thus remedying the deficiency.

Serotonin is also a CNS neurotransmitter. A lack of serotonin in some depressed people correlates with low levels of its metabolite, 5-hydroxyindoleacetic acid (5-HIAA) in the cerebrospinal fluid (CSF). These people have normal or elevated urinary levels of MHPG, but low levels of 5-HIAA in the CSF. They have been shown to respond clinically to amitriptyline, a tricyclic antidepressant that blocks serotonin reuptake by presynaptic neurons and thus increases the amount of serotonin available for neurotransmission.

In summary, then, two types of unipolar depression appear to correlate with CNS neurotransmitter deficiency. One is characterized by a norepinephrine deficiency at nerve synapses, low urinary levels of MHPG, and a good response to imipramine and desipramine. The other is characterized by a serotonin deficiency at nerve synapses, low levels of 5-HIAA in the CSF (but normal or elevated levels of urinary MHPG), and a good response to amitriptyline.

It must be emphasized that many people who are clinically depressed do not have demonstrable norepinephrine or serotonin deficiencies, nor do they necessarily respond to treatment with antidepressants. Thus, neurotransmitter deficiencies do not sufficiently account for all depressive syndromes.

Other biologic factors. Also investigated for possible roles in the etiology of depression are electrolyte disturbances, electroencephalographic (brain wave) abnormalities, and neuroendocrine abnormalities. Hypothalamic, pituitary, adrenal cortical, thyroid, and gonadal functions have been examined for possible clues. Of particular interest at the time of this writing is the pituitary-adrenal axis and the empirical finding that some depressed people cannot suppress cortisol production by the adrenal cortex when challenged with a dose of dexamethasone sufficient to suppress cortisol production in normal individuals (see Chapter 16 for a discussion of the dexamethasone suppression test).

Personality and psychodynamic factors. The literature on the psychodynamics of depression is vast. No single personality trait or group of traits which predisposes one to depression has been identified, nor has a single psychological mechanism by which depression comes about been elucidated.

Many psychodynamic theorists note that those prone to depression are characterized by low self-esteem and a high degree of self-criticism. Some conceptualize depression as anger turned inward. Others write about instability and insecurity in early mother-child interactions as laying the groundwork for later sensitivity to separations from loved ones.

In studying the roots of depression, much attention has been focused on the role of interpersonal loss. Freud and his followers examined the similarities (and differences) between normal bereavement and depression, noting that people commonly seek help for depressive episodes that seem to come on the heels of some setback in personal relationships (e.g., loss of a job, death of a loved one, breakup of a marriage or romance). Researchers have noted an increased incidence of depression among adults who have suffered the loss (by death) of a parent in childhood. Such early losses may make individuals particularly sensitive to losses later in life, and thus more vulnerable to depressive illness. But not all those who lose parents in childhood go on to become depressed as adults, and there seem to be many variables that determine one's response to loss. The variety of psychological factors that contribute to depression is practically infinite.

Treatment

Optimism is usually justified in treating clients with depressive disorders. Currently available therapies have proved effective and afford depressed clients a good prognosis, particularly in cases of acute depressive episodes. A wide range of somatic and psychological treatment modalities is useful in depression. You must be ready to use varying combinations of treatments tailored to each individual client's needs. Basic approaches to the treatment of depression are outlined below.

Treat emergencies first. Suicide constitutes the greatest danger to depressed people, and you must assess the suicide potential of every client who complains of depressed feelings. Suicidal thoughts and

Table 6–5. General indications for hospitalizing a depressed client.

Significant risk of suicide
Significant risk of homicide
Loss of ability to care for oneself, either because of immobilizing symptoms
  or because of psychotic thinking
Acute medical conditions of life-threatening proportion that result from the
  depression (e.g., anorexia, dehydration)
Concomitant medical conditions (e.g., severe cardiac disease) that require
  special diagnostic and treatment considerations

---

actions may be obvious, or clues to self-destructive intent may be subtle. For example, drug abuse, reckless driving, and other "daring" activities often represent disguised suicidal wishes (for the assessment of suicide risk, see Chapter 13).

The danger of homicide must not be overlooked, since people with depression may try to kill others on the basis of deluded beliefs (e.g., the mother who feels her children would be better off dead than growing up in a cruel and heartless world).

Acute psychosis must be treated as an emergency, as must severe starvation and/or dehydration secondary to anorexia. All of the above conditions should prompt you to consider immediate hospitalization to stabilize the client medically and keep the client and others physically safe (Table 6-5).

Somatic Therapies

Medications and ECT are particularly useful in depressive disorders that include psychosis and/or physical symptoms (particularly the classic vegetative signs noted above).

Tricyclic antidepressants (TCAs) are the most widely used medications for depression. Their actions seem to be related to their capacity to potentiate the CNS actions of norepinephrine and serotonin. TCAs are used in the treatment of acute depressive episodes, to alleviate more chronic depressive syndromes, and to prevent recurrent depressive episodes. The indications for the use of TCAs are discussed in detail in Chapter 16, along with the principles that physicians use in prescribing these medications.

Lithium is most widely used as an antimanic drug, but recent studies have shown lithium to be effective in preventing the recurrence of depressive episodes in unipolar depressives. Lithium maintenance is now being used as an alternative to TCA maintenance for the prophylaxis of recurrent depression. However, lithium has not been demonstrated to be useful in treating acute depressive episodes.

The antidepressant action of *monoamine oxidase inhibitors* (MAOIs) is thought to be related to their ability to block the metabolism of norepinephrine and serotonin in the CNS. MAOIs are generally the second-line drugs in treating depression pharmacologically because they are somewhat less effective than TCAs, and adverse reactions are more common with MAOIs than with TCAs. However, MAOIs are useful in treating depression with atypical symptoms, and in cases where TCAs are contraindicated or have not proved helpful (see Chapter 16 for more details).

ECT, sometimes referred to as "shock treatment," involves the induction of a seizure by passing a controlled pulse of electrical energy through the brain. The seizure is induced while the client is partly paralyzed by a muscle relaxant and under general anesthesia. The seizure itself is necessary for the antidepressant effect of ECT, although the operative mechanism is not known. Courses of treatment vary, but clients often receive between six and 20 treatments, given at a rate of three or four treatments per week. ECT is safe and highly effective. It has the advantage of being rapidly effective; response often occurs within days rather than weeks. Thus, ECT is frequently the treatment of choice when depressive symptoms are so severe as to be life-threatening and rapid improvement is essential (see Chapter 16).

Major tranquilizers, also called antipsychotics or neuroleptics, are very useful in depression that is complicated by psychotic symptoms or overwhelming anxiety. They are often used in combination with TCAs or with ECT, since psychotic depression does not generally respond well to antidepressant therapy alone. Symptoms likely to respond to treatment with antipsychotics include delusions, hallucinations, confusion, and overwhelming anxiety.

Sedatives and minor tranquilizers (Valium, phenobarbital, and other sedatives and antianxiety agents) are sometimes used to treat anxiety, restlessness, insomnia, and irritability that are part of depressive syndromes. However, when depression is the basis for these symptoms, they frequently resolve with antidepressant therapy. Like all central nervous system depressants, these drugs can actually cause depression and thereby complicate rather than alleviate the illness.

Note that insomnia associated with a depressive syndrome is best treated by treating the depression itself, not by the long-term use of sedatives or hypnotics.

Psychological Therapies

Individual psychotherapy based on psychodynamic principles is the most widely used psychosocial treatment for depression. Psychodynamic psychotherapy emphasizes the importance of past experiences and unconscious motivation in determining human behavior.

Short-term therapy (roughly five to 20 sessions) is often aimed at support, crisis intervention, and symptom relief for acutely depressed people so that they may cope better with daily activities and in dealing with others. Long-term psychotherapy (several months to several years) allows clients to identify, examine, and resolve intrapsychic conflicts that impair their lives, and to explore ways in which important childhood experiences have served as inadequate models for current relationships. Clients who improve with short-term treatment may or may not need more extended psychotherapy. The decision to continue in long-term treatment is usually based on whether a client's life is chronically hampered by emotional difficulties and the extent to which he or she is motivated to explore these difficulties.

Group psychotherapy can help depressed people improve their social skills and self-esteem. A therapy group provides a mutually supportive environment in which clients can examine their styles of dealing with others and test out new ways of forming relationships.

Cognitive therapy is a specific technique for treating depression and anxiety. It is based on the premise that distorted modes of thinking about oneself and the world in negative and pessimistic terms foster depression and that, by identifying such cognitive distortions and teaching the client to substitute more realistic and self-enhancing thoughts, painful feelings can be reduced. The therapy is short term and sessions are more structured than in psychodynamic psychotherapy.

In clinical studies, cognitive therapy has been shown to be of value to many depressed and anxious clients. Clinicians debate whether the therapeutic effects are due to cognitive therapy techniques per se or to the trust and rapport that develop between client and therapist. Equally controversial is the assumption in cognitive therapy that negative thoughts can actually cause painful feelings rather than simply result from them. Cognitive therapy continues to be a subject of active research (see Chapter 15).

Combining Different Treatment Modalities

Used in combination, somatic and psychosocial treatments are generally more effective than either modality alone. Psychotherapy influences social effectiveness and personality functioning, while medications and ECT affect physiologic functions like sleep, appetite, and sexual drive.

Thus, it is possible that many clients can benefit from both types of treatment. Decisions about treatment must be based on the availability of resources, on the client's willingness to comply with different regimens, and on the client's motivation to engage in self-exploratory work.

No one treatment for depression is universally effective, and none has been shown to be the treatment of choice for all types of depression. Ongoing clinical trials are now attempting to evaluate the relative efficacy of different treatments used alone and in various combinations.

BIPOLAR DISORDERS

Bipolar disorders are illnesses that are characterized by two extremes of mood: elation and depression. Stereotypically, the person with bipolar disorder cycles from wild mania into deep depression and back into mania again. In reality, bipolar illness covers a variety of clinical pictures that will be discussed below.

Depressive episodes in bipolar illness are clinically indistinguishable from those seen in unipolar illness. Thus, the distinctive—and often most dramatic—feature of bipolar illness is elation. Like depression, elation encompasses a broad spectrum of moods, including normal states of euphoria and joy, as well as the pathological elations known as mania and hypomania. *Mania* denotes extreme elation, hyperactivity, agitation, and accelerated speech, often with disordered thinking. *Hypomania* refers to a syndrome similar to, but not as severe as, mania. Many clinicians use *hypomania* to refer to elation without psychosis, and reserve the term *mania* for elation so severe as to include disordered thinking.

The term *elation* warrants an explanatory note. An individual's subjective experience of mania and hypomania can be pleasurable, involving feeling "high," happy, and euphoric, but these mood states are also characterized by extreme irritability, paranoia, and rage. Thus, it would be more accurate to speak of *excited* rather than elated mood states, since the manic person's subjective experience often varies from extreme euphoria to profound dysphoria.

The major syndromes included under bipolar disorders are *manic-depressive illness* and *cyclothymic disorder.* The two are distinguished from each other on the basis of the intensity and duration of symptoms.

Manic-Depressive Illness

Manic-depressive illness (MDI) generally includes full-blown episodes of mania and depression. Manic episodes may alternate one for one with depressive episodes, or one mood extreme may predominate. While people who only experience depressive episodes are categorized as having unipolar illness, those who only experience manic episodes are included in the bipolar category. Such people are quite rare; the rule in MDI is a history of both depressive and manic episodes.

Symptoms of Mania

The symptoms of depressive episodes have already been discussed at length. Since the diagnosis of manic-depressive illness hinges on the recognition of manic episodes, it is essential that you learn to recognize the symptoms of mania and hypomania. The cardinal symptoms outlined in *DSM-III* are listed in Table 6-6 and described below.

Mood disturbance. The manic person commonly experiences euphoria, and this mood can be quite infectious. In fact, you may find yourself smiling and suppressing the urge to laugh when interviewing a euphoric client; a reaction which should prompt you to suspect the diagnosis of mania. Those who know the person well usually recognize that the euphoria is uncharacteristic and excessive. Manic people have seemingly limitless enthusiasm for interacting with others, and commonly seek people out in an intrusive way (e.g., they may call friends to chat at 4:00 A.M., and be oblivious to the others'

Table 6–6. The symptoms of mania and hypomania.

Mood disturbance (euphoria, irritability)
Hyperactivity (motor restlessness, overinvolvement socially, at work, or
  sexually)
Pressured speech
Flight of ideas
Distractibility
Inflated self-esteem
Decreased need for sleep
Lability of mood
Delusions and hallucinations (in mania)

---

wish to sleep). As noted above, the predominant mood in some manic individuals is irritability rather than euphoria. Particularly when their desires are in any way thwarted, people who are manic can respond with extreme annoyance, even rage and violence (whence the term "maniac").

Hyperactivity. This includes motor restlessness and overinvolvement in sexual, recreational, occupational, and other activities. Manic individuals will plan and enter into a variety of projects, overcommitting themselves and using poor judgment. A client may, for example, start to repaint his house, begin to write a novel, and rebuild his auto engine—all in one day. Along with poor judgment, manics commonly demonstrate expansiveness, grandiosity, and unwarranted optimism—and these characteristics lead to many painful consequences.

For example, someone in the throes of mania can give away an entire fortune, amass huge debts on a buying spree, take off impulsively on a trip around the world, drive recklessly, engage in uncharacteristic sexual behavior, or stand on street corners and engage strangers in conversation.

Pressured speech. Manic people speak as if they are under pressure to get the words out. They speak loudly and rapidly and are usually difficult to interrupt. Their speech content may be normal, or full of jokes and puns, or full of hostile accusations and angry tirades. Manics often have a theatrical style and can be quite entertaining. Associations and word choice may be based on sounds rather than ideas, resulting in clang associations (e.g., "talk—tic-toc—what's up doc?").

Flight of ideas. This involves skipping from one idea to another in a continuous flow of accelerated speech. The speaker makes associations that are comprehensible but based on puns, extraneous stimuli, or other chance factors. If it is severe, flight of ideas can make the manic person's speech impossible to follow.

Distractibility. Manic people have difficulty in screening out extraneous stimuli. They often react to noises, sights, or smells, shifting their focus of attention rapidly from one irrelevant stimulus to another (hence, the use of seclusion as a means of calming agitated manics).

Inflated self-esteem. An unrealistic sense of one's own merits and importance often accompanies an elevated mood. Some people simply become overconfident and less self-critical; others develop grandiose ideas of delusional proportions. They may come to believe, for example, that they have a special relationship with God, that they have a plan to save the universe from destruction, or that they have unparalleled gifts they must share with the world.

Decreased need for sleep. Almost all manics experience a decreased need for sleep, feeling full of energy despite little or no rest. Some manic individuals actually go without any sleep for days at a time and do not report feeling tired.

Lability of mood. Some manic people move rapidly from euphoria to anger or depression. Mood swings may last for minutes or even several hours at a time, but rarely longer.

Delusions and hallucinations. The content of delusions or hallucinations is usually consonant with an elevated and grandiose mood. For example, a client may believe that he or she is being persecuted by enemy agents because he or she possesses special powers. Another may believe he or she sees God and speaks directly with Him.

Diagnosis
The diagnostic criteria outlined in *DSM-III* are essentially as follows:

1. An elevated, expansive, or irritable mood.
2. At least three of the following symptoms persisting for at least one week:

   - Increase in activity or physical restlessness,
   - Increase in talkativeness or pressured speech,
   - Flight of ideas or racing thoughts,
   - Inflated self-esteem,
   - Decreased need for sleep,
   - Distractibility,
   - Excessive involvement in activities the person does not realize may have painful consequences (e.g., buying sprees, reckless driving, sexual indiscretions).

3. No psychosis or bizarre behavior during periods of normal mood.
4. Symptoms are not due to another condition, such as schizophrenia or a paranoid disorder or to substance abuse.

Differential Diagnosis

Many clinical studies have concluded that MDI has been under-diagnosed in the United States in recent years because bipolar disorder is frequently mistaken for other mental illnesses, most notably schizophrenia. Although there are many causes of excited and elated states, only a small number of disorders are commonly confused with manic-depressive illness.

Organic affective syndromes. Organic causes of elation and full-blown mania include the use of such drugs as steroids, alcohol, and amphetamines; as well as specific illnesses like cerebral tumors, multiple sclerosis, and dementia. The evaluation of a first acute manic episode should include a thorough physical examination, routine laboratory screening (complete blood count, routine blood chemistries, urinalysis), screening of serum and urine for toxic substances, and a thorough medical and drug history to rule out organic causes of mania (Table 6-7).

Table 6–7. The medical work-up of the manic client.

Medical history—including drug use
Physical examination
Routine laboratory screening
   Complete blood count (CBC)
   Blood chemistries (SMA-12)
   Urinalysis
   Thyroid function tests
Screening of blood and urine for toxic substances

Schizophrenia. Mania and schizophrenia often look very similar. In some cases it is almost impossible to distinguish between them on the basis of presenting symptoms alone. For example, hallucinations, paranoia, grandiose delusions, loose associations, bizarre behaviors, and irritability are common features of both illnesses. Thus, the clinician must frequently rely on factors other than the client's mental status to make as accurate a diagnosis as possible. Table 6-8 outlines historical data that favor a diagnosis of MDI and those that favor a diagnosis of schizophrenia.

Table 6-8. Features which help to differentiate between manic-depressive illness (MDI) and schizophrenia.

Favors MDI	Favors schizophrenia
Previous episode of mania or depression	No previous history of affective disturbance
History of complete recovery between acute episodes of illness	History of residual impairment between acute exacerbations of illness
Good premorbid functioning	Gradual deterioration and poor premorbid functioning
Family history positive for a remitting psychotic illness	Family history negative for remitting psychotic illness
History of favorable treatment response to lithium and/or ECT	Poor response to treatment with lithium and/or ECT

Schizoaffective disorder. This diagnostic category is used for people who exhibit symptoms of a mood disorder (mania and/or depression) but whose chronic impairment of thought and functioning is more consistent with schizophrenia. Many clinicians consider this a "wastebasket" diagnosis, and believe schizoaffective disorder is a variant of MDI or schizophrenia rather than a separate disease entity. The diagnosis is usually made when it is impossible to categorize an illness as MDI or schizophrenia. Lithium and TCAs are often used for schizoaffective clients, but generally with less success than in treating true bipolar or unipolar affective illness. Antipsychotic drugs are also used to treat disordered thinking, and the combination of an antipsychotic and lithium or a TCA is very common in treating schizoaffective illness.

Cyclothymic disorder. Essentially, this disorder involves periods of depression and hypomania, but with briefer mood swings and less severe symptoms than in MDI. This diagnosis will be discussed at greater length below.

Clinical Course
People with MDI may initially present with either a manic or a depressive episode. Obviously, a client who presents with a depressive episode and no history of mania may have either bipolar or

unipolar illness. Only time will tell whether that person will go on to have manic episodes or only experience bouts of depression.

In bipolar illness, the first disturbance of mood is often manic. Manic episodes generally begin suddenly and escalate rapidly over a few days. Mania may persist for several days or several months, but the episodes are generally briefer and occur more abruptly than major depressive episodes. Particularly if it is not treated early, mania generally goes through stages of severity, beginning with a mild syndrome and progressing to a much more dramatic and disorganized clinical picture. Initially, mood is predominantly euphoric, but the manic individual becomes increasingly irritable and finally panicked and/or enraged. What begins as mildly increased psychomotor activity develops into frenzied and bizarre behavior; initial suspiciousness, grandiosity, and racing thoughts give way to frank delusions, hallucinations, and flight of ideas. This increase in severity is followed by a gradual abatement of symptoms and ultimately a return to normal mood in the majority of manic people, but the rate at which they pass through these stages of mania is highly variable.

Almost everyone who has one or more manic episodes will eventually have at least one depressive episode. An episode of either type may be followed immediately by a brief episode of the other kind, but manic and depressive episodes are usually separated by an intervening period of normal mood and functioning. Some people go for many years after an initial mood disturbance without any recurrence; others have clusters of manic and depressive episodes; still others have increasingly frequent manic and/or depressive episodes as they grow older.

There is a subgroup of manic-depressives (estimates range from 10 to 35 percent) who do not return to normal moods or functioning between episodes, but have a chronic course with significant residual symptomatic and social impairment.

Before lithium, ECT, and antipsychotics were used in the treatment of mania, the average duration of a manic episode was three months; with these treatment modalities, that time has been considerably shortened. Since there is marked variation in both the severity and duration of manic and depressive episodes and the length of intervening periods of normal mood, you should develop a profile of mood cycles for each client in order to plan for the most effective treatment.

The most common complications in the course of a manic episode are substance abuse and the consequences (personal, financial, etc.) of poor judgment.

Epidemiology

The annual rate of first hospital admission for MDI in men is eight to 10 per 100,000; in women, it is 15 to 20 per 100,000 population. Between 0.4 and 1.2 percent of the adult population carries the diagnosis. The lifetime risk of developing MDI is roughly 1 to 2 percent.

Age. The first manic episode in bipolar disorder usually occurs before age 30. In fact, a first manic episode in someone over the age of 50 is so rare that you should strongly suspect an organic cause of mania (e.g., drugs or central nervous system tumor).

Sex. MDI is roughly as common in men as in women, although studies suggest a slight preponderance of the disease among women (the male:female ratio is 1.0:1.5). This is in contrast to the unipolar depressive disorders, which are considerably more common in women than in men.

Socioeconomic status. Although there are no sharp distinctions on the basis of social class, there appears to be a somewhat higher incidence of MDI in the higher social strata.

Marital status. There is no appreciable difference in the incidence of MDI on the basis of marital status.

Family history. The frequency of MDI is markedly higher among the biologic relatives of those who have the disease.

Etiology

The cause of MDI is not known. As with unipolar depressive disorders, researchers have looked at a wide variety of biological and psychological variables.

The most substantial information we have to date is about the genetic basis of the illness. Twin studies, family studies, and surveys of the general population support the idea of a genetic predisposition to MDI. Most striking are twin studies that show the concordance rates for MDI to be 68 percent for monozygotic twins and 23 percent for same-sex dizygotic twins. (In other words, among identical twins, if one is manic-depressive the other will be manic-depressive in 68 percent of cases. By contrast, among twins who are not genetically identical, the rate is only 23 percent.)

It is possible that incomplete gene penetrance accounts for the fact that the concordance rate for MDI in monozygotic twins is less than 100 percent. However, it is also possible that other nongenetic factors operate in determining which individuals develop the clinical syndrome of MDI and which do not.

Neurochemical studies of manic-depressive individuals have shown decreased levels of urinary MHPG during depressive episodes, but no similar derangement of the levels of biogenic amines during manic episodes. Investigators have speculated that mania results from an increase in dopamine levels in the brain, but this hypothesis has not been proven in research studies. Investigators have also hoped to solve the mystery of MDI by elucidating the mechanism by which lithium exerts its therapeutic effect, but to date we do not know how lithium works.

Treatment

Acute mania. Depending on its severity, an acute manic episode may constitute a mental health emergency. You must quickly assess the manic client for *self-destructive behaviors, proneness to violence,* and an *inability to care for himself or herself.*

Self-destructive behaviors include not only overtly suicidal behaviors, but also acts involving such poor judgment as to be potentially life-threatening (reckless driving, "daredevil" stunts).

Particularly when paranoia is severe, manic people can be very violent and may even kill others because of a delusional belief that they are acting in self-defense.

In mania, a patient's inability to care for himself or herself often takes bizarre forms, e.g., walking naked outdoors in freezing weather, giving away all one's money to strangers, going on wild spending sprees, not sleeping or eating for many days.

Any of the above warrant hospital admission. Hospitalization should also be considered for a first manic episode, to facilitate a complete medical work-up and planning for adequate ongoing treatment.

Treatment of an acute manic episode generally involves both medication and setting limits on manic behavior. Severe mania is often terrifying to the client insofar as it represents a loss of self-control. Hospital admission to a locked unit can therefore be reassuring, since it conveys the message that others will take control and keep the client safe.

Similarly, many manics initially require locked-door seclusion and physical restraint to keep them from harming themselves or others; this, too, can be reassuring rather than punitive. Physical

Table 6–9. Common therapeutic interventions in manic-depressive illness.

Acute mania
  Setting limits on manic behavior
    Seclusion
    Physical restraints
  Antipsychotic medications
  Lithium
  ECT

Acute depression
  Suicide precautions, assistance with self-care
  Antidepressants
  Antipsychotic medications
  ECT

Prevention of further episodes (maintenance)
  Lithium
  Antipsychotic medications
  Antidepressants
  Education about the illness for clients, families
  Psychosocial therapy

restraint should be used only when other measures have proved insufficient to calm the manic individual. Frequently, unlocked seclusion alone will have a significant calming effect. Manic people are highly excitable and easily distracted, so the simple act of reducing sensory stimulation in a quiet, secluded room can help to ease severe agitation.

Pharmacologic treatment is aimed at both the rapid amelioration of symptoms and long-term reduction in the frequency, severity, and duration of manic episodes.

Antipsychotics are the mainstay of rapid treatment. They have a marked antianxiety effect and can considerably reduce the manic person's terror, combativeness, and confusion. Manic people generally respond to adequate oral or intramuscular doses of neuroleptics (see Chapter 16) within a few hours to a few days, often eliminating the need for seclusion and restraint. Because lithium takes roughly 10 to 14 days to work, an antipsychotic such as chlorpromazine is often the drug that is tried first. Lithium is started in addition to the neuroleptic as soon as the necessary preliminary laboratory work has been completed. In many cases, the antipsychotic may be discontinued once the client has been stabilized on lithium.

ECT has been shown to be a safe and effective treatment for acute mania. It is often used when antipsychotic treatment is either ineffective or, for some reason, contraindicated in a particular case. ECT and lithium should not be used concurrently (i.e., when ECT is administered, lithium should be temporarily discontinued), since there is evidence that this treatment combination may diminish the therapeutic effects of each modality and increase the risk of neuropsychological side effects.

Lithium produces a therapeutic response in roughly 70 percent of acutely manic people in 10 to 14 days. It decreases both the severity and duration of the acute manic episode, and dramatically reduces the rate of relapse. Since mood stabilization is related to the amount of lithium in the bloodstream, serum lithium levels are monitored to titrate the correct dosage of the drug. For a more extensive discussion of indications, contraindications, and guidelines for the use of lithium, see Chapter 16.

Acute depression. There is considerable evidence that lithium is effective in preventing depressive episodes in MDI. However, acute depressive episodes do occur in people who are maintained on lithium, and these often require treatment with antidepressants in addition to lithium. The principles of treatment are the same for acute depressive episodes in MDI and in unipolar depression. However, there is a critical distinction between bipolar and unipolar depression in the use of tricyclic antidepressants, because TCAs can precipitate mania in bipolar people. Thus, the treatment of acute depressive episodes in clients known or suspected to be bipolar must be undertaken with caution, and clients must be carefully monitored for signs of developing mania. If mania develops, TCAs must be discontinued and the mania treated.

Prevention of further episodes (maintenance therapy). Lithium is the mainstay of long-term, as well as acute, treatment of MDI. It has been shown to prevent recurrent mania and depression with moderate, if not total, efficacy. Because such underlying conditions as kidney disease, heart disease, and organic brain syndromes can make lithium administration dangerous, a careful medical screening must be done whenever maintenance therapy is contemplated. In addition, serum lithium levels must be sampled on a regular basis (usually monthly or bimonthly) to ensure that the client is on an adequate dosage. Certain laboratory tests, including serum creatinine levels (to assess kidney functioning) and white blood cell count, must be monitored every few months to prevent possible toxic effects of lithium on the body. Thus, lithium can only be used safely in people who can comply with a precise treatment regimen (see Chapter 16).

In manic-depressive individuals who manifest residual thought disorder between episodes of mood disturbance, antipsychotic drugs are commonly used as treatment on a long-term basis along with lithium.

For some manic-depressives in whom recurrent depressive episodes are severe and frequent, maintenance therapy with tricyclic antidepressants (with or without lithium) may help to prevent cycles of depression. In such cases, the client must be carefully monitored lest the antidepressant precipitate a manic episode.

Education is important to help clients and their families recognize the signs and symptoms of incipient mania and depression, so that they may seek treatment for acute episodes early, and thereby increase the likelihood that a full-scale affective disturbance can be prevented or ameliorated. Clients must have a clear idea of what treatment is available (hospital, emergency room, outpatient clinic) and whom they are to contact when they experience affective disturbances.

There is a good deal of controversy over whether any psychosocial therapy is helpful for manic-depressives. Certainly supportive therapy can be useful in helping people to cope with the devastating social and occupational effects of severe affective illness and in promoting compliance in taking medications. But it has not been demonstrated that insight-oriented, exploratory psychotherapy is useful in treating MDI. Manic-depressive illness can occur in an infinite variety of personality types; some manic-depressives in remission may be psychologically quite healthy and function well, while others may have significant underlying personality disorders. In general, clients who, in remission, manifest personality disturbances that impair their functioning are candidates for psychotherapy, along with routine pharmacologic treatment of MDI.

Cyclothymic Disorder

Clinicians recognize the existence of bipolar affective disturbances that are milder and briefer than those in manic-depressive illness. Cyclothymic disorder describes a syndrome of chronic mood disturbance of at least two years' duration, characterized by numerous periods of depression and hypomania that are less severe and less prolonged than those in MDI. By definition, no psychotic features accompany the affective disturbances in cyclothymic disorder, because the presence of psychosis indicates the full-blown affective syndrome of MDI.

Diagnostic Criteria

The diagnostic criteria for cyclothymic disorder outlined in *DSM-III* are as follows:

1. During the past two years, there have been numerous periods during which some symptoms characteristic of both depressive and manic syndromes were present, but not of sufficient severity and duration to meet the criteria for a major depressive or manic episode.
2. The depressive periods and hypomanic periods may be separated by periods of normal mood lasting months at a time, they may be intermixed, or they may alternate.
3. During depressive periods, there is depressed mood or loss of interest or pleasure in almost all the person's usual activities and pastimes, along with at least three of the symptoms in Table 6-10.
4. During hypomanic periods, there is an elevated, expansive, or irritable mood, along with at least three of the symptoms in Table 6-10.
5. There are no psychotic features such as delusions, hallucinations, incoherence, or loosening of associations.
6. Symptoms are not due to any other mental disorder, such as partial remission of bipolar disorder. However, cyclothymic disorder may precede bipolar disorder.

Cyclothymic disorder usually begins early in adult life, generally with an insidious onset and a chronic course. The degree to which the illness impairs social and occupational functioning is variable, and may range from mild to severe. The disorder was previously assumed to be rare but, as the syndrome has become more clearly defined in recent years, it has been recognized with increasing frequency, particularly among people seeking outpatient treatment. It appears to be more common among women than among men. It is also more prevalent among those who have biological relatives with major depression and bipolar disorder than it is in the general population.

The most common complication of cyclothymic disorder is substance abuse. As in MDI, cyclothymic individuals tend to medicate their depression with stimulants and alcohol, and to abuse stimulants and psychedelics during hypomanic periods.

Table 6–10. Symptoms of depressive and hypomanic periods in cyclothymic disorder.

Depressive symptoms	Hypomanic symptoms
Insomnia or hypersomnia	Decreased need for sleep
Low energy level or chronic fatigue	More energy than usual
Feelings of inadequacy	Inflated self-esteem
Decreased effectiveness or productivity at school, work, or home	Increased productivity, often associated with unusual and self-imposed working hours
Decreased attention, concentration, or ability to think clearly	Sharpened and unusually creative thinking
Social withdrawal	Uninhibited people-seeking (extreme gregariousness)
Loss of interest in or enjoyment of sex	Hypersexuality without recognition of the possibility of painful consequences
Restriction of involvement in pleasurable activities, guilt over past activities	Excessive involvement in pleasurable activities and lack of concern for painful consequences, e.g., buying sprees, foolish business investments, reckless driving
Feeling slowed down	Physical restlessness
Less talkative than usual	More talkative than usual
Pessimistic attitude toward the future, brooding about past events	Overoptimism or exaggeration of past achievements
Tearfulness or crying	Inappropriate laughing, joking, punning

The differential diagnosis of cyclothymic disorder is essentially the same as that for major depressive and manic episodes. Also, MDI may be superimposed on an underlying, more chronic cyclothymic disorder.

Treatment is similar to that of MDI. Many clients experience a stabilization of their moods when they are maintained on adequate amounts of lithium.

A FINAL NOTE ON MOOD DISORDERS

Affective illness is now the subject of intense research in this country and abroad. Exciting data are emerging that suggest the existence of "affective equivalents"—that is, symptoms that do not look like mood disturbances yet respond to antidepressant medications. Among the symptoms thought to be possible affective equivalents are panic attacks and eating disorders. You will undoubtedly hear more about new categories of affective illness in the coming years.

REFERENCES

American Psychiatric Association: Affective disorders, in Diagnostic and Statistical Manual of Mental Disorders, 3rd ed. Washington DC, American Psychiatric Association, 1980, pp 205-224

Appleton WS, Davis JM: Practical Clinical Psychopharmacology, 2nd ed. Baltimore, Williams & Wilkins, 1980, pp 82-136

Bibring E: The mechanism of depression, in Affective Disorders. Edited by Greenacre P. New York, International University Press, 1953, pp 154-181

Carlson GA, Goodwin FK: The stages of mania: a longitudinal analysis of the manic episode. Arch Gen Psychiatry 28:221-228, 1973

Childress AR, Burns DD: The basics of cognitive therapy. Psychosomatics 22:1017-1027, 1981

Freud S: Mourning and Melancholia (1917), in Complete Works, standard ed, vol 14. Translated and edited by Strachey J. London, Hogarth Press, 1957, pp 237-258

Isenberg PL, Schatzberg AF: Psychoanalytic contribution to a theory of depression, in Depression: Biology, Psychodynamics, and Treatment. Edited by Cole JO, Schatzberg AF, Frazier SH. New York, Plenum Press, 1978, pp 149-171

Klerman GL: Affective disorders, in The Harvard Guide to Modern Psychiatry. Edited by Nicholi A Jr. Cambridge, Mass, Harvard University Press, 1978, pp 253-282

Lloyd C: Life events and depressive disorder reviewed, I: events as predisposing factors. Arch Gen Psychiatry 37:529-535, 1980

MacVane JR, Lange JD, Brown WA, et al: Psychological functioning of bipolar manic-depressives in remission. Arch Gen Psychiatry 35:1351-1354, 1978

Pope HG Jr, Hudson JI, Jonas JM, et al: Bulimia treated with imipramine: a placebo-controlled, double-blind study. Am J Psychiatry 140:554-558, 1983

Pope HG Jr, Lipinski JF Jr: Diagnosis in schizophrenia and manic-depressive illness. Arch Gen Psychiatry 35:811-828, 1978

Schatzberg AF: Classification of depressive disorders, in Depression: Biology, Psychodynamics, and Treatment. Edited by Cole JO, Schatzberg AF, Frazier SH. New York, Plenum Press, 1978, pp 13-40

Weiner D: The psychiatric use of electrically induced seizures. Am J Psychiatry 136:1507-1517, 1979

CHAPTER 7

Personality Disorders

The diversity and complexity of human personality are highly cele-
brated in our society. It may seem presumptuous, therefore, to speak
of "personality types" or "character styles"—to try to fit ourselves and
our fellow beings into categories according to the way we behave. Yet
human beings are generally consistent in their ways of dealing with
the world and particularly with other people. Our styles of thinking,
experiencing, and behaving usually remain stable as we meet a variety of new challenges in new settings—hence the concept of character.

Character is reflected in our attitudes, our interests, our intellectual inclinations, our job aptitudes, and our social affinities. We all
know people who fit certain stereotypes of character styles: the hard-
driving unemotional scientist who buries himself in his laboratory
work and is oblivious to life around him, or the dazzling actress who
is the "life of the party." It would be no surprise to hear that the
scientist is fastidious and conservative in dress, or that the actress
wears lavish and seductive clothing. Nor would it be surprising that
the scientist enjoys complex puzzles and mathematical games, while
the actress has little interest in balancing her checkbook. Of course,
these are stereotypes; fortunately, most people are flexible enough to
have a variety of styles in their repertoire. But most of us have a major
personality style that shows itself in many different settings during all

139

sorts of activities—in everything from the hobbies we enjoy to the lovers we choose.

Certainly, the "typing" of personalities does not imply any abnormality. In fact, the traits associated with particular personality types are often highly useful and adaptive, for they allow us to tolerate anxiety, to solve problems, to be creative, and to cope with a variety of life's stresses. For example, students would be in trouble if they did not possess some "obsessional" capacities for organizing and concentrating on a variety of tasks. Yet labels like "obsessive-compulsive" and "hysterical" have taken on very pejorative connotations in our daily language, and it is fashionable to use such terms in a sort of diagnostic name-calling.

When do personality *traits* become personality *disorders?* The boundary is not clear, but—generally—when character traits are so maladaptive and inflexible that they significantly impair one's work life and social life or cause major subjective distress, a diagnosis of personality disorder is warranted.

WHAT ARE PERSONALITY DISORDERS?

Personality disorders are common, they are difficult to treat, and the people who have them typically end up being labeled "bad" or "deviant" by others—even by mental health professionals. With that ominous prelude, let us look at some general characteristics of all personality disorders. The following generalizations may not hold true in every case, but they are good rules of thumb to help you put this category of psychopathology into a larger context:

- Personality disorders involve inflexible and maladaptive responses to stress.
- Personality disorders are global—they affect nearly all areas of a person's life, so that he or she is severely handicapped in working and loving. By contrast, neurotics are people whose problems are confined to discrete aspects of their lives, while other aspects remain relatively free of psychological conflict.
- People with personality disorders commonly feel the problem lies not within themselves but in their environment (e.g., "No one understands me!" or "Everyone thwarts my plans!"). Neurotic people are more likely to locate the source of their problems within themselves.
- Personality disorders do not, for the most part, involve psychosis. Brief psychotic episodes occur, but florid lapses in reality testing (see Chapter 4) are the exception rather than the rule. Most people

with personality disorders are in touch with reality most of the time.

- People with personality disorders are often untroubled by their illness, for they fail to see themselves as others see them. In fact, they may feel themselves to be in the best of emotional health, while others are quite distressed by their behavior. They may be dragged to mental health care facilities by others; the vast majority never seek treatment.
- People with personality disorders have an uncanny ability to get under the skin of others. They are likely, therefore, to be rejected by those close to them. They invariably irritate the mental health professionals who try to treat them. Treatment is difficult, and failure is common.
- The complications associated with personality disorders are many. The most common are depression, suicide, violence and antisocial behavior, brief psychotic episodes, and multiple drug abuse.

From this list of features, you may wonder whether the label of "personality disorder" is simply a technical way of saying that someone is obnoxious. Indeed, the diagnostic label is easy to misuse in this way, as an epithet for any client you do not like. But in fact, individuals with personality disorders have specific and often crippling illnesses, defined not by their unpleasantness but by their social dysfunction and personal inflexibility. They are incapable of responding to life's varied stresses and challenges except in a very rigid manner. They are like musicians who can play only one note.

Causes

Little is known about the causes of specific personality disorders.

Environmental factors have been assumed to play the dominant role in the genesis of these disorders. Psychoanalytic theorists have focused primarily on the significance of childhood experiences within the family. However, few good large-scale studies have correlated early deprived or traumatic childhoods with later personality disorders. To date, there are no hard data to answer the perplexing question of why some people who suffer early emotional trauma develop severe character pathology while others, with equally unhappy childhoods, do not.

Genetic factors are under active investigation as possible contributors to the development of personality disorders. There is some evidence for the heritability of certain character traits—particularly for the heritability of introverted personality traits. Work is also being done on the heritability of obsessive-compulsive traits.

Other constitutional factors, such as physical illness, seem to play a role in the development of personality disorders in some people. Neurologic disorders—particularly birth-related trauma, encephalitis (a generalized infection of brain tissue), and temporal lobe epilepsy—have been found to increase both the incidence and severity of personality disorders. In fact, a history of minimal brain dysfunction (a childhood syndrome which includes such symptoms as learning disabilities and "hyperactivity") or the presence of "soft" (nonspecific) signs of neurologic dysfunction (e.g., abnormal movements of arms or legs, incoordination, left-right confusion) in childhood correlate with an increased incidence of personality disorders in adolescence and adulthood.

Course and Prognosis

Personality disorders usually become evident in adolesence, or sometimes earlier. Clinical lore holds that, once you have a personality disorder, you have it for life. However, surprisingly little is known about the course of these illnesses. It may be, for example, that personality disorders seem intractable because such people frequently fail in psychiatric treatment. Also, it may be that personality-disordered people who "grow up" or "burn out"—or in some way get better—cease to require professional attention, leaving only the truly intractable population in treatment and in correctional facilities. More work needs to be done in charting the course of these illnesses.

Diagnosis

The diagnostic criteria for the personality disorders are described below. Diagnosis is often difficult. The following are points to keep in mind in your assessments:

- Be suspicious of reports by family or friends that the client's personality has changed abruptly. Personality disorders do not begin suddenly. A history of sudden change in character should alert you to the possibility of some other illness, especially a central nervous system disorder (e.g., tumor, stroke), incipient psychosis, or drug or alcohol abuse. Any of these can mimic a personality disorder.
- Be curious why someone with a personality disorder comes to you at a particular time. Look for some change in important relationships that upset the former balance and suddenly made the disordered personality obvious to the client or others.
- Pay attention to your feelings about the client. A person who makes

you feel intensely angry, helpless, powerful, or frightened in the first few minutes of the interview may be showing you the nature of his or her personality disorder.

- Beware of overdiagnosing personality disorders in people who are ethnically and culturally different from you. Behavior is more likely to look abnormal outside its social context.

Eleven personality disorders are described in the third edition of the *Diagnostic and Statistical Manual of Mental Disorders (DSM-III)*. Some of these are new to the third edition. The delineation of the various personality disorders has been a difficult task. First, there is no clear boundary to separate personality disorders from less severe conditions; diagnosis involves a measure of subjectivity. Second, personality is too complex to fit neatly into eleven categories. Many people with personality disorders exhibit features of more than one personality type. Some theorists have suggested that personality disorders are more accurately seen as clusters of pathologic traits that can occur in an almost infinite variety of combinations.

As you read through the following descriptions, remember that these are stereotypes—individual people will have highly individual presentations. *DSM-III* has sorted the personality disorders into three general groups, as shown in Table 7-1.

Table 7–1. Categorization of people with personality disorders.

Those who appear odd or eccentric and who fear social relationships
    Paranoid personality disorder
    Schizoid personality disorder
    Schizotypal personality disorder

Those who appear dramatic, emotional, or erratic and who act directly on their environment
    Histrionic personality disorder
    Narcissistic personality disorder
    Antisocial personality disorder
    Borderline personality disorder

Those who are primarily anxious and careful (rather than fearful) of intimacy
    Avoidant personality disorder
    Dependent personality disorder
    Compulsive personality disorder
    Passive-aggressive personality disorder

PARANOID PERSONALITY DISORDER

Profile

"Paranoid" is a common term in our everyday language, used to describe anyone from a jealous boyfriend to politicians who support a heavy build-up of nuclear armaments. Paranoia refers to a pervasive and unwarranted suspiciousness and mistrust of others. Suspiciousness may be highly justified and adaptive in war and other stressful situations, but paranoid people cannot abandon their suspicions when presented with convincing contradictory evidence. They remain constantly on guard, because for them there is always a war going on.

Paranoid people are keen observers. They search intently for some confirmation that they are in danger. By disregarding facts that do not confirm their suspicions, they invariably find the plots and threats they so ardently seek. They are hypersensitive, they expect trickery and disloyalty from others, and they try to avoid all surprises by anticipating them.

Paranoid people appear tense, guarded, and secretive; they are often litigious and highly moralistic. They are usually humorless and overly serious. They have difficulty expressing warm emotions and tolerating feelings of being dependent on others. They appear cold and may be quite logical. They are often interested in electronics, mechanics, and communication devices. They are also keenly aware of power and rank.

Because paranoid people seize upon irrelevant details to confirm their suspicions, they generally do not see the forest for the trees. They have very poor judgment in matters relating to their fears. They may, under stress, become floridly delusional (e.g., believing themselves pursued by the FBI) or experience ideas of reference. As a rule, however, psychotic episodes are brief and transient. The paranoid individual relies heavily on the defense of projection to maintain a psychological equilibrium. Projection involves attributing one's motives, feelings, or drives to someone else because one finds them unacceptable in oneself. This all happens unconsciously—i.e., individuals who use projection are unaware that the motives they see in others are really their own. They make their inner world safe by making the outer world dangerous. Not surprisingly, paranoid people often bear a striking resemblance to the "demons" they choose.

In interviews, paranoid people are likely to be very businesslike. They may tell you they see no reason why they were referred to you. They may scan the room anxiously and have great difficulty relaxing.

Or their preoccupation with details and constant questions may be the only things that belie their fear and mistrust.

Diagnosis. DSM-III provides a list of items that are characteristic of the paranoid person's current and long-term functioning. These diagnostic criteria are shown in Table 7-2.

Causes. The causes of this disorder are unknown. A genetic predisposition to paranoid personality disorder has been considered, but no substantial evidence has emerged to date to support this hypothesis.

Table 7–2. *DSM-III* criteria for the diagnosis of paranoid personality disorder.

Pervasive, unwarranted suspiciousness and mistrust of people, as indicated by at least three of the following:

Expectation of trickery or harm
Hypervigilance, manifested by continual scanning of the environment for signs of threat, or taking unneeded precautions
Guardedness or secretiveness
Avoidance of accepting blame when warranted
Questioning the loyalty of others
Intense, narrowly focused searching for confirmation of bias, with loss of appreciation of total context
Overconcern with hidden motives and special meanings
Pathological jealousy

Hypersensitivity, as indicated by at least two of the following:

Tendency to be easily slighted and quick to take offense
Exaggeration of difficulties (e.g., "making mountains out of molehills")
Readiness to counterattack when any threat is perceived
Inability to relax

Restricted affectivity, as indicated by at least two of the following:

Appearance of being "cold" and unemotional
Pride taken in always being objective, rational, and unemotional
Lack of a true sense of humor
Absence of passive, soft, tender, and sentimental feelings

Not due to another mental disorder such as schizophrenia or a paranoid disorder

Some psychoanalytic theorists suggest that people who were the objects of irrational and overwhelming parental rage may come to adopt their parents' style and project onto others the rage they believe was once directed toward them. Others have characterized the families of paranoids as overly constricted emotionally.

Epidemiology. Little is known about the incidence or prevalence, because many paranoid people never seek treatment. The disorder is more frequently diagnosed in men than in women. There is no known familial pattern, but the disorder occurs with increased frequency in the biologic relatives of schizophrenics.

Course and prognosis. No good long-term outcome studies have been done on paranoid personality disorder. Some people apparently have the disorder throughout life, while others "grow out of it" as stress diminishes or other life circumstances change. Some people who are diagnosed as having paranoid personality disorder go on to develop schizophrenia.

Differential Diagnosis

There are several conditions from which paranoid personality disorder must be differentiated.

Paranoid disorders. These disorders are characterized by persistent psychotic symptoms (e.g., delusions, hallucinations) that are not present in paranoid personality disorder.

Schizophrenia. Like paranoid disorders, schizophrenia is marked by persistent psychosis, which does not characterize paranoid personality disorder.

Borderline personality disorder. Although borderline individuals may show some paranoid features, they tend to be overinvolved in chaotic relationships with people. Paranoid people, by contrast, remain aloof and distant from others.

Antisocial personality disorder. Both antisocial and paranoid personality disorders involve difficulty with intimacy, but paranoids do not have the lifelong history of antisocial behavior that is found in antisocial personality disorder.

Impulse disorders. These may be distinguished from paranoid personality disorder because they are characterized primarily by difficulty with impulse control rather than by suspiciousness.

Treatment

Because paranoid people are so frightened of intimacy and so reluctant to trust, a relationship with a therapist may be both longed for and dreaded. You must be particularly careful to operate in as open and straightforward a manner as possible in dealing with such people. Use humor sparingly and with great care at the start, for paranoid people are prone to feel that others are laughing at them rather than with them.

You must be careful to assume a professional manner, not one that is overly warm; paranoid people will be suspicious of and frightened by overtures they do not understand. When paranoid clients develop false beliefs about you (e.g., that you are part of a conspiracy to harm them), their accusations can easily become threats. You must limit any threatening behavior, both for your own and the client's safety.

Among the most commonly used treatments, individual psychotherapy is probably the treatment of choice, although no good controlled studies on the treatment of paranoid personality disorder have been done. A primary aim of therapy is to help paranoid clients see how they attribute their own unacceptable thoughts and feelings to others, and the ways in which this distorted perspective hampers their lives. Paranoid people have difficulty tolerating confrontation by others in group therapy, or tolerating the directive techniques used in behavior modification.

SCHIZOID PERSONALITY DISORDER

Profile

The term *schizoid* has long been used to describe people who are socially withdrawn, introverted, eccentric, and uncomfortable with others. If you consider the schizophrenic disorders as a spectrum (see Chapter 5), then schizoid personality disorder—along with paranoid and schizotypal personality disorder, occupies the healthier end of the schizophrenic spectrum. Schizoid individuals resemble schizophrenics in their odd and withdrawn manner but, while schizophrenics have chronically disordered thinking, schizoids do not.

The avoidance of human contact is a way of life for schizoid people, and they show little need or longing for emotional ties to others. Instead, they are likely to be quite absorbed in their own private fantasy worlds, in which they carry on relationships with imaginary friends. Their sex life may exist only in this world of make-believe. While they may have violent fantasies, they usually express little emotion to others.

Schizoid individuals actively pursue isolation, and will therefore choose solitary jobs other people find difficult to tolerate. They are likely to work as night-shift security guards or to bury themselves in the stacks of a library. In fact, schizoid people can be quite absorbed in and successful at such pursuits as mathematics and astronomy, which demand little human contact.

In an interview, you will find the schizoid person to be uncomfortable with you and eager for the meeting to end. He or she will make infrequent eye contact, show little emotion, and offer little in the way of spontaneous comments—answering your questions but not elaborating on answers at all. Occasionally, you may hear odd word usage, but speech and thought content do not generally appear abnormal.

Why does the schizoid person flee from other people? Although he or she is seemingly indifferent to others, the schizoid person usually feels quite vulnerable and finds human interaction confusing, frightening, and painful. The isolation is thus sought in self-defense. One schizoid woman described her situation as that of a tiny, naked baby locked inside a steel drawer (Guntrip 1973, p. 152).

Diagnosis. The diagnostic criteria given in *DSM-III* for schizoid personality disorder are shown in Table 7-3.

Causes. No one knows why some individuals become schizoid and others do not. In psychotherapy, schizoid clients commonly report bleak childhoods devoid of emotional warmth, but no prospective studies have been done to see which factors in childhood can be correlated with schizoid personality traits in adult life. There is also considerable speculation, but no clear evidence, of possible genetic factors in the genesis of schizoid personality disorder.

Epidemiology. The incidence, prevalence, and sex ratio of schizoid personality disorder are not known. Many schizoid people never seek treatment.

Table 7–3. *DSM-III* criteria for the diagnosis of schizoid personality disorder.

Emotional coldness and aloofness and the absence of warm, tender feelings for others

Indifference to praise or criticism or to the feelings of others

Close friendships with no more than one or two persons, including family members

No eccentricities of speech, behavior, or thought that are characteristic of schizotypal personality disorder

Not due to a psychotic disorder such as schizophrenia or paranoid disorder

If under 18, the person does not meet the criteria for schizoid disorder of childhood or adolescence

Course and prognosis. Schizoid personality disorder generally begins in childhood and may last throughout life. Neither the frequency of remission nor the frequency with which schizoid people go on to develop schizophrenia is known.

Differential Diagnosis

Schizoid personality disorder must be differentiated from the following disorders.

Schizophrenia. The presence of a thought disorder at some time during the course of schizophrenia differentiates it from schizoid personality disorder. Also, schizoids usually function better than schizophrenics in work situations.

Schizotypal personality disorder. The schizotypal and schizoid disorders both involve an odd and eccentric manner, but schizotypal personality disorder is closer to schizophrenia in the following respects: poor work history, oddities of perception and communication, and a high frequency of schizophrenic relatives.

Avoidant personality disorder. Individuals with avoidant personalities are similar to schizoid people in that they avoid most human interaction. Unlike schizoid individuals, they profess to long for relationships with others and hang back from them because of extreme sensitivity to rejection.

Paranoid personality disorder. Paranoid personality disorder involves a greater ability to engage others socially. Paranoid people are more verbally aggressive than schizoid people are, and they are less absorbed in fantasy.

Treatment

Individual psychotherapy with schizoid clients is difficult, but by no means impossible. Such people engage in any human interaction reluctantly, and a therapeutic relationship is no exception. However, as schizoid people begin to trust the therapist, they begin to share their fantasy lives, as well as their intense fears about becoming close to the therapist.

The value of group psychotherapy in treating schizoid people has not been established, but some schizoids manage to become involved in and use groups to experiment with interpersonal closeness.

Since schizoids do not have disordered thinking, antipsychotic medication is not likely to benefit them.

SCHIZOTYPAL PERSONALITY DISORDER

Profile

Schizotypal personality disorder is a new diagnostic category, used to describe a condition that is like schizoid personality disorder but characterized by additional symptoms; it is believed to be genetically linked to schizophrenia. Although it is not always easy to differentiate schizotypal from schizoid individuals, schizotypals are likely to look more obviously strange and eccentric, even to those who meet them in passing.

People with schizotypal personality disorder suffer from clear disturbances of thinking and communication. Although they may never have a frank psychotic episode with hallucinations or bizarre delusions, they show milder forms of thought disorder, such as derealization, ideas of reference, and perceptual illusions (see Chapter 4). They are extremely sensitive to others, and so retreat into a world of imaginary relationships and vivid fears and fantasies.

In an interview, you will find schizotypal people to be withdrawn and to have a great difficulty with face-to-face interaction. They show little feeling, and their affects are at times grossly inappropriate to the subject being discussed. Speech is usually peculiar, in that they use words in odd ways and express ideas unclearly; you may often need to ask for clarification. Although schizotypals will be guarded about their inner worlds, they may admit to unfounded beliefs, e.g., that they have special powers, or that they are the focus of special attention.

Diagnosis. DSM-III lists the following characteristics of schizotypal personality disorder. At least four must be present for diagnosis:

- Magical thinking, e.g., superstitiousness, clairvoyance, telepathy, sixth sense, "others can feel my feelings" (in children and adolescents, bizarre fantasies or preoccupations);
- Ideas of reference;
- Social isolation, e.g., no close friends or confidants, social contacts limited to essential everyday tasks;
- Recurrent illusions, sensing the presence of a force or person not actually present (e.g., "I felt as if my dead mother were in the room with me"), depersonalization, or derealization not associated with panic attacks;
- Odd speech (without loosening of associations or incoherence), e.g., speech that is digressive, vague, overelaborate, circumstantial, metaphorical;
- Inadequate rapport in face-to-face interaction due to constricted or inappropriate affect, e.g., aloof, cold;
- Suspiciousness or paranoid ideation; and
- Undue social anxiety or hypersensitivity to real or imagined criticism.

Causes. This diagnostic category was created in *DSM-III* for persons who are believed to share genes with schizophrenics. This disorder is more common among the biologic relatives of schizophrenics than among the general population, but no studies have clearly demonstrated particular causal factors.

Epidemiology. Because schizotypal personality disorder is a classification new to *DSM-III*, no epidemiologic information is available on people who fit into this specific category.

Course and prognosis. The course of people with schizotypal personality disorder is marked by chronic impairment of role performance and social isolation.

Differential Diagnosis

The validity of this new diagnostic category has yet to be confirmed in clinical studies. The three major disorders from which schizotypal personality must be distinguished are schizoid personality disorder, schizophrenia, and borderline personality disorder.

Schizoids do not show the oddities of speech, perception, and behavior seen among schizotypals. Schizotypals are not frankly psychotic, unlike schizophrenics, who have gross psychotic disturbances at some point in their illness. Although many of the cognitive and perceptual oddities of schizotypal personality disorder are also found in borderline personality disorder, borderlines are more likely than schizotypals to have intense, stormy interpersonal relationships.

Treatment

As with schizoid people, schizotypals are absorbed in fantasy and private belief systems that they may share, with great difficulty, in psychotherapy. Therapy is aimed at establishing a relationship and weathering the difficulties these people encounter in dealing with another human being. Exploratory psychotherapy is often resisted; supportive treatment is less threatening to many of these people.

Antipsychotic medication may be of help to diminish disordered thinking in schizotypal personality disorder, but it is not clear that the therapeutic effects of these medications outweigh their side effects in schizotypal people.

HISTRIONIC PERSONALITY DISORDER

Histrionic personality disorder is really a descendent of hysteria, a term used in clinical settings all the time. It is one of the oldest psychiatric diagnoses in Western civilization and has acquired a bewildering variety of uses over the years.

The four most common uses of the term describe 1) a specific personality style, 2) a conversion reaction (e.g., hysterical paralysis), 3) a neurotic illness characterized by phobias and anxiety, and 4) certain pathological character traits. It has also been used in our culture as a term of disapproval, particularly toward women. We will focus here on hysteria as a normal personality style, and then look at histrionic personality disorder as a pathological exaggeration of that style.

Hysterical people are typically warm and imaginative, with well-developed intuition. They tend to look at the world in global, impressionistic terms rather than focusing on details—i.e., they are "head-line readers." They gravitate toward activities that do not require intense concentration on facts but allow for the use of intuitive faculties. Thus, hysterical people are less likely to be technicians and scholars than they are to be actors or artists. Hysterical people tend to see those things in life that are vivid, colorful, and immediately striking; they often overlook more subtle or more neutral details. They are emotive, and often act as the life of the party in groups. Stereotypically, hysterical people are seductive and somewhat superficial in their relationships, getting carried away by exaggerated emotionality that is not founded on deep convictions.

Hysterical people characteristically rely on the defense of *repression* to maintain their psychological equilibrium. Repression is akin to forgetting, in that it involves banishing unacceptable ideas, feelings, or impulses from one's conscious awareness in order to decrease anxiety. Thus, the hysteric might simply repress the fact of upcoming examination and forget to arrive on time. This tendency to "forget" unpleasant facts often makes the hysterical individual appear to be more scatterbrained and less intelligent than he or she really is.

Now let us go on to look at histrionic personality disorder, in which hysterical traits are highly inflexible and maladaptive.

Profile

Although people with histrionic personality disorder may be colorful and outgoing, they are also highly excitable and have great difficulty maintaining deep and lasting attachments to others. They tend to use displays of emotion to control other people—to get attention, to avoid unwanted responsibilities, and to coerce others into taking responsibility for their welfare. Typically, these people can induce guilt in others by throwing temper tantrums or bursting into tears, and their control by these means can be quite powerful. Their affections and loyalties are extremely fickle, and this frustrates those who try to get close to them. While these people are often quite seductive, their purpose in attracting partners is not always sexual—e.g., they may seduce lovers who will then satisfy their wishes to be taken care of and nurtured.

Diagnosis. The diagnostic criteria given in *DSM-III* for histrionic personality disorder are shown in Table 7-4.

Causes. The etiology of histrionic personality disorder has not been demonstrated in any prospective studies.

Table 7–4. *DSM-III* criteria for the diagnosis of histrionic personality disorder.

Behavior that is overly dramatic, reactive, and intensely expressed, as indicated by at least three of the following:

Self-dramatization, e.g., exaggerated expression of emotions
Incessant drawing of attention to oneself
Craving for activity and excitement
Overreaction to minor events
Irrational, angry outbursts or tantrums

Characteristic disturbances in interpersonal relationships, as indicated by at least two of the following:

Perceived by others as shallow and lacking genuineness, even if superficially warm and charming
Egocentric, self-indulgent, and inconsiderate of others
Vain and demanding
Dependent, helpless, constantly seeking reassurance
Prone to manipulative suicidal threats, gestures, or attempts

---

Epidemiology. Little information is available on the prevalence of this disorder, because people with this condition previously were included in the larger and more ambiguous category of hysterical personality. The disorder is diagnosed much more frequently in women than in men, but this may reflect sex-role bias on the part of diagnosticians.

Course and prognosis. Little is known about the outlook for this disorder, but it is thought to improve with advancing age.

Differential Diagnosis

Histrionic personality disorder and borderline personality disorder are quite similar. However, borderlines generally feel chronically empty, lack a sense of identity, experience brief psychotic episodes, and engage in overtly self-destructive acts. Histrionic people do not exhibit these features with any regularity.

Along with histrionic personality disorder, people may suffer from a somatization disorder (akin to the old category of conversion hysteria)—see Chapter 8.

Treatment

Psychodynamic, insight-oriented psychotherapy is the treatment of choice for histrionic personality disorder. Both individual and group therapy have been found useful. The therapist must work on helping histrionic clients to clarify their genuine feelings, since the experience of deeply felt emotion is foreign to them. The therapist must help histrionic clients learn to take responsibility for the consequences of their actions, and to use their rational cognitive abilities rather than remaining "helpless" and "scatterbrained."

NARCISSISTIC PERSONALITY DISORDER

Narcissus, legend tells us, was a beautiful Grecian youth who fell madly in love with his own reflection when he happened upon a pool one day. Realizing that he could never possess what he so ardently desired, he killed himself.

Narcissism has come to represent many things in our culture, including self-centeredness and the ethos of the "me generation." In one sense, narcissism simply refers to self-love, and loving self-regard is both desirable and healthy. Only when self-absorption impairs one's ability to form lasting attachments to others do we term it pathological. Ironically, the crippling self-doubt and insecurity involved in pathological narcissism are a far cry from simple self-regard.

Profile

People with narcissistic personality disorder have severe problems maintaining a realistic concept of their own worth. They generally set goals and make demands of themselves that are utterly unrealistic, and then feel inadequate and helpless when they fail to meet these standards. They constantly crave love, attention, and admiration from other people as a means of bolstering their faltering self-esteem. Their demands for such love and praise can be insatiable, and they are likely to fly into a rage when these demands are not met. They are exquisitely sensitive to perceived slights from others, and approach people expecting to be disappointed. Thus, the narcissist struggles to keep a tenuous balance between the intense need to be admired by an important person and rage at that person's disappointing qualities. This struggle makes intimacy difficult and threatening. The narcissist often idealizes other people, only to come to devalue and despise them when they reveal themselves to be in some way imperfect.

Narcissistic people are preoccupied with fantasies of unlimited success, and tend to overestimate their abilities and their own specialness. This inflated self-importance often coexists with an unrealistic sense of worthlessness. Fantasies of achievement may take the place of actual work, but some people with this disorder are highly successful, pursuing fame and power with a relentless driven quality, never feeling satisfied with their achievements.

People with narcissistic personality disorder have difficulty recognizing how other people feel. They usually expect special favors from others without feeling any need to reciprocate; in this respect, they have a characteristic sense of entitlement. Narcissists are more concerned with how they look to others than with genuine feeling. They often use other people for their own ends.

All of this, it must be remembered, is in the service of protecting the narcissistic person's very fragile self-esteem. Narcissists feel devalued easily, and they may react to perceived slights not only with inappropriate rage, but also with emotional withdrawal, depression, and even suicide. The "insults" that trigger such rage and depression are often as minor as a misunderstood remark or a canceled appointment.

Diagnosis. The *DSM-III* diagnostic criteria for narcissistic personality disorder are shown in Table 7-5.

Causes. No specific genetic or environmental factors have been clearly demonstrated to cause narcissistic personality disorder. Many psychoanalytic theorists believe that the disorder stems from early childhood experiences in which parents did not encourage or appreciate the child's efforts at self-assertion, and did not help the child take pride in accomplishments. The child is left emotionally hungry and unable to maintain a stable sense of self-worth without constant support from important people (see Chapter 2).

Epidemiology. No good data on the prevalence of narcissistic personality disorder are available. Reports in the literature indicate that the diagnosis is made more frequently in men than in women, but it is not yet clear whether men are actually more susceptible to the disorder.

Course and prognosis. No good data are available on the outlook for this disorder.

Table 7–5. *DSM-III* criteria for the diagnosis of narcissistic personality disorder.

Grandiose sense of self-importance or uniqueness, e.g., exaggeration of achievements and talents, focus on the special nature of one's problems

Preoccupation with fantasies of unlimited success, power, brilliance, beauty, or ideal love

Exhibitionism and the requirement of constant attention and admiration

Cool indifference or marked feelings of rage, inferiority, shame, humiliation, or emptiness in response to criticism, indifference of others, or defeat

At least two of the following chracteristic disturbances in interpersonal relationships:

Entitlement: expectation of special favors without assuming reciprocal responsibilities, e.g., surprise and anger that people will not do what is wanted

Interpersonal exploitativeness: taking advantage of others to indulge one's own desires or for self-aggrandizement; disregard for the personal integrity and rights of others

Relationships that characteristically alternate between the extremes of overidealization and devaluation

Lack of empathy: inability to recognize how others feel, e.g., inability to appreciate the distress of someone who is seriously ill

---

Differential Diagnosis

Some theorists have questioned the validity of narcissistic personality disorder as a separate diagnostic category because many people with other disorders have prominent features of pathological narcissism. In particular, it may be difficult to differentiate narcissistic personality disorder from the following:

Histrionic personality disorder. Although both disorders involve seductiveness and self-dramatization, the person with a histrionic personality disorder is generally more playful and warm, while the narcissist is likely to be haughty, cold, and more obviously exploitative in dealings with others.

Borderline personality disorder. As a rule, borderlines show poorer impulse control and are more socially and occupationally dysfunctional than narcissists. Borderlines often appear to be very emotionally needy, while narcissists *appear* to be more self-sufficient.

Antisocial personality disorder. People with antisocial personality disorder are more impulsive than narcissists and show a constant calculated disregard for social standards. Narcissistic people either do not recognize their violations of social norms or else view themselves as deserving to be above society's rules.

Compulsive personality disorder. Both compulsive people and narcissistic people set high standards and pursue perfection with a driven quality. However, the narcissist is haughty and claims perfection to maintain an idealized self-image; the compulsive strives for perfection in order to feel capable and in control.

Treatment

Individual and group psychotherapy are the treatments of choice, but treatment is fraught with difficulties. Narcissistic clients will often idealize you at the outset of treatment and then find it difficult to tolerate later recognition that you are not all-giving, all-knowing, and all-caring. This disappointment may cause disruptions in treatment; you and the client must weather the storms of rage and periods of haughty devaluing that ensue.

In group therapy, the client may act out this scenario with group members or the group leader. The aim of therapy is to provide a consistent, caring relationship in which narcissistic clients can develop more realistic concepts of themselves and of other people as neither perfect nor worthless.

ANTISOCIAL PERSONALITY DISORDER

Profile

The term *antisocial personality disorder* may sound quite judgmental and pejorative, but it is in fact an accurate label for this illness. The most salient diagnostic feature is a long history of antisocial behavior in which the rights of others are repeatedly violated. This is not simply the medical term for criminality, but describes a longstanding illness that impairs the most important areas of the person's life. In clinical settings, you may also hear the more informal term *sociopath* used to refer to people with antisocial personality disorder.

People with this disorder are not usually clients—i.e., they do not commonly appear in mental health care settings—but are more likely to end up in courts, prisons, and welfare offices. When they do appear in mental health clinics, it is often either because they were brought there unwillingly or because they are trying to avoid the legal consequences of some recent act.

By definition, the people with this disorder begin their antisocial behavior before age 15. In childhood, they typically lie, steal, fight, and have pervasive difficulties with authority. In adolescence, sexual behavior begins early and may be unusually aggressive, and there is generally excessive drinking and drug use. By the time they reach adulthood, these people are usually unable to hold a responsible job or maintain family ties; most of them habitually break the law. Alcoholism, vagrancy, and social isolation are common, and a substantial number commit suicide. What is often striking and exasperating about sociopaths is their apparent lack of anxiety or depression in situations where one might expect such emotions.

People with antisocial personality disorder often turn on their charm at will in order to subtly manipulate others. You may find yourself baffled in an interview with somebody who has an antisocial personality disorder, for they can present a charming and strikingly "normal" facade. In fact, if an interview discloses nothing that seems abnormal, think first about the possibility that your client has no disorder, but then consider whether you may have been "conned" by a sociopath.

Obviously the diagnosis of this disorder depends not on the mental status examination but on the person's history. You are more likely to get reliable historical data from the family or from law enforcement officials than from the client. Despite a healthy facade, the sociopath may show you some signs of stress in the interview— complaining of tension, of vague somatic symptoms, of feeling depressed, or of feeling (often correctly) that others are hostile toward him or her.

Diagnosis. The diagnostic criteria for antisocial personality disorder given in *DSM-III* are shown in Table 7-6.

Causes. Both environmental and genetic factors seem to play a role in the genesis of antisocial personality disorder. The main environmental factor seems to be the sustained deprivation in early

Table 7–6. *DSM-III* criteria for the diagnosis of antisocial personality
disorder.

Current age at least 18

Onset before age 15, as indicated by a history of three or more of the following before that age:

Truancy (at least five days per year for at least two years, not including
the last year of school)
Expulsion or suspension from school for misbehavior
Delinquency (arrested or referred to juvenile court because of behavior)
Running away from home overnight at least twice while living in paren-
tal or parental surrogate home
Persistent lying
Repeated sexual intercourse in a casual relationship
Repeated drunkenness or substance abuse
Thefts
Vandalism
School grades markedly below expectations in relation to estimated or
known IQ (may have resulted in repeating a year of school)
Chronic violations of rules at home and/or at school (other than truancy)
Initiation of fights

At least four of the following manifestations of the disorder since age 18:

Inability to sustain consistent work behavior, as indicated by too frequent job changes, significant unemployment, serious absenteeism
from work, or walking off the job without another job in sight (similar
behavior in an academic setting may substitute for this criterion for
those who have not had an opportunity to demonstrate occupational
adjustment)
Lack of ability to function as a responsible parent, as evidenced by
child's malnutrition, child's illness resulting from lack of minimal
hygiene standards, failure to obtain medical care for a seriously ill
child, child's dependence on neighbors or nonresident relatives for
food or shelter, failure to arrange for a caretaker for a child under six
when parent is away from home, or repeated squandering of money
required for household necessities
Failure to accept social norms with respect to lawful behavior, as indicated by repeated thefts, illegal occupation (pimping, prostitution,
fencing, selling drugs), multiple arrests, or a felony conviction
Inability to maintain enduring attachment to a sexual partner as indicated by two or more divorces and/or separations (whether legally
married or not), desertion of spouse, promiscuity (ten or more sexual
partners within one year)
Irritability and aggressiveness, as indicated by repeated physical fights or

Table 7–6. (*Continued*)

assault (not required by one's job or to defend someone or oneself), including spouse or child beating

Failure to honor financial obligations, as indicated by repeated defaulting on debts, failure to provide child support, failure to support other dependents on a regular basis

Failure to plan ahead, or impulsivity, as indicated by traveling from place to place without a prearranged job or clear goal for the period of travel or clear idea about when the travel would terminate, or lack of a fixed address for a month or more

Disregard for the truth, as indicated by repeated lying, use of aliases, "conning" others for personal profit

Recklessness, as indicated by driving while intoxicated or recurrent speeding

A pattern of continuous antisocial behavior in which the rights of others are violated, with no intervening period of at least five years without antisocial behavior between age 15 and the present time (except when the individual was bedridden or confined in a hospital or penal institution)

Antisocial behavior is not due to severe mental retardation, schizophrenia, or manic episodes

---

childhood of any consistent emotional ties with a significant person. The classic example of such deprivation is parents who are inconsistently available to the child and who are impulsive and erratic in their behavior. It is therefore no surprise to find that antisocial personality disorder is frequently found in the parents (particularly among the fathers) of those who have the disorder.

The evidence for genetic factors in antisocial personality disorder comes from studies which show that having a sociopathic or an alcoholic father is a powerful predictor of developing a sociopathic personality, even among children who were adopted at birth and not raised by their biologic parents.

There also appears to be a modest correlation between 1) hyperactive behavior and having "soft" (nonspecific) neurologic abnormalities in childhood and 2) later development of antisocial personality disorder.

Contrary to what you might expect intuitively, antisocial personality disorder is not correlated with such factors as living in a high-crime area, keeping bad company, or being a member of a "deviant" subgroup in society.

Epidemiology. The prevalence of antisocial personality disorder in our society is estimated to be roughly 3 percent for American males and less than 1 percent for American females.

The disorder is more common among lower socioeconomic groups, probably because 1) most people with antisocial personality disorder have very poor work records and, therefore, impaired earning capacity and 2) since the fathers of those who have the disorder frequently had it themselves, many of these people grew up in impoverished homes. However, the disorder is found in all social classes, including the most privileged.

The prevalence of the disorder among prison populations is very high—perhaps as high as 75 percent.

Course and prognosis. Antisocial personality disorder begins in childhood, and antisocial behavior reaches its peak in adolescence and young adulthood. Two changes seem to occur later in life. First, for some people, the disorder seems to remit. Among those who have the disorder, roughly 2 percent improve (i.e., stop their antisocial behavior) each year once they get beyond age 21. Second, many of those who stop their antisocial behavior in their adult years develop hypochondriacal concerns and depression.

Differential Diagnosis

There are several conditions from which antisocial personality disorder must be differentiated.

Criminality. As noted above, antisocial personality disorder is not simply another term for criminality. It is a disorder that impairs all aspects of the individual's life—social functioning, work capacity, and the ability to achieve and maintain intimate relationships. Many people with this disorder manage to keep their actions within the limits of the law but nevertheless violate social norms and harm others by their behavior. Conversely, some people who commit crimes may act with loyalty and a sense of responsibility toward others in their lives (e.g., spouses, parents) and could not be accurately labeled sociopaths.

Borderline personality disorders. Both borderline and antisocial personality disorders may involve impulsive and destructive behavior, directed at the self as well as others. However, borderlines are more likely than sociopaths to behave self-destructively. Also, although sociopaths often act aggressively toward others without anger or guilt, borderlines usually become hostile only when feeling deprived by people who are important to them, and they commonly feel guilty about their anger. Borderline personality disorder is more frequently diagnosed in women, while antisocial personality disorder is more frequently diagnosed in men.

Manic episode. Mania may involve antisocial behavior, but such behavior is clearly episodic rather than chronic and longstanding, and it accompanies a highly altered mood.

Substance abuse disorder. Drug and alcohol abuse can certainly result in global impairment of functioning and chronic antisocial behavior (stealing, lying, etc.) as the individual struggles to maintain and conceal an addiction. In these cases, antisocial behavior stops when the drug abuse stops. Often, however, substance abuse is simply secondary to an underlying antisocial personality disorder, and both diagnoses may be warranted in such cases.

Treatment

Sociopaths look unreachable and untreatable in an outpatient setting. They appear to lack anxiety, to lack any motivation for change, and to learn nothing from experience. However, these are only the characteristics of a sociopath who is in flight. When people with an antisocial personality disorder are immobilized—i.e., when they are held in a treatment or prison facility and can no longer act to avoid unpleasant feelings—a very different picture emerges. Sociopaths begin to experience considerable anxiety and become convinced that this anxiety will be intolerable to others. The fear of getting close to others becomes much more apparent, as does the sociopath's sensitivity to criticism and rejection.

Thus, actual control over the behavior of sociopaths is the cornerstone of treatment. They must be prevented from running away, or from hurting themselves or others, when feelings seem intolerable. This control is usually impossible to achieve on an outpatient basis, and can only be achieved in prison or on a locked inpatient unit. The goal of treatment is to show these people that they and others can tolerate their anxiety. Sociopaths often need much more support than is possible in individual therapy. Peer support groups of all kinds are probably the most effective treatment, since the sociopath can use such groups to identify with others who struggle with similar problems.

You may be tempted to try to rescue charming sociopaths, and to shield them from the consequences of their own behavior (e.g., legal proceedings, prison sentences). This is antitherapeutic. People with antisocial personality disorder cannot be treated without the clear understanding that they are responsible for whatever they do.

BORDERLINE PERSONALITY DISORDER

For many years, psychiatric thinkers taught that an individual could be either psychotic or neurotic, but not both. Yet therapists reported many cases in which people became transiently psychotic under stress, recompensated quickly, and in most situations remained completely in touch with reality. Some thought these people had a mild form of schizophrenia; others called them severely neurotic. Out of this confusion, contemporary theorists developed the concept of the borderline personality—borderline referring to the line between psychosis and neurosis.

Profile

Many borderline people do indeed move in and out of psychosis. When they lose touch with reality it may take the form of frank hallucinations and delusions, but more often the psychosis involves dissociative states, derealization, and depersonalization (see Chapter 4). These episodes are usually brief—lasting several minutes to several days—and generally occur in response to stress (e.g., a break-up with a lover).

But reactive psychosis is by no means the only prominent feature of the borderline syndrome. Intense and persistent anger is one of the hallmarks of this disorder. Borderlines are characteristically rageful and demanding, going to great lengths to get others to feel responsible for their woes and their welfare. They form chaotic relationships with others because they struggle with intense dependence upon and intense hostility toward those to whom they become attached. Borderlines are adept at manipulating others to do their bidding. But their use of emotional blackmail (e.g., suicide threats) and angry outbursts ultimately drive away the people who are important to them.

The borderline individual is easily overwhelmed by anger and frustration, and generally acts impulsively when feelings become intolerable. This usually involves repeated self-destructive acts (e.g., wrist slashing, overdoses, car crashes) and may also include drug abuse, sexual promiscuity, and abrupt changes in job and living situations.

Borderlines usually possess a facade of sociability and adaptiveness that makes them quite engaging in superficial contact. Thus, many borderlines are very good at interviews but function erratically and below their apparent capabilities in work situations.

People with borderline personality disorder chronically experience feelings of emptiness and uncertainty about who they are. This disturbed sense of identity can be seen in a variety of areas—gender identity, personal goals, the difference between their own and others' feelings, their self-image, and their body image. When borderlines complain, "I don't know who I am," they generally reflect a profound sense of internal chaos and confusion. This is particularly acute when there is no one around from whom the borderline can take his or her cues; therefore, the borderline has difficulty being alone and will seek out companionship, at times frantically, in order to avoid it.

Diagnosis. DSM-III gives the diagnostic criteria for borderline personality disorder shown in Table 7-7. In addition to the criteria listed in the table, some clinicians insist that true borderline personality disorder must involve psychotic experiences that are brief, reversible, and stress-related.

Table 7–7. *DSM-III* criteria for the diagnosis of borderline personality disorder.

At least five of the following:

Impulsivity or unpredictability in at least two areas that are potentially self-damaging, e.g., spending, sex, gambling, substance use, shoplifting, overeating, physically self-damaging acts

A pattern of unstable and intense interpersonal relationships, e.g., marked shifts of attitude, idealization, devaluation, manipulation

Inappropriate, intense anger or lack of control of anger, e.g., frequent displays of temper, constant anger

Identity disturbance manifested by uncertainty about several issues relating to identity, such as self-image, gender identity, long-term goals or career choice, friendship patterns, values, and loyalties, e.g., "I feel like I am my sister when I am good"

Affective instability: marked shifts from normal mood to depression, irritability, or anxiety, usually lasting a few hours and only rarely more than a few days, with a return to normal mood

Intolerance of being along, e.g., frantic efforts to avoid being alone, depressed when alone

Physically self-damaging acts, e.g., suicidal gestures, self-mutilation, recurrent accidents or physical fights

Chronic feelings of emptiness or boredom

If under 18, does not meet the criteria for identity disorder

Causes. Most of the major work on the etiology of borderline personality disorder has come from psychoanalytic theorists. They focus on early childhood, particularly between the ages of six months and two years, when the child learns to separate from the mother and gains a sense of himself or herself as a separate being. Many psychoanalysts postulate that disturbances in the mother-child relationship during this separation-individuation phase of development can leave children with a poorly developed sense of self and render them extremely vulnerable to separations from important others. One theorist (Otto Kernberg) has hypothesized that borderlines may have an inborn deficit in their ability to tolerate anxiety.

Empirical studies are now under way to try to validate the theories mentioned above, and to explore possible biologic factors in the etiology of borderline personality disorder.

Epidemiology. Little is known about the prevalence of this disorder, since diagnostic criteria have only been established in the past decade and are still the subject of some debate. In recent years, roughly 10 to 20 percent of hospital admissions have been of patients with this diagnosis. Women are diagnosed as borderline more than twice as often as men, but it may be that clinicians underdiagnose the disorder in men and overdiagnose it in women.

Course and prognosis. There is considerable disagreement about what happens to borderlines over time. While the disorder begins in childhood or adolescence and continues well into adult life, it may be that the disorder remits somewhat after age 40, since the diagnosis is made much less frequently in people over 40. Whether borderlines "burn out," become more stable in their functioning, or simply stop seeking help as they get older is unclear. Further research needs to be done in this area.

Differential Diagnosis

Other personality disorders. Borderline individuals often have features consistent with other personality disorders—particularly histrionic, narcissistic, schizoid, schizotypal, and antisocial personality disorders. If someone meets the criteria for more than one personality disorder, more than one diagnosis is warranted.

Affective disorders. Because the person with borderline personality disorder has intense and highly changeable emotional storms, it is easy to confuse symptoms of the disorder with mood swings due to an underlying affective illness. Recent studies suggest that up to 50 percent of people with borderline personality disorder have a concurrent affective disorder; in such cases both disorders should be diagnosed and treated.

Treatment

While psychotherapy is the treatment of choice for borderlines, treatment is extremely difficult for both client and therapist. Borderlines often cannot tolerate the intense feelings they develop for the therapist, and their responses range from abruptly breaking off treatment to intense verbal abuse to severe self-destructive acts. They frequently threaten and attempt suicide, using this and other maneuvers to try to elicit signs of the therapist's love and concern. This behavior is designed in part to manipulate others, but it is nonetheless quite dangerous. Suicide is common. You may become overwhelmed by your own emotional responses to borderlines. Intense anger is common, as is an unrealistic sense of responsibility for the client's safety.

Two differing views of psychotherapy with borderlines predominate. Some clinicians advocate intensive individual psychotherapy (two or more sessions per week) aimed at in-depth exploration of how clients relate to others in their lives and, most important, how they relate to the therapist. Another view is that such intensive work prompts the borderline to become irreversibly clinging and dependent on the therapist, that treatment should instead be limited to weekly sessions that focus on "here-and-now" issues of improving job performance, stabilizing the client's living situation, etc. Group therapy is often advocated as an adjunct to both intensive and supportive individual therapy, since groups can often confront borderlines with their manipulative behavior quite effectively. Treating borderlines in groups is very difficult because of their wish to have an exclusive relationship with the therapist.

Medication has proved to be of little use in borderline personality disorder. Psychotic episodes are too brief to require antipsychotic medication, and mood swings are too rapid and dependent on life events to be stabilized by antidepressants or lithium. However, people who have an affective disorder in addition to borderline personality disorder often benefit from medication.

Whatever treatment regimen is decided upon, it is crucial that the therapist have support. This should always include the option to hospitalize the client when self-destructive activities or psychosis make it impossible to continue treatment on an outpatient basis. Supervision, peer group support, and consultation with other clinicians can also help the therapist to maintain some perspective on the treatment during particularly difficult periods.

AVOIDANT PERSONALITY DISORDER

Profile

The hallmark of the avoidant personality disorder is extreme sensitivity to rejection. Avoidant individuals stay away from relationships—not because they want to, but because they are so afraid of rejection. Only when guaranteed uncritical acceptance can they feel safe enough to get attached to other people.

Avoidant people generally lack self-confidence, which they attempt to bolster by seeking out unusually supportive companions. They are often afraid to speak up, and feel uncomfortable in the limelight and in positions of authority.

In the interview, people with avoidant personality disorder will be anxious about what you think of them. They may seem fragile and waiflike. If you attempt to clarify something they have said, they are likely to interpret your comments as critical even when you did not mean them to be.

Diagnosis. The diagnostic criteria for avoidant personality disorder given in *DSM-III* are shown in Table 7-8.

Causes. The causes are unknown. Childhood experiences and inborn temperament may exert some influence in the genesis of this disorder.

Table 7–8. *DSM-III* criteria for the diagnosis of avoidant personality disorder.

Hypersensitivity to rejection, e.g., apprehensively alert to signs of social derogation; interprets innocuous events as ridicule

Unwillingness to enter into relationships unless given unusually strong guarantees of uncritical acceptance

Social withdrawal, e.g., distances self from close personal attachments, engages in peripheral social and vocational roles

Desire for affection and acceptance

Low self-esteem, e.g., devalues self-achievements and is overly dismayed by personal shortcomings

If under 18, does not meet the criteria for avoidant disorder of childhood or adolescence

---

Epidemiology. Since the diagnosis is new to *DSM-III*, there is no information on prevalence, sex ratio, or familial patterns of the disorder.

Course and prognosis. The course and prognosis are also unknown.

Differential Diagnosis

Avoidant personality disorder was not included in diagnostic manuals prior to *DSM-III*. There is considerable disagreement about whether the avoidant personality constitutes a true personality disorder or merely represents a trait common to a variety of personality types.

The individual with an avoidant personality disorder longs for and responds to genuine attention and support from others; the person with a schizoid personality disorder expresses no desire for social relations.

Unlike people with dependent, borderline, and histrionic personality disorders, avoidant people suffer quietly and are not demanding of others' attention.

Treatment

Psychotherapy is the treatment of choice. In individual therapy, a strong alliance is difficult to form because it is so easy for the avoidant individual to feel rejected. However, once formed, this alliance can help the avoidant person learn to weather the storms inherent in human interaction.

Group therapy can demonstrate to avoidant individuals the difficulties their hypersensitivity poses for other people. But avoidant individuals are likely to be very reluctant to take the risk involved in entering into group therapy in the first place.

Some clinicians feel that an important distinction between avoidant and schizoid personality disorders is that the avoidant individual is more inclined than the schizoid to seek and profit from psychotherapy.

DEPENDENT PERSONALITY DISORDER

Profile

Dependent personality disorder is another new diagnostic category in *DSM-III*. Clinicians disagree about whether extreme dependence is a trait common to many types of personality disorder or whether it is truly a unique disorder in its own right.

People with dependent personality disorder structure their lives so that other people will take responsibility for their welfare. They feel unable to function on their own, and so seek out lovers, bosses, and friends who will allow them to be passive and who will tell them how to live their lives. They avoid making decisions whenever they can get others to do it for them—e.g., whom to see socially, where to work, and even what to wear.

The person with this disorder will put up with a great deal from others in order to preserve a dependent relationship and avoid having to function autonomously—for example, the wife who puts up with verbal and physical abuse from her husband because she feels incapable of functioning without him. Dependent people lack self-confidence and are preoccupied with fears of being abandoned.

Diagnosis. The diagnostic criteria for dependent personality disorder given in *DSM-III* are as follows:

- Passively allows others to assume responsibility for major areas of life because of inability to function independently (e.g., lets spouse decide what kind of job he or she should have);
- Subordinates own needs to those of persons on whom he or she depends in order to avoid any possibility of having to rely on self (e.g., tolerates abusive spouse); and
- Lacks self-confidence (e.g., sees self as helpless, stupid).

Causes. Most theorists who write about the roots of extreme passivity and dependence emphasize early childhood experiences. One hypothesis is that parents can foster dependent personality traits by giving their children the implicit or explicit message that independent behavior is bad and will lead to abandonment.

Evidence has begun to emerge that suggests that dominant and submissive personality traits may be genetically transmitted. Researchers have found a higher rate of concordance for these traits among identical twins than among fraternal twins. However, submissiveness and dependence are not the same thing, and it is not clear whether these two traits usually coexist in the same person.

Epidemiology. The diagnosis is more often assigned to women than to men, and more often to people who are the youngest children within their family constellations.

Course and prognosis. Functioning depends on the person's maintenance of dependent relationships. When these are disrupted in some way (e.g., the death of a spouse), a person who previously functioned well may seriously decompensate and seek mental health care.

Differential Diagnosis

Dependent traits are common in other personality disorders, particularly in borderline, histrionic, avoidant, passive-aggressive, and schizoid personality disorders. Some diagnosticians believe that masochism—i.e., the pleasure obtained from pain, failure, and disability—is the more central trait in dependent personality disorder than dependence per se. This calls into question whether dependent personality disorder is a valid diagnostic category.

Agoraphobia (Chapter 8) may be mistaken for dependent personality disorder, but the agoraphobic individual is much more active in demanding that others take responsibility for his or her life (e.g., the agoraphobic husband who insists that his wife drive him everywhere). Dependent individuals "can't" do things because of a sense of inadequacy and incompetence, while agoraphobics "can't" do things because of overwhelming fear and anxiety.

Treatment

Psychotherapy can be very helpful for people with dependent personality disorder. In the relationship with the therapist, clients can begin to examine the effects of their passivity, and to recognize their own competence and self-worth. In the beginning, it is important that the therapist respect the client's need for dependent relationships (even abusive ones) and not push the client to give them up until he or she is ready.

COMPULSIVE PERSONALITY DISORDER

The "obsessive-compulsive" is an infamous character familiar to every hard-working student. We often use this label to lampoon ourselves or others for being too careful, too preoccupied with detail, and too diligent or perfectionistic. The terms obsessive and compulsive are used in three major ways: 1) to describe a classic preoccupation with unwanted thoughts or behaviors (obsessive-compulsive neurosis), 2) to describe a general personality style, and 3) to describe a specific personality disorder.

Obsessive-compulsive neurosis. Obsessions are persistent unwanted ideas or images that seem as if they come from outside the mind and force themselves on the victim's thoughts against his or her will. One might, for example, be obsessed with the thought that one has accidentally hurt someone, or be terrified of being contaminated by touching a doorknob. People who suffer from this disorder may be hopelessly preoccupied with obsessions despite realizing that these preoccupations are absurd and irrational. They usually feel powerless to keep obsessive thoughts out of their awareness, and become anxious when they attempt to do so.

Compulsions are the behavioral equivalents of obsessions—repetitive urges to perform acts that are contrary to one's ordinary wishes or standards. Common compulsive acts include hand-washing, counting (e.g., money), and checking (e.g., to be certain the stove has been turned off). The action usually seems senseless; performing the act is not pleasurable, but it does relieve tension. When the problem is severe, people may need to spend most of their waking moments carrying out compulsive acts (e.g., cleaning) to avoid massive anxiety.

According to psychodynamic theory, obsessive thoughts and compulsive acts serve as benign substitutes for more threatening unconscious ideas or impulses (e.g., the wish to kill one's parent). True obsessions and compulsions (i.e., discrete and isolated symptoms) are relatively rare—estimated at 0.05 percent of the general population.

Obsessive-compulsive style. Much more common than true obsessions or compulsions is the obsessive-compulsive personality style, which may be both normal and highly adaptive. Like hysterical traits, obsessive-compulsive traits can be very useful—e.g., when studying for an exam, or organizing a business venture, or even planning a wild party.

Obsessive-compulsive people have the ability to focus their attention and screen out distractions. Thus, they can be skilled at highly detailed work; many obsessive-compulsives are technicians, academicians, and scientists. Obsessive-compulsives are perfectionists and they are list-makers. They are usually intensely and continuously active at some kind of work. Their deliberateness makes them less open than others to spontaneous experiences. Obsessive-compulsives rarely get hunches, and often immerse themselves so completely in small details that they cannot step back and see the "big picture."

In contrast to hysterics, obsessive-compulsives are characteristically serious. They generally apply great pressure to themselves to live up to high standards of performance and morality, for they live according to the dictates of a very demanding conscience. "I should . . ." is their motto. They are their own harshest taskmasters and never feel that they are free. In fact, many obsessive-compulsives are uncomfortable in situations where they are truly free, such as while on vacation.

Decisions are the bane of the obsessive-compulsive's existence, and he or she will try to find a rule or moral dictum to avoid having to exercise free choice. Obsessive-compulsives have difficulty when faced with decisions in which no duty is involved and when they must act wholly according to their own desires, because they are generally unaware of their desires.

Profile

As with other personality types, the line between what constitutes style and what qualifies as a disorder is not at all clear in the case of the obsessive-compulsive. This is a judgment call, based on the extent to which personality traits are inflexible and impair one's ability to love and to work.

Individuals with compulsive personality disorder are very limited in their ability to express warm and tender feelings toward others. Feelings provoke anxiety, and compulsives focus on facts instead of feelings to overcome anxiety. They are preoccupied with the "right" way of doing things, and often alienate others by their insistence on having their own way. They can be moralistic to the point of absurd rigidity and extreme insensitivity to the needs of others.

Lists and routines dominate the lives of people with compulsive personality disorder. They may focus on their bowel habits, for example, to the point that any irregularity leaves them unable to function at other daily activities. Decision making will often be reduced to a "science." When this is not possible, compulsives may be paralyzed by indecision and the fear of making a mistake.

Other compulsive traits include parsimony, extreme cleanliness, and orderliness. At the healthier end of the spectrum, the individual with a compulsive personality disorder may have a stable marriage and hold a responsible job, but is constantly tense and driven, unable to have fun.

When you interview people with compulsive personality disorder, you will most likely find them neatly and conventionally dressed. They may sit stiffly, and will be serious in demeanor. They are likely to drone on and on in a monotonous tone of voice as they give detailed and often circumstantial answers to questions. In fact, when you ask how they feel about something, they will usually give an answer consisting of facts and circumstances instead of emotions. They will be slow to "warm up" to you, and preoccupied with ideas about what you expect of them in the interview.

Diagnosis. According to *DSM-III*, at least four of the following must be present for a diagnosis of compulsive personality disorder:

- Restricted ability to express warm and tender emotions, e.g., the individual is unduly conventional, serious and formal, and stingy;
- Perfectionism that interferes with the ability to grasp the "big picture," e.g., preoccupation with trivial details, rules, order, organization, schedules, and lists;
- Insistence that others submit to his or her way of doing things, and lack of awareness of the feelings elicited by this behavior, e.g., a husband stubbornly insists that his wife complete errands for him regardless of her plans;
- Excessive devotion to work and productivity, to the exclusion of pleasure and value of interpersonal relationships; or
- Indecisiveness: decision making is either avoided, postponed, or protracted, perhaps because of an inordinate fear of making a mistake, e.g., the individual cannot get assignments done on time because of ruminating about priorities.

Causes. Classic psychoanalytic thinking emphasizes the importance of the anal phase of development (age two to four years) in the genesis of compulsive personality disorder. Toilet training is the standard metaphor for this stage: children want to gratify their urges wherever and whenever they occur, but these urges conflict with the desires of parents and society. The tension, then, is between the assertion of autonomy and the development of self-control.

Many therapists write about the role of rigid, controlling parents in fostering compulsive personality disorder in their overdisciplined offspring. However, these ideas have yet to be validated in long-term prospective studies.

Compulsive personality disorder is more prevalent among family members of identified compulsive clients than in the general population, and newer studies suggest that genetic as well as environmental factors play a role in determining which people develop this condition.

Epidemiology. Prevalence is unknown, because much depends on where the diagnostician draws the line between the personality style and the disorder. It is more common in men than in women.

Course and prognosis. The course of the disorder varies tremendously. Compulsives are quite vulnerable to unexpected life changes, and are prone to bouts of depression. However, some compulsive people appear to "loosen up" with age and exhibit fewer symptoms of the disorder as they grow older. Still others develop frankly compulsive behaviors, and a small number appear to adopt compulsive symptoms as a prelude to a schizophrenic break. Unfortunately, many severely compulsive people continue to lead an emotionally barren existence throughout life.

Differential Diagnosis

People with obsessive-compulsive neurosis report being plagued by obsessive thoughts, or of feeling unable to resist performing compulsive acts, and these symptoms are disturbing to those who have them. By contrast, compulsive personality disorder is not characterized by ego-dystonic obsessions or compulsions.

People who fulfill the criteria for compulsive personality disorder may also show features of other personality disorders—particularly schizoid and paranoid personality disorders.

Treatment

Psychotherapy is the treatment of choice; medication has not proved effective in this disorder.

Compulsive people differ from many others with personality disorders in that they often see themselves as troubled and seek help on their own. Therapy is a long and slow process, because the compulsive sees therapy, like every other relationship, as a struggle for control. The therapist must carefully sidestep potential battles and point out the client's extreme sensitivity to issues of power and authority. The focus must be clearly maintained on the client's feelings, because the compulsive tends to use his or her intellect to defend against feelings that are less controllable than ideas and therefore more threatening.

Group psychotherapy has also proved effective, either alone or in combination with individual therapy. Group members can have a powerful influence on the compulsive person, by pointing out the maladaptive ways of dealing with others revealed in the group. They can also reward the compulsive with praise when positive changes are made.

Behavior therapy, while useful for specific compulsive behaviors, has not been shown to be effective for more global compulsive personality traits.

PASSIVE-AGGRESSIVE PERSONALITY DISORDER

Passive aggression is a powerful means of controlling other people. Hunger strikes, sit-ins, and work slow-downs are common examples of how doing nothing can be a highly effective means of gaining attention or power. Where more openly aggressive behavior is impossible, passive resistance may be the only reasonable course of action. Gandhi made masterful use of this technique on a national scale in India. However, as a global and pervasive style of dealing with life, passive-aggressive behavior is usually self-defeating and self-destructive.

Profile

Individuals with passive-aggressive personality disorder spend their lives saying "yes" and behaving as if they had said "no." They fail to live up to demands made on them by their jobs and by people who are important to them. They do not fail directly or deliberately but "by accident"—e.g., by forgetting, procrastinating, or misplacing things. Typically, passive-aggressive individuals are largely unaware of their obstructiveness and feel that they are doing their best. They feel that no one appreciates how hard they try and how many difficulties the world puts in their way. They do not get angry at others directly, nor are they direct about their own needs and desires. People usually experience the passive-aggressive person's behavior as punitive; initial guilty acquiescence gives way to anger and even abandonment. Thus passive-aggressive people are not only underachievers who infuriate their bosses, but they are also tyrants who hold captive those friends and lovers who remain close to them.

Diagnosis. The diagnostic criteria for passive-aggressive personality disorder given in *DSM-III* are shown in Table 7-9.

Causes. There have been no prospective studies of the causes of passive-aggressive personality disorder. Certainly, early childhood experiences seem to be of primary importance in the genesis of the

Table 7–9. *DSM-III* criteria for the diagnosis of passive-aggressive personality disorder.

Resistance to demands for adequate performance in both occupational and social functioning

Resistance expressed indirectly through at least two of the following: procrastination, dawdling, stubbornness, intentional inefficiency, and "forgetfulness"

As a consequence of the above, pervasive and long-standing social and occupational ineffectiveness (including roles of housewife or student), e.g., intentional inefficiency that has prevented job promotion

Persistence of the behavior pattern even under circumstances in which more self-assertive and effective behavior is possible

Does not meet the criteria for any other personality disorder and, if under age 18, does not meet the criteria for oppositional disorder

disorder, particularly in conveying the message to the developing child that the direct expression of aggression is in some way taboo.

Epidemiology. The prevalence, sex ratio, and familial patterns of this disorder have not been well studied.

Course and prognosis. People with this disorder are prone to depression and to alcohol and drug abuse.

Differential Diagnosis

Borderline and histrionic individuals may use a great many passive-aggressive maneuvers, but they are more flamboyant and more openly aggressive than people with passive-aggressive personality disorder.

Because passive-aggressive behaviors are used defensively in a wide range of disorders, many clinicians question the validity of passive-aggressive personality disorder as a separate diagnostic category.

Treatment

Psychotherapy is the treatment of choice for passive-aggressive personality disorder. Clients invariably attempt to put the therapist in the same bind that they put others in their lives: If the therapist gratifies the client's covert demands for assistance, the client will make further and more unreasonable demands. However, the client will take a refusal to honor these requests as rejection. The therapist must constantly try to sidestep this dilemma by bringing the client's covert aggression out into the open. This means confronting veiled threats and minipulative efforts, and asking what the client hopes to gain by such tactics.

SOME FINAL THOUGHTS ON TREATMENT

People with personality disorders are notoriously difficult to treat. Their pathological ways of dealing with the world are deeply ingrained, yet they act as if the problem lies with the world and not with them. They are often angry, demanding, and abusive toward therapists and have an extraordinary capacity to home in on the weaknesses and vulnerabilities of those who try to help them. They will attempt to form the same type of pathological relationship with you that they form with others in their lives. They are generally reluctant to see their behavior as a problem and are likely to blame you when their wishes are not fulfilled in therapy.

You may become so angry at such clients that you will unwittingly retaliate when they are abusive. You may, for example, withdraw your emotional investment from your work with them in subtle ways, prompting them to feel increasingly worthless. You must pay close attention to the hostile feelings that invariably arise toward the client with a personality disorder; by being aware of these feelings and tolerating them, you can avoid acting on them.

The following ground rules may be helpful to you in dealing with a personality-disordered client, whether you are doing a single interview or embarking on long-term therapy:

- Focus on the client's behavior, not on his or her explanations of that behavior.
- Do not listen to repetitious complaints. When clients recount the supposed injustices the world has dealt them, direct the focus to their own role in these events.
- Maintain the stance that you and your clients are collaborating— i.e., that you are doing something with them rather than for them or to them.
- Pay close attention to your own fantasies of "rescuing" the client. You are bound to be disappointed.

- Set limits on any behavior that threatens your safety, the client's safety, or the future of the treatment. This may range from ending your meeting early to putting the client in the hospital. When clients try to push you into the role of savior, friend, or co-conspirator, show them what they are doing.
- Scoldings and guilt trips are of no use to your clients. You must simply hold them responsible for their behavior, rather than making any moves to shield them from its consequences.
- Provide yourself with support. Seek supervision from a more senior person, or "let off steam" with a peer. Use all the help available to you to weather the difficult times that are unavoidable in treating people with personality disorders.

REFERENCES

Akhtar S, Thompson JA: Overview: narcissistic personality disorder. Am J Psychiatry 139:12-20, 1982

American Psychiatric Association: Diagnostic and Statistical Manual of Mental Disorders, 3rd ed. Washington, DC, American Psychiatric Association, 1980, pp 305-330

Chodoff P, Lyons H: Hysteria, the hysterical personality, and "hysterical" conversion. Am J Psychiatry 114:734-740, 1958

Frances A: The *DSM-III* personality disorders section: a commentary. Am J Psychiatry 137:1050-1054, 1980

Frosch JP (ed): Current Perspectives on Personality Disorders. Washington, DC, American Psychiatric Press, 1983

Gunderson JG: Borderline Personality Disorder. Washington, DC, American Psychiatric Press, 1984

Gunderson JG, Singer MT: Defining borderline patients: an overview. Am J Psychiatry 132:1-10, 1975

Guntrip H: The schizoid problem, in Psychoanalytic Theory, Therapy, and the Self. New York, Basic Books, 1973, pp 145-173

Kernberg O: Borderline personality organization. J Am Psychoanal Assoc 15:641-685, 1967

Shapiro D: Neurotic Styles. New York, Basic Books, 1965 (An excellent and highly readable discussion of personality styles.)

Stanton AH: Personality disorders, in The Harvard Guide to Modern Psychiatry. Edited by Nicholi AM Jr. Cambridge, Mass, Harvard University Press, 1978, pp 283-295

Vaillant GE: Sociopathy as a human process: a viewpoint. Arch Gen Psychiatry 32:178-183, 1975

Vaillant GE, Perry JC: Personality disorders, in A Comprehensive Textbook of Psychiatry, 4th ed. Edited by Kaplan HI, Sadock BJ. Baltimore, Williams and Wilkins, 1985, pp 958–986

Chapter 8

Anxiety, Phobias, Somatoform Disorders, Dissociative Disorders, and Eating Disorders

ANXIETY

What is anxiety? Each of us has experienced it, and ours has been called "the age of anxiety." Yet precise definition of the term is difficult, for it has been applied to a wide range of emotional responses.

Fear is a normal reaction to a consciously recognized external source of danger. It is appropriate to the source of danger, both in its intensity and in its duration, and it dissipates when action is taken that leads to escape or avoidance. Fear involves both subjective feelings of apprehension and objective physiological changes that usually include rapid heartbeat, rapid respiration, muscle tremor, and redistribution of blood from the skin and internal organs to the large muscle groups. These changes prepare the body for the violent muscular activity (fight or flight) that may be necessary in responding to a threat.

Anxiety, by contrast, involves tension, apprehension, or even terror about danger, the source of which is largely unknown or unrecognized. Like fear, anxiety is accompanied by increased activity of the sympathetic nervous system, which is manifested by such physical signs as sweating, rapid heartbeat, tremor, rapid breathing, and gastrointestinal distress. But, unlike fear, anxiety stems from sources that are not obvious to the one who suffers, or that seem minor compared with his or her intense emotional reaction. Anxiety is common, and in many instances consists of an overreaction to mildly stressful events (e.g., excessive concern over a relatively unimportant examination). We regard anxiety as pathological when it interferes with daily functioning, the achievement of desired goals, or reasonable emotional comfort.

Situational anxiety occurs in response to a specific stress and ends shortly after the stress is removed. *Free-floating anxiety,* by contrast, involves apprehension that is not clearly linked to a specific situation.

What Causes Anxiety Disorders?

Anxiety disorders do not have a single cause—there are both psychological and somatic factors that foster the development of anxiety.

Psychological factors. Psychoanalytic theorists postulate that anxiety stems from intrapsychic conflict. When a young child's wishes come into conflict with parental expectations and the realities of the world, the child may imagine being punished for these wishes (e.g., a youngster who harbors murderous wishes toward his little brother may fear that he will be severely punished for these feelings). These conflicts may be within a young child's awareness, but they are repressed as children grow up. In adulthood, circumstances may reactivate an unconscious conflict and foster anxiety. Typical childhood fears that may be repressed and lead to anxiety disorders in adult life are listed below:

- Loss of, or separation from, a parent or other caretaker on whom one depends.
- Loss of love through anger or disapproval of an important person.
- Damage to or loss of the genitals (also called *castration anxiety*).
- Loss of self-esteem when one fails to live up to one's moral standards adopted from early caretakers.

Thus, for example, a woman may become terrified when her husband leaves on a business trip, not on the basis of any actual danger to herself or her husband, but because the separation revives her early fears of separation from her parents.

Biologic factors. Genetic predisposition to anxiety disorders is now the subject of intense research. Specific syndromes like panic attacks (discussed below) have been shown to be familial diseases,

Table 8–1. Somatic illnesses that are commonly accompanied by anxiety.

Cardiovascular	Neurologic
Angina pectoris	Partial complex seizures
Cardiac arrhythmias	
Mitral valve prolapse	Toxic metabolic
Hyperkinetic heart syndrome	Medication side effects
Recurrent pulmonary emboli	Substance abuse
	Withdrawal states

Endocrine
  Hyperthyroidism
  Pheochromocytoma
  Hypoglycemia
  Hypoparathyroidism
  Cushing's syndrome

and researchers are currently looking for possible biological markers of panic and other anxiety disorders.

Underlying somatic illnesses. Many organic disorders are accompanied by symptoms of anxiety. Some of the most common of these are listed in Table 8-1. For descriptions of these disorders, refer to any general textbook of medicine.

Among people who come to health care facilities complaining of anxiety, medical illness is found in only a minority of cases. Nevertheless, the possibility of underlying somatic disease must not be overlooked when you evaluate anxious clients, and everyone who is being evaluated for anxiety for the first time should have a thorough medical evaluation as well as a mental health assessment.

Generalized Anxiety Disorder

The system of classification outlined in the third edition of the *Diagnostic and Statistical Manual of Mental Disorders* (*DSM-III*) divides the anxiety disorders according to whether the symptoms are nonspecific (generalized anxiety disorder) or specific (phobic disorders, panic disorders).

Generalized anxiety disorder, also called "anxiety neurosis," is characterized by persistent anxiety for at least one month without specific phobias or panic attacks. The symptoms of the disorder vary greatly from person to person, but usually include the following manifestations:

- *Motor tension:* trembling, muscle aches and tension, easy fatigability, inability to relax, and restlessness;
- *Autonomic hyperactivity:* sweating, palpitations, rapid respirations, rapid pulse, dry mouth, clammy hands, dizziness, paresthesias (tingling in hands or feet), nausea, stomach pain, frequent urination, diarrhea, hot or cold spells, flushing, pallor;
- *Apprehensiveness:* continual worry and anticipation that something bad will happen to oneself or another; and
- *Vigilance:* hyperattentiveness, impatience, irritability, distractibility, difficulty concentrating, insomnia, and fatigue on awakening.

Generalized anxiety often accompanies other psychiatric disorders, particularly depressive syndromes, schizophrenia, and various personality disorders. The diagnosis of generalized anxiety disorder is not made when another mental disorder or an underlying organic disorder is responsible for the client's distress.

People commonly attempt to medicate their anxiety by abusing such drugs as alcohol, barbiturates, and antianxiety agents. In such cases, substance abuse often stops when the anxiety disorder is treated. The extent to which anxiety interferes with work and social life varies greatly among individuals with this disorder, but impairment is usually mild.

Treatment may employ a variety of modalities. *Antianxiety medications* (e.g., benzodiazepines) are used to relieve symptoms and improve functioning. However, these are prone to abuse, and dependence on them is a common problem among anxious clients. Thus, their use must be closely monitored, and the prescribing physician will want to limit their administration to short periods of time (see Chapter 16). *Psychotherapy* is effective in helping some people understand and master the underlying conflicts that prompt anxiety; a therapeutic relationship provides much-needed emotional support to anxious clients. *Behavior therapy* can teach patients techniques of relaxation that they can use in anxiety-provoking situations to overcome fears and decrease symptoms (see Chapter 15).

PHOBIAS

A phobia is a persistent and irrational fear of a specific object, activity, or situation that results in a compelling desire to avoid what is feared. Even though the afflicted person recognizes the fears as excessive or unrealistic given the actual dangerousness of the object, activity, or

Table 8-2. Major categories of phobias.

Social phobias
Fear of embarrassment or humiliation in public situations

Simple phobias
Fear of specific objects or situations (other than being alone, being away
from home, or embarrassment in public)

Agoraphobia
Fear of being alone or in public places from which escape might be difficult or help unavailable in case of sudden incapacitation

situation, he or she nevertheless goes to some lengths to avoid it. If this avoidant behavior has no major effect on the person's life, the phobic behavior does not constitute a disorder (e.g., being afraid of spiders). However, when the phobia impairs one's ability to function at normal daily tasks, the diagnosis of a phobic disorder is warranted.

Phobias are generally divided into three major categories, as shown in Table 8-2. *Agoraphobia* involves a fear of being alone or in public places from which escape might be difficult (e.g., crowds or closed spaces) and where help might not be readily obtainable. *Social phobias* involve a fear of embarrassment or humiliation in situations in which one must interact with other people (e.g., fear of speaking in public, using public lavatories, or eating in public). *Simple phobias* involve fear of specific objects or situations other than being alone, being away from home, or embarrassment in public (e.g., fear of snakes, fear of heights). For most people with phobias, anxiety occurs not only when they are faced with the dreaded stimulus, but even when they anticipate encountering it (anticipatory anxiety).

Psychoanalytic theory holds that phobias begin as perceived dangers from within—that one's own fears of forbidden sexual or aggressive impulses become transposed onto some external object (e.g., snakes). Internal dangers cannot be avoided but a danger in the external world can be; thus, by using the defense mechanism of *displacement*, the phobic person achieves a partial solution to the problem.

Behavioral treatment of simple and social phobias is often quite successful in alleviating the symptom and restoring the client's lost ability to function at daily tasks. *Systematic desensitization* is a widely used behavioral technique that involves the creation of a hierarchy of anxiety-producing stimuli (e.g., thinking about a snake, then looking at pictures of snakes, and finally watching a live snake). The therapist uses this hierarchy of stimuli to desensitize the client, presenting them to the client gradually until they no longer produce anxiety (see Chapter 15). Psychotherapy that focuses on the childhood origins and symbolic meanings of the client's fears has also been found to be helpful in some cases. Benzodiazepines and other antianxiety drugs can alleviate anticipatory anxiety, but are generally not suitable for long-term treatment. Some clinicians have found the phobic anxiety itself to be responsive to treatment with imipramine or phenelzine (see Chapter 16). At present, behavior therapy is the mainstay of treatment for simple and social phobias.

Since agoraphobia is usually associated with panic attacks, the treatment of agoraphobia will be discussed in the next section.

PANIC DISORDER

Panic disorder is a dramatic syndrome characterized by discrete spontaneous panic attacks—crescendos of fear and apprehension—associated with multiple physical symptoms. Attacks resemble the body's normal physiologic response to a life-threatening situation or extreme physical exertion. However, in panic disorder, attacks come on suddenly and unpredictably without provocation.

Panic attacks are characterized by feelings of fear, extreme tension, and a sense of impending doom. Various physical symptoms accompany these feelings, most commonly the following:

- Shortness of breath;
- Palpitations;
- Chest pain or discomfort;
- Choking or smothering sensations;
- Dizziness, vertigo, or unsteady feelings;
- Feelings of unreality;
- Paresthesias (tingling in hands or feet);
- Hot and cold flashes;
- Sweating;
- Faintness;
- Trembling or shaking;
- Fear of going crazy, dying, or doing something uncontrolled during an attack; and
- Nausea, vomiting, and diarrhea.

Attacks commonly last for several minutes or, more rarely, for an hour or more. They recur with varying frequency. Psychotic disorders, medical illnesses (listed above), and substance abuse and withdrawal can all produce symptoms of panic and must be ruled out before you make this diagnosis.

Conversely, because the symptoms of panic attacks mimic many organic disorders, people often consult internists for these symptoms and may have extensive medical work-ups and numerous consultations before the idea of a panic disorder is considered. The disorder is common; it occurs in an estimated 1 to 2 percent of the general population, although it frequently goes unrecognized. It is diagnosed more often among women than men, and typically begins in late adolescence or early adulthood. Panic disorder tends to run in families, and an accumulating body of evidence suggests both that biochemical factors play a crucial role in the etiology of this condition and that there may be a genetic vulnerability to it.

Panic disorder may be limited to one brief period of illness lasting several weeks or months, it may recur several times, or it may become chronic. People with this disorder usually develop nervousness and apprehension between attacks; when this is severe, agoraphobia ensues.

Agoraphobia with panic attacks. Agoraphobia and panic attacks are so frequently encountered together that you are unlikely to encounter them separately in your clinical work.

How do the two go together? Many clinicians postulate that panic attacks come first, and that the fear of being alone and in public places where help is unavailable develops in response to these terrifying episodes of panic. People who experience recurrent symptoms of panic become preoccupied with a fear of developing subsequent attacks and develop an increasing number of phobias about the settings in which they have experienced attacks in the past (e.g., in the supermarket, while driving a car). The number of situations they avoid increases until they are considered truly agoraphobic—afraid of being on their own in public places or of staying alone at home. Between panic attacks, they develop chronic anticipatory anxiety about having another attack.

They often do not seek professional help until they have had symptoms for many years, and by that time they may have agoraphobia with multiple particular phobias, and chronic anticipatory anxiety in addition to the panic attacks themselves. Sadly, some people with this syndrome become shut-ins, unable to leave the house or stay alone for even short periods of time.

Treatment must be aimed at each of the three aspects of this syndrome: panic attacks, anticipatory anxiety, and agoraphobia. It begins with a careful history, physical examination, and laboratory studies to rule out underlying organic illnesses. Panic attacks can be blocked effectively by maintaining clients on an antidepressant such as imipramine or on a monoamine oxidase inhibitor. Anticipatory anxiety and free-floating anxiety can be treated with selective intermittent use of a benzodiazepine (e.g., diazepam). Some clinicians have advocated the use of the benzodiazepine alprazolam (Xanax) alone, since it is thought to have properties that both reduce anticipatory anxiety and block panic attacks.

Agoraphobia may be treated with behavior therapy designed to expose clients gradually to feared experiences, so that they can slowly master their fear of recurrent attacks in specific situations (e.g., in supermarkets, at parties). Dynamically oriented psychotherapy may be necessary when anxiety is due to conflicts or to reactions to the environment that must be explored before symptoms will resolve.

POST-TRAUMATIC STRESS DISORDER

Post-traumatic stress disorder occurs among people who have survived traumatic events that are outside the realm of normal human experience—e.g., rape or assault, physical injury, military combat, bombings, torture, and floods or earthquakes. The afflicted person reexperiences the traumatic event through painful, intrusive recollections of nightmares. Episodes may last from several minutes to several days. During an episode, the person may behave as if he or she were reliving the event.

This disorder also involves a kind of "psychic numbing" or decreased responsiveness to the environment, which may be experienced as decreased ability to receive pleasure from life's activities, or diminished capacity to feel interest in and tenderness toward other people. Anxiety and depression commonly occur with this disorder.

People who experienced traumatic events with others may also feel guilty about having survived when others did not (e.g., concentration camp survivors). Some people are only minimally impaired by this disorder, but others are severely incapacitated by phobic avoidance of all situations that might remind them of the traumatic event and trigger further episodes. This disorder has received increasing attention in the United States in recent years because of its prevalence among those returning from the Vietnam War.

Psychotherapy, antianxiety agents, and antidepressants have all been used in the treatment of this disorder. Group psychotherapy with survivors of the same traumatic situation has been found useful, particularly for war veterans.

SOMATOFORM DISORDERS

Somatoform disorders are, quite literally, mental disorders that assume the form of somatic illness. As any internist will tell you, these disorders are very common in general medical practice. People afflicted with them are often called "doctor-shoppers" or "hypochondriacs." They go from one medical facility to another, seeking help for an illness for which physicians can find no organic basis. It is a frustrating situation for clients, their families, and their physicians. They are told that there is nothing wrong, or that it is "all in their heads," yet they remain convinced that their pain and physical symptoms are real.

In fact, their symptoms and concerns *are* real—as real as if there were visible physical lesions to account for them. People with these disorders do not experience their symptoms as being within their control—i.e., they do not feel that they have voluntarily produced these problems. Yet the symptoms are linked to psychological factors that these people are generally reluctant to explore, and so they persist in searching for an organic cause.

The somatoform disorders fall into the four major categories outlined below and in Table 8-3. All are characterized by physical symptoms that cannot be accounted for by any demonstrable physical findings or known physiological mechanisms.

Table 8–3. Major categories of somatoform disorders.

Somatization disorder
　Multiple recurrent somatic complaints of several years' duration which
　　are not due to any physical disorder

Conversion disorder
　Sudden, dramatic loss of physical functioning that has no known pathophysiological cause and appears to be a manifestation of psychological
　　need or conflict

Psychogenic pain disorder
　Pain in the absence of adequate physical findings or pathophysiologic explanations, and in association with psychological factors that seem to
　　play an etiological role

Hypochondriasis
　Unfounded fears of having serious illness

Somatization Disorder

This disorder, also called *Briquet's syndrome* or *Briquet's hysteria*, is characterized by multiple somatic complaints that are recurrent and of several years' duration, for which medical attention has been sought but for which no physical cause can be found. Complaints are often general, vague, and dramatically presented. Any or all body systems may be involved, but the most common complaints are neurological (e.g., pseudoseizures), gastrointestinal, gynecologic, sexual, and cardiopulmonary. Chronic pain is generally present (e.g., back pain, joint pain), and abdominal pain is probably the most frequent specific complaint encountered among people with this disorder.

Somatization disorder begins before age 30 and has a chronic course, usually involving consultation by many physicians and frequently complicated by multiple hospital admissions and unnecessary surgical procedures. Abuse of both prescribed and nonprescribed substances is common. Anxiety and depression often accompany this disorder. When afflicted individuals seek mental health care, it is often for symptoms of depression, or after suicide threats or gestures. The disorder is much more commonly diagnosed among women than men, with estimates that 1 percent of women in the general population suffer from it.

Before you make this diagnosis, you must be sure that medical evaluation has excluded organic illnesses (e.g., multiple sclerosis, systemic lupus erythematosus) that can present with vague and diffuse symptomatology. Also, some schizophrenics suffer from somatic delusions as part of their illness (e.g., "my insides are rotting"); it is important to differentiate such psychotic individuals from people with somatization disorder, who are, by definition, not psychotic and do not benefit from treatment with antipsychotic medication.

Conversion Disorder

Also called *conversion hysteria*, this is the "classic" disorder that fascinated Freud and other pioneers in the field of psychoanalytic psychiatry. It typically involves the sudden and dramatic onset of blindness, paralysis, seizures, or other symptoms that seem to suggest neurological disease but that have no known pathophysiological cause. It is different from somatization disorder in that it generally involves a single symptom during any one episode, and this symptom results in the loss or alteration of a particular physical function.

In addition to the symptoms mentioned above, typical conversion symptoms include loss of speech, involuntary movements, inability to walk, loss of coordination, tunnel vision, and numbness or tingling sensations in a body part. Although symptoms appear to be neurological, careful examination and tests reveal discrepancies between the loss of function and known anatomical distribution of motor and sensory nerves. For example, numbness of a hand typically occurs over a "glove" distribution (a common-sense notion of how the hand *ought* to be innervated), rather than according to the actual patterns by which nerves carry sensory impulses to and from the hand.

Conversion symptoms are not under the person's voluntary control, yet they appear to be the expression of a psychological conflict or need. These symptoms are thought to provide "sufferers" with two sorts of gains. The *primary gain* from the symptom is thought to be relief from an emotional conflict and the reduction of anxiety. The symptom actually represents the conflict and achieves a partial solution to it. In such cases, there is usually a temporal relationship between an event that provokes conflict and the onset of the symptom (e.g., conflict about expressing overwhelming rage at a spouse, which results in loss of speech).

The *secondary gain*, common to all somatoform disorders, is that, by assuming a sick role, the disabled person can avoid unwanted responsibilities and get support from others that would not otherwise be forthcoming. Because the conversion symptom diminishes anxiety and intrapsychic conflict, clients may be blind or paralyzed and yet seem relatively unconcerned about their severe physical disability—a phenomenon called *la belle indifference.*

Conversion disorder usually begins in adolescence or young adulthood. Episodes of conversion begin suddenly during times of severe stress and resolve abruptly. Functioning may be greatly impaired, and the client may develop physical complications (e.g., muscle weakness and atrophy) due to prolonged loss of function. Unnecessary medical procedures can also produce serious complications. Although it was more common several decades ago, the disorder is now relatively rare in clinical practice in industrialized nations.

Psychogenic Pain Disorder

Psychogenic pain disorder involves the predominant complaint of pain in the absence of any physical findings or pathophysiologic explanation. It differs from somatization disorder in that pain, rather than a variety of symptoms, is the primary presenting complaint. Pain generally does not follow the anatomical distribution of motor and sensory nerves, and laboratory studies reveal no underlying lesions. There is usually a relationship between the exacerbation of psychological conflict or need and the onset of or increase in pain. Secondary gain is generally an important motivating force in the illness (e.g., the man whose chronic back pain worsens every time his wife plans an outing with friends). However, the person with this disorder does not experience the pain as being within his or her voluntary control.

The disorder typically begins in adolescence or early adulthood, but it can occur at any age and may remit spontaneously or become chronic. It is more common in women, but the reasons for this are not clear. As you might expect, frequent medical consultations, unnecessary surgery, and abuse of analgesics are common complications of this disorder.

Hypochondriasis

Unlike the other somatoform disorders, hypochondriasis involves unfounded *fears* of having serious illness. It is based on a preoccupation with body functions and the unrealistic interpretation of physical signs or sensations as abnormal, e.g., an occasional cough may be interpreted as a sign of lung cancer. Although these concerns are not frankly delusional, people with this disorder cannot shake their fears of physical illness despite repeated reassurance from physicians and persistently negative physical and laboratory findings.

Hypochondriasis is equally common in men and women. It begins most frequently among men in their thirties and among women in their forties. It is quite common in general medical practice, and its chronic course invites extensive work-ups and unnecessary surgery. Although some people can continue to function with only mild impairment at home and at work, others become invalids. One danger in this disorder is that real organic pathology may go unnoticed because of repeated "false alarms."

Treatment of Somatoform Disorders

The treatment of somatoform disorders is dificult. Clients usually refuse to accept the possibility that the roots of their problems are psychological. Insight-oriented psychotherapy can help some explore and resolve conflicts that foster physical symptoms; with conflict resolution, symptoms often disappear spontaneously. However, many of these people are particularly resistant to exploratory psychotherapy. Biofeedback and other behavior modification techniques can help clients to relax and control pain and anxiety.

Antianxiety medications are helpful for some clients on a short-term basis, but the potential for abuse and dependence on such drugs limits their value in the treatment of these disorders. Antidepressant medication has been found to be helpful for clients who have prominent symptoms of depression along with somatic complaints.

One great service a therapist can provide people with somatoform disorders is to coordinate their care, so that "doctor-shopping" ends and unnecessary surgical procedures are avoided. This requires a good working relationship between the psychotherapist and physicians responsible for the client's medical care.

DISSOCIATIVE DISORDERS

Dissociative disorders are relatively rarely encountered in mental health settings. The discussion here will therefore be brief. They are, however, quite dramatic and have received much publicity in literature, in films, and on television. The four major disorders are described below and in Table 8-4.

Psychogenic Amnesia

This disorder is a sudden inability to recall important personal information (e.g., name, occupation, family). This may be amnesia for one's entire life up until the moment of onset, or it may be amnesia for a circumscribed period of time (e.g., for the events surrounding a car crash). Amnesia may be selective; that is, some events during a

Table 8–4. Major categories of dissociative disorders.

Psychogenic amnesia
  Sudden inability to recall important personal information

Psychogenic fugue
  Amnesia combined with sudden travel away from home, usually in flight from an intolerable situation

Multiple personality
  The existence of two or more distinct personalities within an individual, each of which is dominant at a particular time

Depersonalization disorder
  Feelings of self-estrangement or unreality that impair social or occupational functioning

specified period of time are forgotten, while others are still subject to recall.

Unlike amnesia that is due to organic mental disorders, psychogenic amnesia usually has an abrupt onset following a traumatic or unusually stressful experience. It generally resolves abruptly as well, and recurrences are rare.

Psychogenic Fugue

In this disorder, amnesia is combined with physical flight, usually from an intolerable situation. The individual assumes a new identity and is unable to recall his or her previous one. This is generally a short-lived phenomenon, involving a minimal amount of travel, but it may be quite prolonged and may result in the assumption of a whole new life in another locale (e.g., a man may leave his family, move to another city, get a new job, and make a new set of friends).

Recovery is usually as abrupt as the onset, and recurrences are rare.

Multiple Personality

Multiple personality involves the existence within the individual of two or more distinct personalities, each with its own unique set of memories, attributes, and social relationships. Each is dominant at different times, and the transition from one personality to another is often abrupt.

The personalities are usually distinct and represent different unintegrated aspects of the person's identity. For example, an individual may have one shy and inhibited personality, another that is gregarious and promiscuous, and a third that is hostile and suspicious. The personalities may call themselves by different names. Each one may be unaware of the existence of the other personalities, and aware only of lost periods of time when the other personalities are dominant.

This disorder is exceedingly rare, and its course is generally more chronic than those of the other dissociative disorders mentioned. Intensive psychotherapy is usually the treatment of choice, with the goal of helping the client to integrate the different personalities into one cohesive self.

Interesting case studies of multiple personality in the popular literature include *The Three Faces of Eve* and *Sybil* (see References at the end of this chapter).

Depersonalization Disorder

This disorder involves the occurrence of one or more episodes of depersonalization, manifested by feelings of self-estrangement or unreality. Clients often report feeling as if they were watching a play rather than participating in real life, or as if they were watching themselves from a distance.

Such episodes are extremely common in normal persons, especially young adults during times of stress. They only constitute a disorder when they impair social or occupational functioning. The disorder is often chronic, commonly waxing and waning as the person's degree of anxiety or depression increases or decreases.

EATING DISORDERS

Eating disorders have become the focus of much interest among mental health professionals in recent years. An increasing number of people (predominantly women) report gross disturbances in their eating behavior. The two most prevalent syndromes are *anorexia nervosa* and *bulimia*. Although these eating disorders are described as primary—i.e., as not resulting from some medical illness—a great many patients with anorexia and bulimia also suffer from other diagnosable mental disorders. In fact, eating disorders occur in people who span the entire range of psychopathology, from psychosis to anxiety disorders and neurosis. In particular, many people with severe disturbances in their eating behavior suffer from personality disorders.

Thus, when you see people who report eating problems such as binge eating and vomiting, or who engage in self-starvation, you should look carefully for underlying psychosis, affective disturbances, and personality disorders before assuming that the eating disorder is an isolated problem. The major categories of eating disorders are outlined below and in Table 8-5.

Anorexia Nervosa

Anorexia nervosa is a syndrome of self-starvation in which the individual willfully restricts food intake and overexercises in an effort to ease the intense fear of becoming obese. Anorectics report feeling fat when they are at normal body weight and even when they are emaciated, because weight loss does not decrease their fear of obesity. They suffer from a distorted perception of their bodies, and have

Table 8–5. Major categories of eating disorders.

Anorexia nervosa
  Intense fear of becoming obese and a disturbance of body image that
  leads to willful restriction of food intake, significant weight loss, and
  refusal to maintain a minimal normal body weight

Bulimia
  Recurrent episodes of binge eating accompanied by a fear of not being
  able to stop eating, and followed by depressed mood and self-
  deprecating thoughts

Bulimarexia
  Features of both bulimia and anorexia nervosa—particularly binge eating
  and refusal to maintain a minimal normal body weight

difficulty identifying bodily sensations, including the feeling of hunger. However, anorexia nervosa is not primarily a disturbance in appetite. Rather, it is related to disturbances in the sense of self, identity, and autonomy. The anorectic struggles desperately to control appetite and weight, often to combat an underlying and global sense of helplessness.

Anorectics are almost exclusively female (95 percent)—most commonly adolescent girls and young adults. The syndrome often begins unnoticed by others, as the anorectic goes on a diet "to slim down." But as weight loss progresses and food intake decreases, family and friends gradually become alarmed, while the anorectic remains adamant in her desire to lose weight because she is fat. Many anorectic teenagers give histories of being overly compliant "model children," who become angry and negativistic as the syndrome develops and they begin to struggle with their families over eating practices. Besides using diet and exercise to accomplish their starvation, anorectics also use self-induced vomiting, laxatives, and diuretics. Weight loss, by definition, amounts to at least 25 percent of the anorectic's original body weight (or projected normal body weight in growing teenagers), and may go well beyond this mark to total emaciation.

Anorectics typically deny that they have a problem and profess that they do not want treatment. Anorectic adolescents often manifest delayed sexual development, and adults show little interest in sex. (Amenorrhea, or loss of menstrual periods, is often one of the earliest results of the anorectic's stringent dieting.) Many theorists postulate a fear of sexuality as contributing to the anorectic's drive to become emaciated.

Fortunately, most anorectics experience a single episode of the eating disorder and then recover completely without recurrence. However, some people have recurrent periods of anorexia, and a sizable proportion take an unremitting course, with progressive starvation. Factors associated with a good prognosis include onset of the problem before age 15 and weight gain within two years after treatment is begun.

If weight loss becomes profound, physical signs ensue, including low body temperature, swelling of the ankles, slowed heart rate, low blood pressure, and lanugo (fine, soft body hair). Medical complications include severe disturbances of blood chemistry (electrolyte imbalances), coma, and death. *Anorexia nervosa is a potentially lethal disease:* mortality ranges from 15 to 21 percent. Hospitalization and forced feeding are often necessary to prevent starvation, and forced feeding procedures often come to be the focus of the severely anorectic person's angry struggles to maintain rigid control over her body.

Treatment of anorexia nervosa is extremely difficult. The first goal must be improvement of the person's nutritional status, both to stabilize her medical condition and to reverse the psychological disturbances (such as difficulty in assimilating new information) that specifically result from starvation. Only when the worst malnutrition is reversed can you get an accurate picture of the person's baseline psychological condition (e.g., the presence of a thought disorder or severe personality disturbance). Underlying illness must be treated with psychotherapy and, where indicated, medication.

Clinicians have reported some success in treating anorexia nervosa with a combination of behavior therapy aimed at maintaining weight at an adequate level and insight-oriented psychotherapy aimed at elucidating and correcting anorectics' inner confusion and misconceptions about their own feelings and needs, their self-worth, and their ability to control their lives. An important adjunct to this treatment is family therapy aimed at decreasing the family's characteristic overinvolvement with the anorectic, and helping the family to allow the anorectic more autonomy.

Bulimia

Bulimia is a disorder characterized by recurrent episodes of binge eating that are frequently associated with self-induced vomiting or laxative abuse. Binge eating involves rapidly consuming large amounts of food in a short period of time. In contrast to people with anorexia nervosa, bulimics are generally aware that their eating patterns are abnormal, and they fear not being able to stop eating voluntarily. Bulimics often become depressed after binges and frequently berate themselves for their behavior.

Binges commonly consist of high-calorie foods, many of which are sweet and can be eaten quickly. Eating is usually done secretively, and the binge eater often stops only when abdominal pain becomes severe, sleep intervenes, or social circumstances make it impossible to continue gorging. Bulimics frequently vomit after binges to relieve abdominal pain, reduce guilt, and control their weight. Their weight may fluctuate widely, because of alternating periods of binge eating and fasting, or it may remain stable. When it is severe, bingeing may disrupt bulimics' social and occupational lives, since they may spend hours secretly procuring food, gorging themselves, and rushing to a bathroom to induce vomiting after each binge.

Bulimia typically begins in adolescence or early adulthood. It is much more common in women than in men. It generally follows a chronic course, occurring intermittently over many years, and episodes of binge eating are often precipitated by life stresses. The etiology of bulimia is not known but, in many cases, the eating disorder is related to more global psychopathology (e.g., an underlying personality disorder).

A variety of treatment modalities have been used with bulimics, including behavior modification techniques, insight-oriented psychotherapy, and cognitive therapy—all with limited success (see Chapter 15). Recently, research has focused on a possible link between bulimia and affective disorder, and new studies suggest a possible role for antidepressant medication in the treatment of bulimia.

Bulimarexia

This term is used to describe a disorder which includes features of both bulimia and anorexia nervosa—i.e., binge eating, vomiting, and self-starvation with severe weight loss. The overlap between the two syndromes is significant; it is estimated that between 40 and 50 percent of people with primary anorexia nervosa exhibit bulimic behavior.

REFERENCES

American Psychiatric Association: Diagnostic and Statistical Manual of Mental Disorders, 3rd ed. Washington, DC, American Psychiatric Association, 1980, pp 225-252

Bruch H: Anorexia nervosa: therapy and theory. Am J Psychiatry 139: 1531-1538, 1982

Bruch H: Eating Disorders: Obesity, Anorexia Nervosa, and the Person Within. New York, Basic Books, 1973

Dietch JT: Diagnosis of organic anxiety disorders. Psychosomatics 22:661-669, 1981

Garfinkel PE, Moldofsky H, Garner DM: The heterogeneity of anorexia nervosa: bulimia as a distinct subgroup. Arch Gen Psychiatry 37:1036-1040, 1980

Pope HG, Hudson JI, Jonas JM, et al: Bulimia treated with imipramine: a placebo-controlled, double-blind study. Am J Psychiatry 140:554-558, 1983

Schreiber F: Sybil. New York, Warner Books, 1974 (An account of the psychotherapy of a woman with multiple personalities.)

Shader RI, Goodman M, Gever J: Panic disorders: current perspectives. J Clin Psychopharmacology 2(Suppl 6):2S-10S, 1982

Shader RI, Greenblatt DJ, Ciraulo DA: Benzodiazepine treatment of specific anxiety states. Psychiatr Ann 11:16-20, 1981

Sheehan DV: Current concepts in psychiatry: panic attacks and phobias. N Engl J Med 307:156-158, 1982

Thigpen CH, Cleckley HN: The Three Faces of Eve. New York, Popular Library, 1974 (A highly readable case study of a woman with multiple personalities.)

CHAPTER 9

Dementia and Delirium

Dementia and delirium are conditions characterized by *global* intellectual impairment. People with these disorders commonly suffer from deficits in memory, in abstract thinking, in the ability to learn new tasks and solve problems, and in orientation to time, place, and person. These syndromes generally result from diffuse disease of the brain and consequent loss of function of large numbers of neurons.

Delirium is commonly referred to as an *acute organic brain syndrome*. It is characterized by a clouded state of consciousness, often with rapid onset, a fluctuating course, and short duration. In addition to diffuse intellectual deficits, the delirious person is likely to suffer from hallucinations, delusions, and increased motor activity (see Table 9-1).

Dementia, by contrast, is often called a *chronic organic brain syndrome*. Consciousness is not usually clouded in dementia until the end stages of the dementing process. The onset of dementia is usually insidious, the course is one of slow but persistent deterioration, and the demented person is much less likely than the delirious person to manifest hallucinations or other signs of disordered thinking. The demented individual is not generally agitated or hyperactive; rather, motor activity is usually normal or slow.

Table 9–1. Comparison of dementia and delirium.

Dementia	Delirium
"Chronic organic brain syndrome"	"Acute organic brain syndrome"
Consciousness unimpaired (until late in the course of disease)	Consciousness clouded
Normal level of arousal	Agitation or stupor
Develops insidiously over months or years	Develops rapidly
Often chronic, progressive	Often reversible
Common in nursing homes, psychiatric hospitals	Common on medical wards in general hospitals

Table 9–2. *DSM-III* diagnostic criteria for dementia.

A loss of intellectual abilities of sufficient severity to interfere with social or occupational functioning

Memory impairment

At least one of the following:

> Impairment of abstract thinking, as manifested by concrete interpretation of proverbs, inability to find similarities and differences between related words, difficulty in defining words and concepts, and other similar tasks
> Impaired judgment
> Other disturbances of higher cortical function, such as aphasia (disorder of language due to brain dysfunction), apraxia (inability to carry out motor activities despite intact comprehension and motor function), agnosia (failure to recognize or identify objects despite intact sensory function), "constructional difficulty" (e.g., inability to copy three-dimensional figures, assemble blocks, or arrange sticks in specific designs)
> Personality changes, i.e., alteration or accentuation of premorbid traits

State of consciousness not clouded (i.e., does not meet the criteria for delirium or intoxication, although these may be superimposed)

Either (a) evidence from the history, physical examination, or laboratory tests of a specific organic factor that is judged to be etiologically related to the disturbance or, in the absence of such evidence, (b) an organic factor necessary for the development of the syndrome can be presumed if conditions other than organic mental disorders have been reasonably excluded and if the behavioral change represents cognitive impairment in a variety of areas

Both dementia and delirium are included under the general diagnostic category of *organic brain syndromes*. But the term is not particularly useful, for it is nonspecific and conveys little information about the conditions it is meant to describe. It is also somewhat misleading, in that it implies that we can neatly separate disorders that have "organic" causes from other mental illnesses that are functional in origin. It makes more sense to refer to dementia and delirium, as well as other "organic" syndromes (such as those caused by drugs and alcohol), by their specific names.

Dementia and delirium are *not* diseases—they are conditions that can result from a large number of underlying organic processes affecting brain tissue. A vast array of underlying somatic illnesses can give rise to them. Stereotypically, delirium is reversible, while dementia is irreversible. However, there are remediable causes of both dementia and delirium, and you must diligently search for such treatable illnesses whenever you encounter someone with global cognitive deterioration.

You need not memorize all the possible organic causes of dementia and delirium, but it *is* important that you:

- Learn to recognize the signs of dementia and delirium, so that you will not overlook these syndromes.
- Be aware of possible underlying causes that are treatable.
- Understand the need for careful medical examination and laboratory work-up of every client who presents with altered cognitive functioning.
- Understand the course and treatment of those common syndromes that are not reversible.

DEMENTIA

Dementia is defined as a deterioration in intellectual abilities that is of sufficient severity to interfere with social or occupational functioning. The deficit involves many aspects of cognition—particularly memory and judgment. Higher cortical functions such as language, abstract reasoning, and the ability to follow directions are also commonly impaired. Although dementia is most common in the elderly, it is *not* synonymous with old age, nor is it a normal part of the aging process; rather, it implies diffuse disease of the brain that has impaired the functioning of large numbers of nerve cells in the cerebral cortex of the brain. The criteria given in the third edition of the *Diagnostic and Statistical Manual of Mental Disorders* (*DSM-III*) for the diagnosis of dementia are shown in Table 9-2.

Clinical Picture

As noted above, dementia normally has an insidious onset, evolving over many months or even many years. It often begins with vague, nonspecific physical complaints, increased moodiness or irritability, and subtle withdrawal of interest from life. People often seem to be "not themselves," and their personalities appear to lose their sparkle. The early symptoms are so subtle that families often cannot identify any specific disorder, and instead are likely to be hurt by the seemingly willful moodiness and emotional withdrawal of their loved one. Demented people begin to have trouble with any activity that requires new or original thought or learning. Dementia may thus be apparent earlier in those who are involved in more intense creative and intellectual endeavors.

Early memory loss may go unnoticed by the affected individual and his or her family. For example, demented people may begin to forget dates or telephone numbers, but may compensate for this quite well by writing things down. They may forget instructions or directions, and may need to ask that these be repeated several times before they can commit the information to memory. Some demented people notice such deficits in memory themselves, while others remain oblivious to them even when they become obvious to family and friends. Demented people may even fabricate false details (*confabulation*) to fill in gaps in their memory. As the dementia progresses, they become increasingly distractible. They may, for example, begin tasks but forget to return to them after an interruption. People who live alone may forget to turn off the stove and thereby put themselves in danger.

Demented people eventually begin to lose more skills, and their deficits become more obvious. They commonly become lost on their way to familiar places, and it is then that their condition may begin to seem more serious to those around them. Language initially remains unimpaired but, as other intellectual functions deteriorate, language usually begins to become more stereotyped and to convey less and less information. Demented individuals may perseverate in speech (i.e, repeat the same word or phrase over and over again) or may continue to perform work, such as arranging chairs, long after the task has been completed. Although they normally become more quiet and socially withdrawn, some demented people become more active in socially inappropriate ways, such as by going on spending sprees or becoming physically assaultive.

When dementia becomes severe, people are unable to perform such simple tasks as feeding themselves, despite the fact that motor functions remain intact. They forget the names of friends, are unable to recognize even close relatives, and finally forget their own name and date of birth (although this information is usually the very last to be forgotten). They increasingly neglect their personal hygiene and begin to disregard normal rules of social conduct. More infantile behaviors, such as incontinence and extreme emotional lability (fits of laughing and crying) may appear. Finally, many people become totally mute and unresponsive to the environment. At this stage, death often occurs within a few months, but people with end-stage dementia may linger on in this stage for several years.

Although dementia occurs most frequently in the elderly, the age at which it develops and the course it takes depends on the underlying cause. Demented people may remain unaware of and unconcerned by their growing deficits, or they may recognize them and react with anxiety, depression, or paranoia. When personality changes occur, they are usually exaggerations of preexisting character traits (e.g., a man who has always been somewhat suspicious by nature may become floridly paranoid as dementia progresses). People with dementia sometimes develop hallucinations, delusions, hypochondriacal concerns, and even suicidal ideation as a result of such personality change and deterioration. All of the symptoms of dementia can be exacerbated by stress, such as a move to unfamiliar surroundings, hospitalization, loss of a loved one, or concurrent medical illness. Dementia is not a lethal condition in and of itself, but the inability to care for oneself predisposes people to malnutrition, decubitus ulcers ("bed sores"), and pneumonia caused by inhalation of saliva, food, or stomach contents. (This type of pneumonia, called *aspiration pneumonia*, is the most common cause of death in dementia.)

Irreversible Causes

Alzheimer's Disease

Senile and presenile dementia (*Alzheimer's disease*), the most common form of dementia, accounts for roughly half of all cases. It is of unknown etiology and is associated with diffuse loss of brain tissue, specifically in the cerebral cortex. Clinicians have traditionally made a distinction between senile and presenile dementia, based on whether the disease began before or after age 60, but there is in fact little clinical or pathological basis for such a distinction. The illness is very similar, whether it begins at age 45 or at age 95. The term *Alzheimer's disease* was once synonymous with presenile dementia, but you will now hear it used to describe dementia of unknown cause without reference to age of onset.

Alzheimer's disease usually begins after age 60, but it is seen as early as age 40. Estimates of the prevalence of Alzheimer's disease among those in the general population over age 65 range from 5 to 12 percent, and it is a leading (although often unreported) cause of death among the aged.

Its symptoms begin very gradually and progressively worsen, often over several years. At present, the disease process is irreversible. Afflicted individuals may live as long as 10 years after the onset of the disease, but they eventually require total care and succumb to secondary illnesses, e.g., aspiration pneumonia.

Physical findings are generally absent in Alzheimer's disease, or are present only in the end stages of the illness, when there may be changes in the person's reflexes on neurologic examination (hyperactive deep tendon reflexes; positive Babinski signs; and snout, suck, and rooting reflexes—all signs of frontal lobe release). People with Alzheimer's disease often have normal computed tomography (CT) scans of the brain, although they typically show some tissue loss in the cerebral cortex and enlargement of the cerebral ventricles, particularly if the disease is far advanced. Electroencephalogram (EEG), or brain wave, abnormalities are present in about 80 percent of patients (usually diffuse slowing and decreased alpha rhythm), but these changes are not diagnostic. Thus, *there are no diagnostic laboratory studies; the clinical diagnosis of Alzheimer's disease is made only when the history, physical examination, and laboratory work-up have ruled out other causes of dementia.*

At autopsy, people with Alzheimer's disease have characteristic changes in brain tissue that include the following:

- *Senile plaques:* Microscopic abnormalities of the cerebral cortex, consisting of nerve cells tangled around a core of protein material called "amyloid."
- *Neurofibrillary tangles:* Filaments tangled inside nerve cells throughout the cortex of the brain.
- *Granulovacular degeneration of nerve cell bodies:* Under the microscope, brain cells appear to have "holes" in them.

Such changes occur in normal aging brains, but much less extensively than they do in the brains of people with dementia.

Despite recent intensive research into the causes and treatment of this devastating and common illness, its etiology remains a mystery. Several hypotheses about the cause of Alzheimer's disease have received a great deal of public attention. In particular, the theory that Alzheimer's disease is caused by abnormally high levels of aluminum in the central nervous system has not been sustained by empirical research, nor has the notion of a viral etiology. Much attention has recently been focused on the hypothesis that people with Alzheimer's disease have abnormal (decreased) activity of the chemical acetylcholine in the central nervous system, but at present this too remains unproven.

Pick's disease is similar to Alzheimer's in its clinical manifestations and pathology, but does not involve changes in the parietal lobes of the brain. Since this incurable familial disorder is rare and almost impossible to differentiate clinically from Alzheimer's, it need not be discussed in detail.

Cerebrovascular Dementia

"Hardening of the arteries" in the brain was once thought to be responsible for most cases of dementia. Alzheimer's disease has since been recognized as the major dementing illness in the elderly, but cerebrovascular disease is thought to account for a significant number of cases as well (perhaps 15 to 25 percent).

Atherosclerosis, or "hardening" of blood vessel walls by the accumulation of fatty deposits, does not—in and of itself—result in dementia. Rather, it predisposes people to brain damage from *blood clots*, which block arteries and thereby starve brain tissue of oxygen, and *hemorrhage*, or bleeding into brain tissue resulting in tissue death. In fact, it appears that multiple small clots and hemorrhages in brain tissue produce dementia, and the condition often has a fluctuating, "stuttering" course with stepwise deterioration in functioning. People with this disease commonly have high blood pressure or diabetes, two conditions which predispose people to atherosclerosis. Some people give a history of several strokes in the past, but many have had "silent" strokes and have no awareness of discrete episodes of neurologic illness. There are usually specific neurological signs (e.g., weakness of one limb). In some cases, cerebrovascular disease and Alzheimer's coexist, and both contribute to the picture of dementia.

Although atherosclerosis in major arteries (e.g., narrowing of the internal carotid artery) may be surgically correctable, much atherosclerosis occurs diffusely among smaller vessels and is therefore not treatable with surgery. High blood pressure can be controlled in most cases, and early treatment of hypertension in people who have no symptoms of dementia can help to prevent or arrest the development of cerebrovascular dementia. People who have had or are at risk for strokes may benefit from the administration of anticoagulants or aspirin, which may prevent abnormal formation of blood clots.

Treatable Causes

Tumors

Most brain tumors cause specific neurological signs (e.g., weakness on one side of the body) and are therefore not likely to be confused with Alzheimer's disease. However, depending on their anatomical location, tumors may initially present with psychiatric symptoms and no other obvious disturbances, and so may be mistaken for signs of "senility." The most common forms of brain tumors are gliomas (which constitute 30-50 percent of all brain tumors), meningiomas (20 percent), and secondary metastases (20 percent), most often from lung or breast cancer or malignant melanomas. Tumors of the frontal lobe, thalamus, and corpus callosum, as well as olfactory groove meningiomas, are particularly likely to present with psychiatric symptoms but no neurologic findings. Thus, it is generally recommended that every person with dementia (indeed, everyone who has undergone a major personality change) have a CT scan of the brain to rule out a tumor. Obviously, how treatable tumors are depends largely on the location of the tumor and whether it is malignant or benign, but in some cases intellectual impairment can be completely reversed by successful surgical intervention.

Brain Trauma

Trauma to any part of the nervous system usually results in maximal impairment immediately after the event. Victims of brain injury continue to recover lost function for up to a year. Such obvious cases of trauma are not generally mistaken for Alzheimer's disease or other forms of primary dementia. However, the clinical picture of *chronic subdural hematoma* is easy to confuse with that of Alzheimer's disease, and the consequences of failing to recognize this life-threatening problem may be disastrous.

Subdural hematoma denotes a collection of blood that is outside the brain but within the skull. It often results from head trauma but, particularly in elderly people, the trauma may be minor and not recalled at all. When blood collects slowly and puts gradually increasing pressure on the brain, the person may become demented over days or even weeks without specific neurological signs or impaired consciousness. A CT scan will generally reveal these masses of blood (which are often on both sides of the head). Surgical evacuation of the hematoma may be life-saving, and will frequently reverse the intellectual impairment.

Normal-Pressure Hydrocephalus

A small subgroup of people who present with dementia have been found to have hydrocephalus (an excessive accumulation of cerebrospinal fluid [CSF] that enlarges the ventricles of the brain) with normal cerebrospinal fluid pressure. The flow of CSF from the ventri-

cles to its usual site of absorption in the subarachnoid space surrounding the cerebral cortex is somehow obstructed, so fluid collects
within the ventricles and causes the characteristic syndrome of
dementia, gait apraxia, and *urinary incontinence.* (Gait apraxia is a particular abnormality of locomotion in which the person has normal
strength and coordination, but literally loses the intellectual ability to
organize the act of walking, and therefore has difficulty in lifting each
foot in succession.)

Although some people with normal-pressure hydrocephalus
have a history of meningitis, subarachnoid hemorrhage, or trauma
that might account for the obstruction of the normal flow of CSF, in
many cases there is no apparent cause for this abnormality. The
syndrome develops gradually, often over six to 12 months. A CT scan
reveals dilated ventricles, out of proportion to the degree of loss of
brain tissue.

Treatment is surgical: a shunt allows CSF to flow from the cerebral ventricles to another body cavity, such as the abdominal cavity. In
cases that are accurately diagnosed, this procedure can result in dramatic improvement in symptoms. However, in some cases no improvement ensues—perhaps because of misdiagnosis—and the
shunt procedure has many potential complications. Although normal-pressure hydrocephalus occurs infrequently, it must be considered in the differential diagnosis of dementia because it is potentially
treatable.

Dementia Secondary to Systemic Illness

As noted above, a great many systemic illnesses—including metabolic disturbances, infections, and exposure to toxins—can present
with gradual intellectual deterioration. These conditions run the
gamut from porphyria to pellagra, from lead poisoning to tuber-
culous meningitis. It is therefore critical that each demented client is
carefully screened for these disorders so that you will not overlook
treatable causes of dementia. These illnesses are well described in
general medical texts. Table 9-3 lists some of the most common diseases that may present with dementia.

Pseudodementia

Despite the implication of its name, this condition is a true
dementia, but it is due to a functional psychiatric disorder—depression. When dementia is seen in elderly people, it is often assumed to
be due to Alzheimer's disease. In fact, many older people who present with a deterioration in personality, retardation of thought and

Table 9–3. Some diseases that may present with dementia.

Metabolic disorders
  Hepatic encephalopathy (liver failure)
  Wilson's disease
  Uremia (kidney failure)
  Hypoxia (congestive heart failure, anemia)

Deficiency diseases
  Wernicke-Korsakoff syndrome (thiamine)
  Pernicious anemia (vitamin B_{12}, folate)
  Pellagra (niacin)

Endocrine disorders
  Thyroid disease (hypothyroidism, thyroid storm)
  Hypercalcemia (parathyroid disorders)
  Cushing's disease
  Pancreatic disease (diabetes, hypoglycemia)

Toxins (exogenous)
  Drugs of abuse: amphetamines, cocaine, alcohol, LSD
  Medications: bromides, steroids, reserpine, methyldopa, L-dopa, pro-
    pranolol, scopolamine, atropine
  Industrial toxins: lead, mercury, manganese, carbon monoxide, organic
    solvents

Infections
  Chronic meningitis (tuberculosis, cryptococcosis)
  Viral meningitis
  Syphilis
  Creutzfeld-Jakob disease (slow virus)

Neurologic diseases (often accompanied by movement disorders)
  Huntington's chorea
  Parkinson's disease
  Spino-cerebellar degeneration

Tumors

action, apathy, disorientation, sleep disturbance, and global loss of intellectual functions are not demented, but depressed.

It may be impossible to differentiate depression from dementia on the basis of clinical findings, but if you take a careful history from family or close friends, you are likely to find that people with pseudodementia have not deteriorated over many months or years, but have been "demented" for only a few weeks. Moreover, you are likely to see that this deterioration is associated with feelings of sadness. Be particularly alert to pseudodementia in anyone with a family history of depression or manic-depressive illness.

Differentiating between dementia and depression is extremely difficult, because demented people who recognize their growing deficits may react with depression, and depressed people may also have mild dementia. The important point is that, when there is a depressive component to the illness, such "demented" people may benefit from a trial of antidepressant therapy or electroconvulsive therapy (ECT). In fact, some people who appear floridly demented recover all their lost mental abilities when the underlying depression is treated. If pseudodementia goes undetected, it may be fatal, because the person may lapse into total self-neglect or attempt suicide.

Interview and Evaluation

Demented people are often brought to physicians by family members when they can no longer tolerate such symptoms as increased emotional outbursts, socially embarrassing or dangerous behavior, and suspiciousness. Demented people are less likely than delirious ones to be psychotic or to appear medically ill. They are often quite alert, neatly dressed, and socially appropriate when they meet you. Evidence of dementia in the course of conversation may be difficult to find, and may only take the form of an apparent hesitancy in answering questions. People may cover their memory deficits by dismissing a question as unimportant (e.g., "I don't need to know the date any more since I retired") or by giving a tangential answer.

Only by performing a careful mental status examination (Chapter 4) will you pick up early signs of dementia. People with dementia will have difficulty with tests of recent memory, and so be unable to remember three unrelated objects (e.g., apple, tree, chair) several minutes after they are given the task. Their interpretations of proverbs will be concrete if their abstract thinking is impaired, and they will have difficulty naming objects, doing simple calculations, following directions, or copying geometric patterns.

If dementia is more advanced, signs of memory impairment, distractibility, and other cognitive difficulties will be readily apparent in conversation before you get to the mental status examination.

A word of caution in interviewing demented people: It is important to be particularly gentle in testing cognitive functioning. A person who is suddenly forced to confront his or her intellectual deficits during the interview may become acutely embarrassed, anxious, depressed, or agitated. Such "catastrophic reactions," as they are called, can sometimes be avoided if you proceed slowly, respectfully, and with tact in conducting a mental status examination.

Taking a History

As you do a general evaluation, keep the following in mind:

- *Document the course of the illness.* When did problems first begin? What were the earliest changes noted? What intellectual functions seem to have deteriorated? Was deterioration rapid or slow, step-wise or gradual? Has the client become unable to care for himself or herself, and in what ways?
- *Note any accompanying symptoms of mental illness.* Have there been mood changes (depression, sadness, elation)? Has the client shown signs of disordered thinking (e.g., hallucinations, paranoia)?
- *Note accompanying physical symptoms.* Have there been vegetative signs (sleep disturbance, weight loss) or other signs of systemic illness (e.g., fever)? Has the client suffered from headaches, sei-zures, or paralysis? Has he or she begun to make any involuntary movements?
- *Take a medical history.* Note major medical or neurological illnesses. Be sure to document any history of mental illness as well (e.g., affective illness, psychotic episodes).
- *Note all medications, drug use, and possible exposure to toxins at home or work (and their relationship to the onset of symptoms).* Do not forget over-the-counter preparations.
- *Obtain a careful family history.* Has anyone else in the family been demented or suffered from other neurologic disease? Is there a family history of depression or mania?
- *Pay attention to the client's social supports.* How much can the client do for himself or herself? How much assistance is required? Who is available to assist? Have the client's support systems been stressed beyond their limits, or can the client continue to receive adequate care at home if the condition is not reversible?

The Mental Status Examination

Take particular care in performing a mental status examination (MSE) on a person who presents with suspected dementia, for it is essential that you document the nature and extent of the existing cognitive deficits. The MSE is discussed at length in Chapter 4.

In examining demented people, be sure to proceed gingerly, to minimize anxiety as you ask about intellectual impairment. Focus on cognitive functions, particularly the following:

- Orientation;
- Memory—immediate, recent, and remote (be careful to test concentration as well, and note attention span);
- Fund of information;
- Calculations;
- Abstraction;
- Judgment; and
- Language—spontaneous speech, naming objects, reading and writing.

Physical Examination
A physician should perform a thorough physical examination on every client who presents with intellectual deterioration. This should include particular attention in the neurologic examination to the following:

- Focal neurologic signs (weakness, sensory loss);
- Papilledema (swelling and blurring of the borders of the optic disc);
- Frontal lobe release signs (snout, suck, palmomental, and rooting reflexes); and
- Hyperreflexia and Babinski signs.

Laboratory Studies
Basic laboratory studies should include the following:

- Urinalysis;
- Chest x-ray;
- Blood studies—complete blood count (CBC) with differential blood count, metabolic screening battery (e.g., electrolytes, glucose, blood urea nitrogen [BUN], creatinine, liver function tests, serum calcium), serological test for syphilis, thyroid function tests, and serum levels of B12 and folate;
- CT scan of the brain; and
- Electrocardiogram (EKG).

Other studies that may be indicated, on the basis of the client's history and physical examination, include the following:

- Lumbar puncture,
- Toxic screen,
- Arterial blood gases, and
- EEG.

Treatment of Dementia

Treatment is likely to be most successful when there is an underlying remediable cause. Whether treatment will result in reversal of the cognitive deficits depends on the underlying illness and how far it has progressed before the initiation of therapy.

In more than three-quarters of all cases of dementia, no treatable cause exists, and therapy is designed to provide symptom relief and support. Such therapy can be remarkably effective in helping clients and their families deal with the stresses of dementing illness. Individual psychotherapy and family therapy can help clarify many of the problems the illness presents, and they can help clients and families find ways of dealing with this chronic debilitating illness. Intervention in the client's environment may be necessary, e.g., arranging home care by professionals or care in a nursing home.

Drug treatment has been helpful in treating specific symptoms in many cases of progressive dementia. Depressive symptoms often respond to treatment with antidepressants (e.g., a tricyclic antidepressant such as desipramine). Anxiety, insomnia, and agitation are commonly alleviated by minor tranquilizers (particularly the benzodiazepines), although these drugs may cause paradoxical agitation in some people. In cases of severe agitation and psychosis, antipsychotics (e.g., haloperidol) are often effective. Drug treatment in elderly clients must be undertaken with caution, for they generally require smaller doses than younger adults and are more prone to such side effects as postural hypotension (a drop in blood pressure which occurs with postural change [e.g.,standing up, lying down]). However, medication need not be avoided, for it can provide them with considerable relief from the symptoms that accompany the dementing process.

The initial evaluation of a demented client may be done on an outpatient basis, but hospitalization often allows for a more thorough work-up and enables the client to be monitored more carefully if a trial of medication is indicated. The decision to hospitalize a person with dementia will depend on the severity of the condition, the social supports available to the individual, and whether serious systemic illness is suspected.

A Word About Aging

The notion that "senility"—or dementia—is an inevitable part of the aging process pervades our youth-oriented culture. In reality, among more than 25 million Americans over the age of 65, only 1 to 2 million suffer from significant intellectual impairment. The overwhelming majority of the elderly care for themselves and live outside of institutions.

The majority of older people maintain their intellectual competence as they age, although the speed with which they perform mental functions (e.g., recalling names or dates) declines somewhat. While mild or "benign" impairment in memory is common among the elderly, this is easily compensated for by keeping notes and establishing routines. The notion that dementia is synonymous with old age is a myth. Dementia is a pathological state, *not* a part of the normal human life cycle.

DELIRIUM

Delirium is a syndrome in which consciousness is clouded, the attention span is shortened, sensory misperception is common, and thinking is often disordered. Like dementia, delirium involves global cognitive deficits but, in addition, there is a change in the person's level of arousal and marked disorientation. Delirious people often present to emergency rooms or on hospital wards with extreme agitation and disordered thinking, while demented people more often come to medical attention in less dramatic ways and hide their deficits rather well in the early stages of the condition.

Delirium develops over hours or days, rather than over months or years. The delirious person may initially show only mild symptoms of sleeplessness, anxiety, depression, irritability, forgetfulness, nightmares, or incoherent speech. More severe delirious states often include florid hallucinations, rapid or slowed thoughts, severe agitation or stupor, extreme distractibility, and fits of uncontrollable crying or laughter. The *DSM-III* criteria for the diagnosis of delirium are shown in Table 9-4.

Underlying medical illness is almost always identifiable in cases of delirium. Illnesses that can produce delirium include virtually all of those listed as causes of dementia. Such acute medical conditions as infection, anemia, hypertensive encephalopathy, cerebral edema, and dehydration and fluid and electrolyte imbalance commonly cause delirium. A long list of medications and street drugs (see Appendix B) can cause this condition—not only through intoxication but also during withdrawal. Alcohol withdrawal resulting in delirium tremens (DTs) is discussed in Chapter 12.

Delirium often occurs in hospitalized patients, particularly among patients in intensive care units. Almost all patients undergo-

Table 9–4. *DSM-III* diagnostic criteria for delirium.

Clouding of consciousness (reduced clarity of awareness of the environment), with reduced capacity to shift, focus, and sustain attention to environmental stimuli

At least two of the following:
    Perceptual disturbance: misinterpretations, illusions, or hallucinations
    Speech that is at times incoherent
    Disturbance of sleep-wakefulness cycle, with insomnia or daytime drowsiness
    Increased or decreased psychomotor activity

Disorientation and memory impairment (if testable)

Clinical features that develop over a short period of time (usually hours to days) and tend to fluctuate over the course of a day

Evidence, from the history, physical examination, or laboratory tests, of a specific organic factor judged to be etiologically related to the disturbance

---

ing open-heart surgery with cardiac bypass become at least temporarily delirious sometime after they awaken from anesthesia. Renal dialysis patients frequently become transiently delirious because of toxic metabolic products or electrolyte imbalance. Refer to a general medical text for a more detailed discussion of the various medical conditions that can cause delirium.

The elderly are more prone to develop delirium than younger people. Nearly one-third of those over 65 who are hospitalized for any reason become delirious at some point during their stay. You are likely to encounter this on general medical wards, where older people often experience transient confusion at night ("sundowning").

The treatment of delirium usually involves discovering the underlying cause and remedying it. A thorough history is essential to your evaluation, and often must be obtained from those who accompany the client. Careful physical and mental status examinations are also part of the work-up. You may learn a great deal about the client's condition by simply observing at the bedside. If the cause of the condition is not obvious, laboratory studies (as noted for dementia above) are indicated and should include a toxic screen. Not all delirium is reversible, but a great many cases resolve completely when the acute medical condition is effectively treated.

Managing the Delirious Client

You may encounter delirium in a wide variety of clinical situations (e.g., in a hospital, in a nursing home, or in an outpatient clinic). Regardless of the setting and the underlying cause of the syndrome, there are certain interventions that can help ease a delirious client's agitation and disorientation:

1. Establish structure for the client. Delirious people are confused and often combative. They may tend to wander from place to place, particularly in unfamiliar locales. Therefore, set clear physical boundaries for the client so that he or she feels contained (e.g., in one particular room). With someone who is combative, physical restraint may not only be necessary for safety, but may also be a relief to a client who feels out of control.

2. Orient the client to time, place, and person. Disorientation can be quite frightening to delirious people. Introduce yourself and all other staff members by name and professional title, stating the purpose of your interaction with the client. Address the client by name and remind the client of where he or she is, what day it is, and what time it is. Your repeated reminders to the client of this information will, in and of itself, help the person calm down.

3. Control the client's sensory input. Disorientation can be made worse by too much or too little sensory input. The sights and sounds of a busy clinic or emergency room may overwhelm a distractible client. Conversely, the silence and darkness of a hospital room at night may add to the confusion and disorientation of a delirious person. Therefore, it is important to work with delirious people in relatively quiet, secluded places where there are a limited number of staff, but where there are constant visual and verbal reminders of time, place, and person.

4. Stay with the acutely disoriented person at all times. Someone should remain with the acutely delirious client at all times to prevent the client from harming self or others, from wandering off, or from becoming more disoriented and frightened.

5. Present your treatment plans firmly and repeatedly. Remind the client of what you are doing and why. Enlist the help of accompanying family and friends in this endeavor.

A word of caution: Delirium may look like an acute episode of a functional psychosis (e.g., a schizophrenic or a manic episode). *Anyone who presents with an acute psychotic episode and no prior history of psychotic illness must have a thorough medical work-up.* Otherwise, you may miss life-threatening and potentially treatable medical conditions that masquerade as mental disorders.

REFERENCES

Adams RD, Fischer CM, Hakin S, et al: Symptomatic occult hydrocephalus with "normal" cerebrospinal fluid pressure. N Engl J Med 273:117-126, 1965

American Psychiatric Association: Diagnostic and Statistical Manual of Mental Disorders, 3rd ed. Washington, DC, American Psychiatric Association, 1980

Caine ED: Pseudodementia: current concepts and future directions. Arch Gen Psychiatry 38:1359-1364, 1981

Hoffman RS: Diagnostic errors in the evaluation of behavioral disorders. JAMA 248:964-967, 1982 (An enlightening survey of patients on medical and surgical wards who develop behavioral disturbances. Many of these are of organic etiology, but are misdiagnosed as primary psychiatric disorders.)

Kaufman DM: Clinical Neurology for Psychiatrists. New York, Grune and Stratton, 1981, pp 89-111 (A clear and highly readable textbook of neurologic disorders, including a discussion of the neurologic aspects of dementia.)

Lipowski ZJ: Organic brain syndromes: overview and classification, in Psychiatric Aspects of Neurologic Disease. Edited by Benson DF, Blumer D. New York, Grune and Stratton, 1975

Schneck MK, Reisberg B, Ferris SH: An overview of current concepts of Alzheimer's disease. Am J Psychiatry 139:165-173, 1982

Wells CE: Chronic brain disease: an overview. Am J Psychiatry 135:1-12, 1978

Chapter 10

Children and Adolescents

THE IMPORTANCE OF DEVELOPMENT

Growth and change are an integral part of human existence. Each person is involved in a life-long process of development, and each of us continually attempts to master developmental tasks, whether we are eight months or 80 years old. It is easy to forget the fact that development does not stop in adulthood, because change in adult life is less dramatic, less rapid, and more easily overlooked than that of the childhood years.

Child development proceeds with incredible speed. Consider, for example, the difference between a three-month-old child who has just begun to laugh and roll over; and a three-year-old who runs, pedals a tricycle, speaks in full sentences, and follows complicated verbal directions. Given the rapidity with which children change, their mental health can have no meaning outside of the context of development. The child's physical, emotional, and intellectual capabilities are in constant flux, and with them our expectations about what is normative and what constitutes pathology.

Behaviors that are the norm in one age group become worrisome when we see them in another. For example, the child who wets the bed repeatedly at age three is not considered abnormal, but the seven-year-old who exhibits the same behavior is likely to be given a diagnosis. Separation anxiety and panic at mother's departure is normal in a 15-month-old, but is more worrisome in an eight-year-old.

Similarly, psychiatric symptoms that seem rather mild in one age group may be much more ominous in another. The well-trained four-year-old who, during a stressful time, reverts to bedwetting and soiling, is usually suffering from a mild reaction to disturbing events. However, the appearance of bedwetting and fecal incontinence in an adult is a troubling sign that often suggests severe mental illness (such as psychosis).

Health professionals who work with children must not only understand what is normative for a child at a given age, but must also look at the child's unique developmental pace and judge the presence and severity of symptoms against the child's own developmental standard. Growth does not occur along a single line. In fact, children develop intellectually, physically, emotionally, and socially at varying rates. The boy who is ahead of his peers in physical growth may be several months behind in cognitive development; the girl who is intellectually precocious may throw tantrums of a type that are more common among children two years her junior. Moreover, development does not follow a straight path forward, but involves both progression and regression. For example, a toilet-trained three-year-old may regress to bedwetting temporarily when a sibling is born, and such short-lived backsliding is expectable and normal.

Anna Freud (1965) is noted for her concept that each child grows along distinct developmental lines. She described six such lines of psychological development as follows:

1. The move from total dependency on caretakers to participation in adult relationships;
2. The shift from suckling to rationally controlled eating;
3. Progression from wetting and soiling to bladder and bowel control;
4. Progression from lack of responsibility for care of one's own body to voluntary endorsement of principles of health and hygiene;
5. The shift from egocentricity to the capacity for companionship, sharing, and empathy; and
6. The progression from play with one's own body to play with toys and then to the capacity for work.

Many schemes of physical, intellectual, and emotional development have been devised by those who study children. The following are brief summaries of several of the most widely discussed developmental models. Each describes growth along a particular developmental line. While the table of motor milestones provided below is fairly straightforward and noncontroversial, the schemes of cognitive and psychological development included here represent particular views of individual theorists. They are not meant to be taken as "gospel," but are presented in order to familiarize you with concepts that you are likely to hear about in the course of your clinical work, and to give you a sense of the many variables that must be taken into account in assessing the mental health of children.

MOTOR AND BEHAVIORAL DEVELOPMENT

Table 10-1 contains a summary of normative behavior for infants and children at specific ages. This information is the result of empirical work by observers of child development. Remember that children do not grow according to any rigid timetable, so the numbers in this table are averages.

COGNITIVE DEVELOPMENT

The Swiss psychologist Jean Piaget (1896-1980) has made profound and fundamental contributions to our understanding of human intellectual functioning and how it develops. Piaget concerned himself with the structure of human thought rather than the content—that is, *how* we think as opposed to *what* we think. Moreover, he concerned himself with the aspects of thinking that are common to all mankind, rather than with the differences among individuals. He started with the hypothesis that heredity endows us with the capacity to organize our mental processes into coherent systems of thinking, and also to adapt our mental processes to the realities of the environment. We assimilate data from the environment using the mental structures that we have developed for understanding the world, and we accommodate those mental structures (that is, modify them) in response to the environment.

Piaget did extensive studies of children at various ages to determine how and in what sequence they develop basic modes of thinking. He organized the development of cognition into a sequence of stages, and he was more concerned with the order in which this sequence occurred for all children than he was with different degrees of intelligence or the different paces at which children passed through this sequence. Piaget thought that mental capacity was not a matter of quantitative growth (e.g, being able to think more quickly). Rather, he believed that, as we mature, the form of our thought changes. Piaget's theories are complex, and what follows is a very brief summary of the most salient points regarding his stage sequence.

Table 10–1. Normative motor and behavioral development.

Age	Motor Behavior	Learning and Adaptive Behavior	Language	Self-Care and Social Behavior
Under 4 weeks	Makes alternating crawling movements Moves head to one side when place in prone position	Responds to sound of rattle and bell Regards moving objects momentarily	Small, throaty, undifferentiated noises	Quiets when picked up
1 month	Can hold head erect for a few seconds	Shows no interest and drops objects immediately	Beginning vocalization such as cooing, gurgling	Regards faces Responds to speech
4 months	Holds head balanced Rolls over	Follows a slowly moving object visually Reaches for objects	Laughs aloud Sustained cooing and gurgling	Spontaneous social smile Begins to recognize familiar people
28 weeks	Sits steadily, leaning forward on hands	One-hand approach and grasp of toy Bangs and shakes rattle Transfers toys from hand to hand	Vocalizes "m-m-m" when crying Makes vowel sounds such as "ah"	Pats mirror image Expectantly awaits feeding
40 weeks	Sits alone with good coordination Pulls self to standing position	Attempts to imitate scribble	Says "da-da" or equivalent Responds to name	Responds to social play such as "pat-a-cake" and "peek-a-boo" Feeds self cracker and holds own bottle

Age	Gross Motor	Adaptive	Language	Personal–Social
1 year	Walks with one hand held / Stands alone briefly		Uses one or two words / Gives a toy on request	Cooperates in dressing
18 months	Walks, unassisted, seldom falls / Throws ball	Builds a tower of three or four cubes / Scribbles spontaneously and imitates writing motion	Says 10 words, including own name / Names a ball and carries out two directions with it—for example, "give to daddy," "put down."	Feeds self in part, spills / Pulls toy on string / Carries or hugs a special toy, such as a doll
2 years	Runs well, no falling / Kicks large ball / Goes up and down stairs alone	Builds a tower of six or seven cubes / Imitates vertical and circular strokes	Uses three-word sentences / Carries out four simple directions	Puts on simple clothing / Refers to self by name
3 years	Rides tricycle / Jumps / Alternates feet going up stairs	Builds tower of nine or 10 cubes / Copies a circle and a cross	Gives sex and full name / Uses plurals / Describes what is happening in a picture book	Puts on shoes / Unbuttons buttons / Feeds self well / Understands taking turns
4 years	Walks down stairs, one step per tread / Jumps over a rope / Catches ball in arms	Copies a square / Repeats four numbers / Counts three objects with correct pointing	Names colors, at least one correctly / Understands prepositions (e.g. "on," "under," "in,") and adjectives (e.g. "cold," "tired")	Washes and dries own face / Plays cooperatively with other children
5 years	Skips using feet alternately / Usually has complete sphincter control / Catches a bounced ball	Draws a recognizable man with a head, body, limbs / Counts 10 objects accurately	Names the primary colors / Names coins: pennies, nickels, dimes / Asks meanings of words	Dresses and undresses / Prints a few letters / Plays competitive exercise games

Infancy: The Sensorimotor Stage (Birth to Two Years)

Freud saw infants as passive beings who seek to avoid stimulation and maximize soothing, while behaviorists see infants as passively shaped by environmental forces. Piaget's work was revolutionary in characterizing the human infant as an active and competent learner. According to Piaget's empirical studies and those of subsequent investigators, infants seek out stimulation, exploring the world visually, tactilely, and motorically and practicing schemes for manipulating objects. In contrast to adults, infants do not possess a sense of object permanence; that is, they do not behave as if they are aware of the existence of objects with which they are not immediately involved. (This is strikingly demonstrated by placing an infant's toy behind a screen and noting that the baby behaves as if the toy no longer exists.) Because memories require the ability to know that objects still exist when not immediately present, Piaget postulates (in contrast to Freud) that there can be no true memory of one's infancy. This hypothesis is at odds with empirical observations that an infant below the age of 18 months commonly reacts with distress to mother's absence and even searches for her—implying the capacity for some awareness of mother when she is not present. At about 18 months of age, children achieve a developmental breakthrough when they begin to develop mental representations (e.g., the mental image of a ball when no ball is in the child's immediate environment). They can then use words and visual images to represent real objects. Thus, they are no longer confined to acting on things in their immediate environment, but can recall the past and think about objects that are not present.

Preoperational Thought (Two to Six Years)

Thinking in this age range is "egocentric" in that the child is not introspective about his or her own mental operations, and judges everything from his or her own point of view. It is difficult for children in this period to see another's point of view. The child is capable of dealing with only a limited amount of data and ignores the rest. Piaget conducted his famous conservation experiments to demonstrate that children in this age range will only focus on one dimension of any available stimulus. For example, a child presented with two identical sets of objects—say, two sets of seven rubber balls—will tell you that the sets are identical when the balls are laid out in two rows of even length. However, when one set of balls is spaced more widely to lengthen one of the rows, the child will tell you that the row of widely spaced balls is more numerous because it is longer. Thus, the child has focused on the dimension of line length, ignoring the dimension of number of balls.

Concrete Operations (Seven to 12 Years)

During this period, the child can deal with several dimensions of a problem at once and process them mentally, so that the conservation problem described above can be solved correctly. Children begin to focus on changes rather than simply on states, so they would attend to the act of altering the state of the widely spaced balls in the conservation experiment. Children capable of concrete operations have flexible thinking—i.e., they can mentally perform an operation to change the state of an object, and then reverse the operation to return the object to its original state.

Formal Operations (Adolescence Onward)

Adolescence heralds the beginning of the capacity for abstract thought. Adolescents can deal with complex problems of reasoning, they can formulate hypotheses, and conceive of many different interpretations of the same events. This capacity for abstraction allows the adolescent to become involved with religious, political, and philosophical doctrines, and to become passionate about ideals and causes. This is the final achievement in Piaget's sequence of the development of cognitive structures.

PSYCHOLOGICAL DEVELOPMENT

The following are three theories of how human beings develop psychosocially. They are not mutually exclusive, but are in many respects complementary schemes. Mahler's ideas about separation and individuation focus on the experience of infants and toddlers, while the developmental stages of Freud carry the child into adolescence, and Erickson's stages encompass birth through old age.

Mahler's Concept of Separation-Individuation

Margaret Mahler has made major contributions to our understanding of infant development. Her ideas are based on data she has gleaned from years of careful observation of infants and mothers in the nursery. She hypothesizes that each child goes through stages of separation and individuation from the mother or other primary caretaker, and that the way in which children negotiate these stages influences the development of personality traits such as the capacities for trust, empathy, and emotional stability in interpersonal relationships. The infant starts out in a state of total helplessness, and lives in what Mahler has called a "symbiotic" relationship to the mother (or other primary caretaker). Mahler (1974) defines mother-infant symbiosis as the human infant's prolonged, absolute dependence on the mother, which results from the infant's biological unpreparedness to maintain life separately. According to Mahler, the infant in this symbiotic phase has no awareness that infant and mother are two different beings, or that infant and environment are not one. The process of separation-individuation, as charted by Mahler in her observations of infant-mother interactions in the nursery, takes the infant from this state of symbiosis to the point where he or she recognizes the self as separate from mother, and recognizes mother's continued existence even when she is away from the child and when the child is in distress.

Differentiation (five to 10 months). Mother satisfies the baby's needs for care, and the infant does not differentiate between self and other. However, as the infant begins to be less physically tied to the mother (developing the ability to crawl), and as the sensory apparatus matures, the infant achieves a growing awareness of being separate from the mother. The infant begins to compare the familiar (mother) with the unfamiliar (other people), and in this phase stranger anxiety first appears.

Practicing (10 to 15 months). The infant uses increasing motor skills to practice leaving mother's side to go off and explore the environment, in what has been called a "love affair with the world." The infant crawls and then walks away from mother but repeatedly comes back to her for "emotional refueling," to be reassured of her continued presence.

Rapprochement (15 to 22 months). The toddler's increasing motor and cognitive abilities prompt further recognition of separateness from the mother. This awareness becomes surprising and frightening, particularly in times of stress (e.g., when the toddler falls down and mother is not nearby to respond to the cry for help). The toddler struggles with the desire to be autonomous and the equally intense desire to have mother always available to magically fulfill the child's every wish. Thus, the toddler's behavior in this phase often alternates rapidly between rejecting mother and clinging to her.

Object constancy (two years and beyond). The infant develops the ability to evoke a memory of mother's comforting presence even when she is not physically nearby. Delay of gratification becomes possible, and the assertion of autonomy (with the frequent use of the word "no") announces to the world the child's acceptance of his or her separateness.

Mahler's work has been particularly important in thinking about older children and adults who show marked difficulty in forming stable trusting relationships with others, and whose capacity to soothe themselves in the absence of important others is limited. It has been hypothesized that people with Borderline Personality Disorder suffered severe disturbances in the mother-child relationship during the rapprochement subphase of the separation-individuation process. However, no causal connection has been established between such early developmental disturbances and subsequent manifestation of severe personality disorders.

Freud's Psychosexual Stages

This scheme of psychosexual development, which underlies so much of psychodynamic thinking, has been described in Chapter 2. It is based on a theory of sexual and aggressive drives and it limits itself primarily to the influences of the nuclear family on the child's emotional growth.

Erickson's Developmental Tasks

Erik Erickson brought Freud's psychosexual stages out of the confines of the family and took into account the interaction between the child and the society in which he or she lives. Moreover, while Freud's psychosexual stages focus on pathology and follow the process of development only through puberty, Erickson's theories start with an assumption of psychological health and the idea that the human personality continues to change and to be molded by the environment throughout life into old age.

Erickson focuses his attention on the ego (see Chapter 2) as the primary agent through which we organize perceptions, govern actions, and adapt to the environment. He writes that the ego is in a state of well-being when we live as we both wish to and feel we ought to. The pull between wishes (e.g., for instant gratification) and the internalized restrictions of parents and society (what we "ought" to do) constantly forces the ego to negotiate between conflicting demands. The ego grows stronger when it can meet new life situations in such a way as to find creative and adaptive ways of bringing personal wishes and social expectations into harmony.

Sensory-oral stage: trust versus mistrust (birth to 18 months). If the child's needs for care and sensory stimulation are met by the mother, the child develops basic trust in the self and the world. However, if the mother-child interaction is somehow disturbed (e.g., if the child is deprived or unduly frustrated, or if care is inconsistently available), the child develops a fundamental mistrust of the world and the sense that he or she will lose what is wanted or needed. Weaning can take place without great trauma to the child's sense of well-being if the child has developed the basic trust that his or her needs will be met.

Muscular-anal stage: autonomy versus shame and doubt (18 months to three years). As the child learns to develop control over more aspects of life, including bladder and sphincter muscles, the choice becomes whether to keep or to let go. If parents allow the child to function with some autonomy around issues such as toilet training—if they are supportive without being overprotective or punitive—the child gains confidence in his or her autonomy by age three, feeling the capacity to control the self and, to some extent, the environment. However, if the child is overrestrained and made to feel ashamed and foolish, he or she mistrusts his own rightness and becomes plagued by self-doubt.

Locomotor-genital stage: initiative versus guilt (three to six years). The child's new-found capacities for locomotion and learning increase curiosity about the outside world. The child can now initiate physical and intellectual activity. The child's independent initiatives are reinforced if the environment allows for physical freedom and satisfaction of curiosity, but initiative is stifled when the child is made to feel bad about new behaviors and interests. The child begins to develop an intense interest in the parent of the opposite sex, and may compete with the same-sex parent and siblings for affection. The division between what a child wants (e.g., to murder little brother and sleep in mommy's bed) and what he "ought" to do (e.g., be nice to little brother and sleep in his own bed) becomes greater. Parental values and societal values are gradually internalized as self-guidance, but if the child incorporates rigid and punishing standards, initiative is inhibited and guilt predominates.

Latency stage: industry versus inferiority (six to puberty). The child develops confidence in abilities to function in the adult world—to master physical tasks, to reason deductively, and to use intellectual skills in comprehending the world outside of the home. Peer relationships and school become important. Peers comprise a reference group in which the child can test ideas and behaviors, and competence relative to others takes on new importance. The child can become confident of his or her industriousness and capacity to function in the adult world or, if mastery is somehow thwarted, can come to feel inferior.

Puberty and adolescence: ego identity versus role confusion (teen years). In the struggle to develop a personal identity, the teenager falls in love with heroes, ideologies, and members of the opposite sex. The adolescent is "suspended between" the morality learned as a child and the ethics to be developed as an adult. In this confusion, adolescents cling to each other, and peer groups become of central importance. Teenagers must undergo further psychological separation from parents in order to prepare for intimate relationships with peers, and as part of this process, children commonly "de-idealize" parents who were once thought to be "perfect" or "heroes." The teenager's ability to develop a stable sense of identity (social and sexual) depends on how successfully he or she has negotiated previous developmental stages, and on the teenager's position in his or her society.

Young adulthood: intimacy versus isolation (18 to 34 years). The young adult who has successfully weathered the identity crisis of adolescence emerges with a sense of self that is firm enough to make intimacy possible without the fear of losing one's own identity. Emotional and sexual closeness involves mutuality. The person who is not capable of sharing love and friendship in long-term relationships becomes self-indulgent and isolated.

Adulthood: generativity versus stagnation (35 to 60 years). During the middle years, adults choose between becoming involved in meaningful and socially useful tasks and the stagnation of satisfying only personal needs and pursuing personal pleasures. Generativity refers not to bearing children, but to the investment of the self in an endeavor outside of the home: parents can stagnate, and people who have no children can be generative.

Maturity: ego integrity versus despair (60+ years). According to Erickson's schema, the person who, in old age, can look back on a life in which intimacy has been achieved and generativity expressed feels a sense of satisfaction and ego integrity. By contrast, those who have never developed beyond narcissistic self-absorption look back in despair upon a life which has been lived to little purpose.

Figure 10-1 is a comparison of the developmental stages of Freud, Erickson, and Piaget.

Age	Freud	Erickson	Piaget
1	Oral	Trust vs. Mistrust	Sensorimotor
2	Anal	Autonomy vs. Shame/Doubt	
3	Phallic	Initiative vs. Guilt	Preoperational Thought
4			
5	Oedipal		
6			
7			
8		Industry vs. Inferiority	Concrete Operations
9	Latency		
10			
11			
12			
13			
14		Identity vs. Role Confusion	Formal Operations
15	Adolescence		
16			
17			
18			
Early Adulthood		Intimacy vs. Isolation	
Midlife		Generativity vs. Self-Absorption	
Old Age		Integrity vs. Despair	

Figure 10–1. The Developmental Theories of Freud, Erickson, and Piaget

THE "NORMAL" CHILD AT VARIOUS STAGES OF DEVELOPMENT

What do children look like at various phases of development? The following are brief descriptions of what is considered normative. Keep in mind, however, that the "normal child" is a fictional character, and that these descriptions are only meant to serve as crude guides to what is to be expected in healthy children.

Early Infancy (Birth to Four Months)

The infant's main task during these early months is to adjust to extrauterine life. The child is born with sucking and crying reflexes, and is programmed to respond positively to human stimuli. The infant at first only stares at the surroundings, but by the age of four months can follow moving objects visually, reach for objects, and roll over. By age three to four months, the baby can smile when talked to, will babble and coo, and can respond to human sounds by turning the head and vocalizing socially. Interest in people is general, and the baby does not differentiate among individuals.

The healthy baby copes well with the mechanics of life, including eating and sleeping. Bodily needs are urgent, and the baby is totally dependent on caregivers and has a low tolerance for frustration. Over this period, the infant cries less, develops increasing periods of wakefulness, and responds to feeding and oral sensations, as well as sound, light, and touch. The baby begins to develop trust in the caretaking adult and to respond expectantly to caretakers.

Minor problems at this stage include feeding and digestive difficulties, sleep problems, and excessive crying or irritability. More extreme problems include an inability to be comforted when crying, extreme lethargy (often secondary to deprivation of care and affection), failure to gain weight, and infantile autism.

Infancy (Four to 18 months)

The infant must begin to differentiate himself or herself from the mother and to develop some degree of self-reliance and self-control (including self-feeding and self-soothing). This is a period of growing social attachment.

As the sensory organs mature, the baby begins to have coordinated movements, including binocular vision and hand-to-mouth coordination. Over this period, the baby learns to sit up, to crawl, and to pull up. Many children walk unassisted by age 10 to 14 months. Grasp becomes much more precise, and the baby can manipulate objects by age 10 months. Infants at this stage put any object they can find into their mouths.

Babbling resembles one-syllable words by age six months. At 10 months the infant can respond to his or her name and shows signs of understanding some words and simple commands. By 12 months, the child can usually say one or two words.

Socially, the baby begins to recognize familiar people and is more responsive to them than to strangers. During this period, playful reciprocal interactions between the infant and primary caregivers foster the development of a deep emotional bond.

The typical seven-month-old plays with toys and feet and expectantly awaits feeding. By 10 months, the baby can play simple nursery games (peek-a-boo) and feed himself or herself a cracker. Self-feeding continues to improve over this period. The baby also learns to cooperate in dressing by age 12 months. The baby begins to have more patience (e.g., while a bottle is heated), develops stranger anxiety at six to 10 months, and has a strong selective tie to the mother. The infant demonstrates joy in play during this period, and begins to show outbursts of negativism and anger.

Minor problems at this stage include excessive crying, anger, and irritability. Finicky eating and disturbed digestion and elimination are also common, as is sleep disturbance (failure to sleep through the night). More serious problems include tantrums, obsessive head-banging or rocking, extreme apathy and lack of interest in the environment, anorexia with failure to gain weight, lack of social discrimination or tie to the mother, and wariness of all adults.

Toddler (18 to 36 Months)

The toddler's tasks during the second 18 months of life include further development of motor capacities, toilet training, differentiating the self from others and developing a secure sense of autonomy, tolerating separations from caregivers, beginning cooperative relationships with peers, and learning gender distinctions.

Maturation of the infant's nervous system allows the toddler to achieve sphincter control and to improve fine motor movements and gait. Children can climb stairs and run unsteadily by two years of age, and by 2½ they can jump and possess good hand and finger coordination. Speech includes a definite repertoire of words and marked increase in understanding (e.g, "no" and "come here") by 18 months. By two years, the child spontaneously puts together two-word phrases to communicate needs and wishes (e.g., "want mommy"). By 30 months, the toddler can make three-word sentences, understands most of what is said to him or her, and ceases babbling so that all speech has communicative intent. During toddlerhood, the child develops what Piaget calls object constancy (i.e., the capacity for mental representation of objects).

The toddler continues the process of separation-individuation (see the preceding discussion of Mahler), so that the child's sense of individuality is consolidated around 24 months of age. The toddler may meet parents' efforts at toilet training and discipline with marked resistance, and may throw temper tantrums when wishes and aims are frustrated by others.

Toddlers learn to play "in parallel" with other children (as opposed to engaging in truly cooperative play), and they usually play with great energy. They are constantly "on the go" and strongly resist any interference from others. They are very concerned about power and "who-bosses-whom," as is evident in their play. They show dependence on their caregivers and are anxious about separations from them. They also demonstrate marked ambivalence, showing extremes of love and anger toward those who care for them. They get pleasure from exercising their new motor skills. Masturbation is common among three year-olds, as are imaginary companions. By 3½, the child talks appropriately of self and others, and learns to take turns with others.

Minor problems in this age group include poor motor coordination, speech difficulties (e.g., stammering), timidity, night terrors, sleep disturbance, difficulty with toilet training, difficulty weaning, temper tantrums, inability to leave mother without panic, lack of interest in other children, and temporary regression to more infantile manners (e.g., bedwetting). Major problems include extreme lethargy, uncommunicative speech or no speech, desperate clinging to mother, impulsive destructive behavior, phobias, lack of play, psychosis, and autism. Toddlers sometimes develop a variety of somatic illnesses that may be a manifestation of emotional distress, including vomiting, diarrhea, constipation, rashes, and tics.

Preschool (Three to Five Years)

The preschool child learns to master internal impulses and social skills, as the focus of life begins to shift away from parents toward peers and life outside of the home. Motor coordination continues to be refined, so that by age four most children can catch a ball in their arms, jump over a rope, walk a line, and copy a square. Five-year-olds can balance on one foot and catch a bounced ball, while six-year-olds can tie a knot in a piece of string. Speech becomes almost entirely intelligible and the child can use plurals appropriately by age three. By age four language is well established, including comprehension of adjectives (cold, tired) and prepositions (under, over).

The preschooler's relationships with parents change with the development of sexual feelings for the parent of the opposite sex. The child's close physical attachment to the opposite-sex parent is given up to some extent, and the same-sex parent is seen as both a rival and as someone to be emulated (see Chapter 2). Resentment of the same-sex parent is often displaced to less threatening people (e.g., siblings, teachers). Relationships with other children become more important than in previous periods, dependence on the mother lessens, and the child spends increasingly long periods of time in activities away from the mother. Separation anxiety is finally mastered to the extent that the child can attend school.

Preschoolers typically shift back and forth between aggressive and regressive behavior as they struggle with conflicting wishes to be dependent and independent. Little boys often appear confident and little girls flirtatious, but these bold fronts collapse easily, particularly in the face of perceived threats or criticisms. Play is physically active, and boys may have particularly violent and cruel fantasies incorporated into their play. Children are inquisitive and imaginative at this age, and ask many questions (e.g., "Where do babies come from?"). Children commonly identify with and imitate parents, teachers, and peers in their behavior as they attempt to try on new roles (e.g., sex roles).

Minor problems at this age include those listed for toddlers. In addition, reluctance to go to school is common at this age but normally resolves quickly. Major problems are also similar to those encountered among toddlers, but in addition, prolonged school phobia and school refusal indicate significant emotional distress (see discussion of school refusal below).

Latency (Six to 10 years)

The latency period, which encompasses the primary school years until the onset of puberty, is marked by greater awareness of the world at large, increased importance of peer relationships, and the mastery of new physical and intellectual skills. This is the period that Erickson characterized as representing a crisis of industry versus inferiority, as the child's sense of self is increasingly bound up with his or her developing competence at physical, intellectual, and social tasks.

Maturation of the central nervous system allows the child to perform complex motor movements and to develop what Piaget terms concrete operational thinking (see discussion above). Language is fully developed by this period.

Social relationships are characterized by same-sex groups and clubs. The child identifies strongly with the same-sex parent and turns to others (e.g., teachers) as role-models. Parents are no longer seen as all-knowing or all-powerful, and the ideas and behavior of people outside the home take on new interest and importance for the latency age child. Aggression is channeled into healthy competition at school and at play. Latency age children are preoccupied with mastering sexual and aggressive impulses, and hence their play commonly involves games with an abundance of rules. Fair play is of paramount importance.

Children in this age group develop pride and self-confidence as they master new tasks and become less dependent on their parents. They are very concerned with sex roles and strongly identify with children of the same sex. Peer interaction and organized play are very important, as is exploration of the environment (school, community, nature). Children achieve better control of their impulses during this period and are better able to channel their energies into learning.

Minor problems at this stage include anxiety and oversensitivity to new experiences (at school, with peers, around separations), learning difficulties, lying, and temper tantrums. Children are often afraid of illness or bodily injury, and somatic complaints (e.g., stomachaches) may be expressions of emotional distress, as in school phobia. More serious problems include social withdrawal, failure to learn, speech difficulties (especially stuttering), uncontrollable antisocial behavior (e.g., chronic bullying or lying or stealing), or self-destructive behavior (frequent "accidents," self-mutilation, suicide attempts). Other serious problems encountered in this age group include obsessive-compulsive rituals (e.g., severe hand-washing), phobias, anorexia or severe obesity, complete absence of or deterioration of peer relationships, and inability to distinguish fantasy from reality.

Adolescence (11 to 18 Years)

The onset of puberty brings about dramatic physical, emotional, and intellectual changes. No longer a child and not yet an adult, the adolescent must negotiate the transition into adult life. This involves coping with body changes and markedly increased sexual drives, consolidating one's sexual and personal identity, and struggling for emancipation from the child's role in the family. This is a time when the teenager develops more collaborative peer relationships, begins heterosexual relationships, and prepares for major educational and occupational choices.

Puberty initiates adolescence. The physical changes of puberty almost always occur in the same sequence, but their onset, speed, and age of completion vary considerably from one person to another. For girls, the spurt in height may begin at age nine or 15, but on average starts at 10½. Similarly, menarche begins anywhere from age 10 to 16½, with average onset at 12½. Breast development may start at age eight or at 18. The sequence of changes for girls is as follows: breast enlargement, appearance of straight pubic hair, growth spurt, appearance of kinky pubic hair, menarche, growth of axillary hair, and maturity of full reproductive function.

For boys, the developmental timetable may also vary greatly. Testes enlarge at anywhere from 9½ to age 17, with the average onset at 11½. Similarly, a boy's height spurt and penis enlargement may begin at 10½ or 16½ but on average begins at 12½. The sequence of pubertal changes for boys is as follows: growth of testes, appearance of straight pubic hair, penile enlargement, early voice changes, first ejaculation, appearance of kinky pubic hair, growth spurt, growth of axillary hair, marked voice changes, and beard development.

Physical development is not confined to sex characteristics and height. Musculature develops rapidly during this period; more so for boys than for girls. Thus, for example, boys are on average twice as strong at age 16 as at age 12. Cognitively, adolescents develop the capacity for formal operational thought (see discussion of Piaget above), so that they have the capacity to deal with abstract concepts such as moral values and political ideals.

This is an exciting and tumultuous time, in which the adolescent pushes more rapidly for independence from parents and becomes keenly interested in other adults as role models and "heroes." The adolescent's primary allegiance shifts between parents and peers, as peer group values and ideals take on a new importance. Peers help validate the adolescent's push for separation from home, and in negotiating this shift, the adolescent commonly engages in battles with authority figures. Exclusive boy-girl relationships begin during this period, as does sexual activity. Aggression may be channeled into destructive rebellion against parental figures, or into more constructive means of achieving independence from parents and into healthy competitive activities (e.g., sports, academics).

In the struggle between the wish to satisfy new sexual urges and the wish to control them, adolescents often vacillate between hedonism and asceticism. Their capacity for self-observation and insight becomes much greater, and the adolescent begins to think about who he or she is in new ways.

Adolescents are often inconsistent, moody, and unpredictable. This is evident in work, at play, and in their relationships with peers and adults. They try on a variety of roles and experiment with themselves and the world. They are eager for peer acceptance and approval, as evidenced by clothing fads and hero worship. They can be highly critical of themselves and others (particularly parents), as they struggle to develop moral and ethical ideals. They are at once anxious about losing their parents' nurturance and eager to be independent of parental ties. Confusion and insecurity are often covered over by false bravado, particularly in early adolescence. Teenagers can fall in and out of love rapidly, and constant experimentation in peer relationships helps the adolescent to form his or her own identity. In later adolescence, the hold of the peer group loosens, and the adolescent moves toward taking his or her place in adult society.

Minor (and common) problems seen in adolescence include apprehensions, fears, and guilt about sex, health, peer relationships, and school; defiant, impulsive, and depressed behavior; frequent physical complaints; dysmenorrhea; sexual preoccupation; excessive masturbation; poor relationships with peers or adults; unwillingness to assume greater responsibility or autonomy; unresponsiveness to parental discipline; and experimentation with drugs or alcohol. Major problems include complete social withdrawal, major depression, delinquency, phobias, compulsions, persistent hypochondriasis, anorexia nervosa (see Chapter 8), complete inability to function at school or work, suicide attempts, drug or alcohol abuse or addiction, and psychosis.

Factors Influencing Development

The above developmental schemes and descriptions attempt to describe a fictional creation known as the "normal child." In reality, each child's development is unique, because development is a constantly changing relationship between a highly particular set of variables within the child and another equally individual set of variables in the child's environment. Prenatal influences on the child's intrauterine growth, genetic endowment, and inborn temperament are but a few of the "internal" variables which each child brings to the world. Environmental variables include the temperaments and expectations of parents, the quality and quantity of caretaking the child receives, the socioeconomic group into which the child is born, life events, and the child's constellation of siblings. Biological and environmental variables influence each other reciprocally.

Psychopathology in children may be thought of in terms of failures in development. How is it possible to take so many variables into account in determining what has gone wrong in the growth of a particular child? It is easiest to think of the child's development in terms of systems as discussed below:

Inborn characteristics. The child's inherited traits, including everything from intelligence to eye color, from shape of the nose to temperament, will affect the child's acceptance by parents and within various cultural groups. This, in turn, affects self-image and self-esteem. Inborn traits also affect the child's ability to adapt to the environment into which he or she is born. In recent years, work has been done on characterizing types of inborn temperament among newborn infants. Thomas et al. (1968) (see also Thomas and Chess 1984) are among the most prominent researchers in the area of inborn temperament. They have looked at variables such as distractibility, activity level, persistence, and adaptability in newborns. Most newborns can be described as having particular temperaments, such as "easy," "slow-to-warm-up," or "difficult." It is not so much the inborn characteristics of the infant that are crucial determinants of later development, as the "fit" between the temperament of the child and the temperaments and expectations of the parents.

Organic impairment. Children who are born with or acquire physical conditions that handicap their functioning will almost always have psychological reactions to such impairment, and the impairment (e.g., an obvious handicap) will elicit reactions from the environment. Consider, for example, the child with an attention deficit disorder (discussed more fully below), a condition with a neurologic basis that involves difficulty paying attention to tasks. Such a child is often labeled "bad," "disruptive," or "stupid" by exasperated parents and teachers, and these labels have a profound effect on the child's sense of self. Learning disabilities, seizure disorders (epilepsy), and other conditions with neurologic components may prompt the child to receive and process environmental stimuli abnormally, and there is a high correlation between such organic disorders and emotional and behavioral symptoms. Chronic ailments, such as asthma, and physical deformities affect the child's ability to function in and be accepted by the world, as well as the child's self-image.

Family environment. Freud was intensely concerned with each person's "family drama" as a means of understanding individual development. Indeed, family members are the center of the young child's world prior to going to school, and in this respect, an understanding of the child's home life is essential to any assessment of psychological distress. Caretaking by parents or others will have a profound influence on the child's development. Caretaking refers not only to whether the child is fed, clothed, and sheltered. It includes also the provision of sensory stimulation and the creation and maintenance of an emotional bond between the primary caretaker and the child. Infants who are offered an adequate diet but deprived of love and affection commonly "fail to thrive" and may literally die because they are unable to grow and gain weight.

Parental expectations of the child and parental values play a formative role in all aspects of development. Because they are dependent on parents for physical survival, love, and protection, children both consciously and unconsciously pay close attention to parents' signals about what they expect and value. Even a process that seems "biologically programmed," such as the acquisition of motor skills, may be greatly enhanced or inhibited, depending on the parents' comfort with a child's physical assertiveness and initiatives in exploring the environment. Similarly, children may develop language skills precociously or late, depending on the extent to which their parents value verbal ability and how parents react to the child's attempts at verbal mastery.

Children develop some personality traits and suppress others based on what is reinforced by parents. For example, a little girl whose father sees her as dainty and ultrafeminine may suppress her wishes to engage in rough-and-tumble play with boys. A boy who is named after a much-loved grandfather may be subtly encouraged by parents to take on grandfather's traits (e.g., an "artistic temperament" and interests). While these influences occur in every parent-child relationship, the self-fulfilling prophecies which result can sometimes be quite destructive. Consider, for example, the father who was himself quite an impulsive adolescent, and who "fears" that his son will grow up to be a "hoodlum." By treating his son with suspicion and taking an intense interest in any mild misbehavior, the father communicates to his son that he is not trustworthy, and also that father will be attentive and intensely interested whenever the boy misbehaves. Such a situation encourages a child to act out a parental wish of which the parent may be totally unaware. (For an excellent discussion of this process, see Johnson [1952].) Families who need to see one member in a certain way (e.g., as the one with all the bad traits or as the "little angel") may stereotype a child in an attempt to maintain some emotional balance within the family system. Such stereotyping usually has a stifling effect on a child, as it fosters the suppression of some aspects of the self and exaggerates others.

Relationships with siblings are of central importance to a child's development, although this is a somewhat neglected area of research. Children spend at least as much time with their siblings as they do with parents. Siblings vie with one another for parental time and attention, and it is generally with siblings that the child first learns to share and to compete. Older siblings may actually parent younger ones or may introduce younger children to the world outside of the family (e.g., school, peer relationships). Siblings can be important sources of learning as well as nurturing in a child's development.

Major life events. Both intellectually and emotionally, children have limited resources with which to cope with and make sense of major life events. Thus, changes such as the birth of a sibling, illness of the child, separation from or death of a parent, or even a move to a new neighborhood may affect the child more profoundly and adversely than the same events would affect an adult. For example, the birth of a sibling may be both exciting and troubling to a young child. A newborn infant demands total care, and so the child must compete with the new arrival for the parents' time and attention. Often more troubling for the child is the separation from mother that usually occurs when mother must be in the hospital around the time of childbirth. Prolonged separation from one or both parents can exert a profound effect on the child. Death, divorce, separation, or the illness of a parent leaves the young child both bereft of a parent and confused about why this event came about. Because young children make sense of the world in self-referential terms, they commonly blame themselves for traumatic life events ("If I had been a better boy, daddy would not have gone away"). When children are seriously ill and require hospitalization, the trauma of medical procedures, combined with periods of separation from parents, can seriously disrupt the child's sense of well-being and his or her body image.

Peers and community. Children are strongly influenced by the communities, cultural groups, and economic groups into which they are born. This influence is mediated by the parents in the first years of life, but as the child reaches school age and spends much of each day outside of the home, the influence of the larger community becomes more direct. School functioning is of central importance in assessing any older (age six and up) child's state of psychological health. The child's occupation is as a student, and like an adult who is having problems at work, the school-age child's problems in school should be taken very seriously. School performance not only gives an indication of possible learning disabilities and cognitive deficits, but gives some indication of emotional health and social development, particularly as reflected in the child's relationships with teachers and peers. For this reason, it is essential that you obtain information from the school about every child whom you see for psychiatric assessment.

THE DIAGNOSTIC EVALUATION OF THE CHILD

If we think of mental illness in children as an absence of growth, a failure to change or a retreat from critical developmental steps, then an initial goal of a psychiatric assessment is to determine where the child should be developmentally and where he or she deviates from this. Making accurate and informative psychiatric diagnoses is even more difficult with children than it is with adults. There are several reasons for this: First, children develop so rapidly that symptoms may not remain stable over even a very short time, and diagnoses may change. Secondly, each child develops at a unique pace, and so what may seem like a developmental "failure" (e.g., a child who does not walk at 18 months of age) may in fact be a developmental lag that will be followed by a "catch up" period of rapid development. Finally, the diagnostic systems used for children are imprecise and inadequately developed, although vigorous efforts continue to be made toward making our diagnostic nomenclature clearer and more precise. In particular, the section of the third edition of the *Diagnostic and Statistical Manual of Mental Disorders* (*DSM-III*) that is devoted to the psychiatric disorders of children represents an important attempt to base diagnostic categories on observable empirical phenomena.

How Do Children Come to the Attention of Mental Health Professionals?

Unlike adults, children rarely ask directly for mental health care. They will usually show the world that they are in distress through some aspect of their dealings with family and peers, or in their school behavior. Achenbach (1966) found that most children who come to the attention of mental health professionals can be grouped into three categories:

1. Overcontrolled children, who are inhibited, shy, and anxious.
2. Undercontrolled children, who are impulse-ridden, create behavioral disturbances, and act with undue aggression toward others.
3. Pathologically detached children, who lack interest in things around them, seem confused and withdrawn, and/or manifest bizarre forms of thinking.

Boys more commonly show their distress in undercontrolled ways, by acting on their environment (e.g., by throwing tantrums, behaving destructively), while girls more often manifest emotional difficulties by becoming more withdrawn or inhibited. Not surprisingly, undercontrolled children cause more distress to their parents than do overcontrolled children, so boys are referred for mental health care over girls by a ratio of nearly 4 to 1. In addition to parents, others who commonly request mental health care for children include siblings, teachers, pediatricians, and court officials. Adolescents are often referred by others as well, but they will sometimes seek help on their own initiative.

Children do not come alone to mental health facilities. They are usually accompanied by parents, guardians, or some other person who wishes the child to have treatment. A mental health assessment should involve family members as well as others who care for, observe, and work with the child. This means that multiple interviews are usually involved—interviews with the child, with the entire immediate family (when possible) to observe family interactions, with parents as a couple or individually, and with teachers or other professionals.

INTERVIEWING PARENTS

Parents are likely to approach you with some guilt, for they have invariably asked themselves, "What did we do wrong?" They will usually be concerned about what you think of them as people and as parents, and may be reluctant to expose "family secrets." You must try to enlist the parents as allies from the beginning, preferably by informing them of how the evaluation process works, of the way in which recommendations are likely to be made, and about ways that they can help you in your work.

You may want to interview the child's parents prior to your first meeting with the child, so that you can get some sense of why the child has been brought to you and what the parents' concerns are. Your task during the evaluation is not only to gather information from the parents about the child's past and present life, but also to learn more about the parents themselves—their personality styles, their own family backgrounds, and their ways of interacting with their child.

Taking a History

You can use the outline for a psychiatric history found in Chapter 3 to organize the information you gather about the child, for the basic data you need is essentially the same for children as it is for adults. However, you will want to pay special attention to the following areas in the child's life.

Developmental phases. Ask about phases of infancy and childhood in greater detail than you might in taking the history of an adult. Focus specifically on each of the major periods of childhood: prenatal events, birth history, infancy, toddlerhood, preschool, elementary school, puberty, and adolescence. Ask about the child's temperament at each stage, motor and intellectual milestones (see Table 10-1), as well as social and emotional development that would be appropriate for each stage.

Specific Symptoms and Behaviors. You may want to ask about the child's fears and inquire about the presence of tics, obsessions (e.g., handwashing), head banging, nightmares, tantrums, or violent outbursts. You might also want to note whether the child has had unduly prolonged separation anxiety from parents (often around starting school) and whether there have been problems with bedwetting (enuresis) or retention and incontinence of feces (encopresis). School performance and behavior and relationships with peers should be explored in detail. Drug and alcohol use should be carefully documented. (Do not forget to ask about this, even in children of primary school age.) Also, be sure to ask about eating problems, such as anorexia, bulimia, or obesity (for a discussion of anorexia and bulimia, see Chapter 8).

Medical History. This should be detailed, and where physical abnormalities are suspected or in cases where it appears that routine medical care has been neglected (e.g., no physical examination in the previous year), the child should be referred to a pediatrician. Pay attention to chronic illnesses, hospitalizations, and surgery. In particular, note whether there have been any major separations from parents due to hospitalization, and ask about the child's reactions to illness and treatment. Be sure to ask about any medications the child is taking, as these can have side effects that mimic psychiatric disorders.

Home Environment. You should spend a considerable amount of time obtaining a picture of the child's home and family life. This will involve taking a family history that is more detailed than that usually documented in adult cases. Try to obtain information about three generations of the family: the grandparents, the parents and their siblings, and the child and his or her siblings. It is often helpful to draw a family tree when you record this information. For each family member, try to document the following:

- Age,
- Marital Status,
- Living situation (with the child or elsewhere),
- School and work history,
- Health (including any medical or psychological problems),
- Relationship with the child (quality and quantity of time spent), and
- Death or other separations from the child.

In addition, inquire about who the primary caretakers for the child have been, what the child's relationships to these people are like, and any changes in these relationships over time (e.g., a transition from full-time care by mother to participation in a day care program). Also, ask about other problems in the child's home life (neighbors, other relatives, step-siblings from parents' previous marriages, etc.). Be sure to ask parents what they think are the possible causes of their child's difficulties. (Often, as you establish rapport with parents, much of this information will emerge spontaneously without your needing to ask long lists of specific questions.) Finally, remember to get an idea of the family's financial resources and social supports (e.g., availability of relatives, community agencies, church facilities), as these will be important factors to consider in developing a treatment plan for the child.

INTERVIEWING THE CHILD

The basic principles of clinical interviewing described in Chapter 1 apply to children as well as adults. However, work with children often requires a whole additional set of tools for understanding clinical material, because children will usually rely more heavily than adults on nonverbal modes of showing you their concerns, and they are likely to display their troubles in their play activities and in their behavior with you. Play is both a diagnostic and a therapeutic tool in working with children. Thus, an hour-long interview with a troubled four-year-old might involve drawing a picture, playing "house" with a set of dolls, and/or making up stories using animal puppets.

When you first meet a child, it will most likely be in a waiting room with the parent or other responsible person who has accompanied the child. Note how the child behaves with the parent, and how he or she separates from the parent. Great difficulty in leaving the parent to go into your office may suggest some specific fears about the meeting with you, or more general problems with separation.

The child needs to understand who you are and why he or she is seeing you. Even small children can understand that your office is a "place to talk about worries." Notice how the child deals with you in the first few minutes of the interview. Does the child warm up to you easily? Can you engage him or her in conversation or play easily, or does the child remain aloof, guarded, or withdrawn? You may want to start talking with the child about something that he or she is likely to be interested in—e.g., pets, sports, hobbies, or favorite foods. Or, particularly with older children and adolescents, you might begin with a direct question about what has been on the child's mind, or what the child understands about why he or she was brought to see you.

The Importance of Play

Young children cannot be expected to sit still and talk throughout an interview. In fact, you would not want them to, because in most cases the child provides you with invaluable information by being active with you and with toys and other objects in your office.

Play allows children to live out and rework problems that are bothering them, to recreate family situations, and to express feelings and impulses that might be "forbidden" in real life. In the stories they create, children can tell you what is on their minds even when they do not have the capacity to verbalize these concerns. For example, a boy of five may not be able to tell you how angry he is at his father (the conscious experience of anger at a loved and needed father may be too threatening), but he may play out scenes over and over again in which big abusive fathers are beaten by small but powerful little boys. A girl of seven is not likely to be conscious of her belief that her parents got a divorce because she was a bad little girl, but in her play she might create stories about bad girls who get punished and daddies who come home again.

Your office should be equipped with materials that will allow for fanciful play: drawing materials, clay, dolls and a doll house, puppets, and other toys that might interest children of various ages. Children will often begin to play with toys in your office spontaneously. You may invite a child to play and then watch for a time, joining in when you feel it is appropriate.

The interpretation of the form and content of play is a complicated and fascinating skill which is well worth study. A discussion of this aspect of working with children is beyond the scope of this chapter. It is best learned by watching experienced professionals play with children (often while observing from behind a one-way mirror) and then talking to these professionals about their understanding of what transpires.

In addition to toys, you can use verbal techniques to help children warm up to you and engage in fantasy and play. You can, for example, make up stories together. Or you might ask the child which animal he or she would most like to be. The choice of animal, and what the child describes about the creature will give you information about self-image. Similar information can be obtained by having the child draw a person and then tell you about the person in the drawing (what the person is feeling, doing, etc.). You might also ask the child to make three wishes (e.g., to change something, to be something, and to do something).

Be sure to give children the opportunity to talk about their strengths. Such information is important in assessing the child's self-esteem, but also in helping to convey the message that you are an ally who wants to hear about what the child feels proud of as well as those aspects of life that are more troublesome. You might get at strong points with a question like, "What things are you good at?" or "What do you like most about yourself?"

Remember that in dealing with children, you may have to be more parental than you would with an adult. For example, children need to know where the bathroom is, and you may have to escort them there during the session. You must set limits on destructive and disruptive behavior in your office, as this will reassure the child that you will not allow his or her impulses to get out of control and will allow the session to proceed.

The above discussion about play may not apply to older elementary school children (e.g., age 10 and up) and adolescents, who may wish to sit and talk as an adult might, or who prefer to talk over a game such as checkers. Children in these age groups can often be quite open and direct in the expression of their concerns.

When interviewing adolescents, it is especially important to respect their autonomy and their right to decide whether to participate in the interview with you. Some adolescents will be very reluctant to talk. In such cases, a passive stance on your part is not as likely to be as helpful as active attempts to engage in discussion. Initially, you might ask about neutral topics of interest such as sports or music or clothes.

Adolescents are likely to have concerns about controlling their impulses, about their sexuality and sexual identity, about intimacy, and about peer relationships. Many teenagers will be worried about some aspect of their sexuality ("Am I developing right?" "Am I gay?"). You might open the way for discussion of these matters with a general comment such as, "Many kids your age have questions about sex and their sexual feelings. Have you had any thoughts like that?" Since peer relationships are of the utmost importance during this period, you will definitely want to discuss friendships and the adolescent's concerns (if any) about social acceptance as part of your assessment interview.

The psychiatric evaluation of the child is recorded in much the same way that it is in the case of adult evaluations. Thus, in preparing a written case report, you can follow the format outlined in Chapter 3. Moreover, your observations of the child in your office should be recorded in the mental status examination, according to the format discussed in Chapter 4.

PSYCHIATRIC DISORDERS OF CHILDHOOD

Children suffer from many of the same disorders that are found in the adult population. Some disorders such as schizophrenia, bipolar illness, and depression are less frequently encountered among children; others (e.g., phobias) are just as common in children as in adults. Disorders such as attention deficit disorder and functional enuresis are diagnosed more frequently among children than adults. And still others, like antisocial personality disorder, are by definition not diagnosed in children at all.

One of the best predictors of psychiatric problems in adulthood is a severe behavior disturbance in childhood. However, mental disorders in childhood do not invariably lead to the same disturbances in adult life. Moreover, some emotionally disturbed children grow up to have no diagnosable mental disorders whatsoever. Thus, for example, personality disorders are diagnosed infrequently and conservatively in children and adolescents, because the plasticity and instability of the personality during these developmental phases makes it impossible in most cases to see any personality patterns as enduring and stable. Despite active research efforts in recent years, we still know very little about the relationship between psychopathology in childhood and mental illness in adult life.

What follows are brief discussions of the disorders that are most commonly encountered among children and adolescents. Some disorders listed in *DSM-III* are not included here, due to the infrequency with which these diagnoses are made. For more detailed discussions of various clinical syndromes, you might wish to consult *DSM-III* and a general child psychiatry text (e.g., Noshpitz and Cohen, *Basic Handbook of Child Psychiatry*, 1979).

As noted in the first section of this chapter, you must be sure to assess the presence and severity of psychiatric disorders in the context of what is developmentally appropriate for each individual child.

ATTENTION DEFICIT DISORDER

Attention deficit disorder (ADD) has been known by a variety of other names, most notably *hyperactive child syndrome* and *minimal brain dysfunction*. Estimates of the prevalence of ADD range from 3 to 10 percent of elementary school children, and ADD is as much as five times as common in boys as in girls. The impulsivity and difficulty in paying attention to tasks that are usually involved in this syndrome are frustrating for parents, teachers, and children alike. The disorder usually appears by age three, but often goes undiagnosed until the child enters school.

The hallmark of ADD is inattention, which usually involves the child's failing to finish things that he or she starts (e.g., schoolwork, household chores, play activities), not seeming to listen to others, and easy distractibility. The second major characteristic of ADD is impulsivity. Children act before thinking, have difficulty organizing their work, shift excessively from one activity to another, often call out in class or have trouble waiting their turn in group situations, and require more supervision than other children.

The third major characteristic, hyperactivity, is seen in a great number of ADD children but not all of them. Symptoms include excessive running and climbing, difficulty sitting still, moving about excessively during sleep, and being always "on the go" as if driven by a motor.

Children with ADD commonly throw temper tantrums and generally have a low tolerance for frustration. They are often socially immature and, although sociable, lose the friends they make because of a need to dominate play situations. They often end up with compliant friends who are younger than they. Relationships with adults also tend to be poor, because behavior problems cause these children to be labeled "bad" or "unruly." Needless to say, ADD usually results in academic difficulties, as children who are of normal intelligence cannot pay attention to tasks and organize their work, thus becoming underachievers. Many of these children also have specific learning disabilities (see below). The severity of the ADD syndrome varies from one child to the next.

ADD children commonly suffer from low self-esteem, secondary to their difficulties in relating to adults and peers, and secondary to school failures. This can result in significant emotional problems, and some of these children begin to exhibit antisocial behavior (e.g., lying, stealing, drug abuse) in adolescence.

The etiology of ADD is an area of active research in child psychiatry. Maternal deprivation, environmental toxins (e.g., lead poisoning), genetic predisposition, severe early malnutrition, and intrauterine or postnatal brain damage are among the factors that have been implicated as possible contributors to the development of the syndrome. To date, evidence is lacking that would conclusively establish any of these as causes of ADD. The course of the disorder is variable. As they move through puberty into adolescence and adulthood, some people retain all of the symptoms of ADD, while others become free of the disorder completely. In a third group, the symptoms of hyperactivity disappear, but the attention deficit and impulsivity persist.

Diagnosis

The symptoms described above are listed in *DSM-III*. Signs of inattention, impulsivity, and hyperactivity must be judged on the basis of what is developmentally appropriate for a child at any given age. It is important to rule out other conditions that might be mistaken for ADD. The differential diagnosis includes medical illnesses, such as constipation and hyperthyroidism; neurologic conditions such as behavioral syndromes resulting from trauma, infection, or lead poisoning; and other psychiatric conditions, including anxiety disorders, parental abuse or neglect, major depression or mania, and manipulative behavior.

History. In many cases, the most reliable reports of abnormalities come from teachers rather than the child's parents, because teachers have greater familiarity with age-appropriate norms and a much larger comparison group on which to base their judgments.

Neurologic examination. The presence of "soft" neurologic signs (e.g., poor coordination, left-right confusion) is often a clue to ADD, although only about 50 percent of children with the disorder have neurologic abnormalities. Electroencephalograms are usually normal.

Psychological testing. Children with ADD show standard patterns of deficits on routine psychological tests, particularly in areas of sustaining attention and organizing information. In addition to standard psychological tests, including IQ tests, the child should be tested for specific learning disabilities, as these often coexist with ADD.

Treatment

The treatment of ADD involves not only the child, but also the child's family and school. Family members need to be educated about the disorder and about what to expect from their child. Parents who feel frustrated and guilty about their problems in dealing with their child often find supportive psychotherapy helpful both in alleviating some of their own distress and in teaching them to respond to their child in ways that promote better functioning and less family strife. Individual psychotherapy is not often useful in younger children, but for older children and adolescents psychotherapy can help the child with the secondary problems of ADD, such as low self-esteem, depression, and poor social skills.

Children with ADD commonly benefit from reducing sensory and emotional stimulation in their environments. This can be done with simple measures, like creating quiet spaces with subdued colors and simple furniture in which the child can play, putting toys away in a closet when they are not in use, allowing only one friend to visit at a time, avoiding crowded places like supermarkets, and putting the child in a small classroom.

Special academic placement is often indicated for children with ADD if they disrupt the learning process for others and cannot learn well in a traditional classroom setting. Consultation with teachers is especially important, both to determine what sort of academic program would be most helpful to the child, and to enlist the teachers' help in monitoring the child's behavioral responses to various treatment interventions.

Attention deficit disorder is one of the few mental disorders of childhood for which the use of medication is clearly indicated in many cases. Roughly 75 percent of children with ADD and hyperactivity respond to some form of somatic treatment. Chemotherapy is not curative but suppresses the symptoms of the disorder (particularly behavioral impulsivity), and many children benefit from the medication for as long as 10 years or until they reach puberty.

The most commonly used medications are stimulants, particularly amphetamine and methylphenidate (Ritalin). These medications exert a seemingly paradoxical effect, in that they do not heighten most children's level of arousal, but instead tend to improve concentration and performance, calm restlessness, improve impulse control, and make the child more responsive to reward and punishment. The mechanism by which stimulants produce these effects in children is not known. Side effects may include loss of appetite, irritability, headache, gastrointestinal distress, and insomnia. Also, many children experience some reversible growth retardation during the first year or two in which the medication is administered. "Drug holidays" (medication-free periods) during school vacations allow the child time to catch up in growth and give the clinician an opportunity to observe whether medication is still necessary for the child.

Tricyclic antidepressants (TCAs) have also been found useful in treating ADD, but children are more sensitive than adults to the cardiac side effects of these medications (see Chapter 16). For this reason, TCAs are not as safe as stimulants for younger children but are sometimes used for adolescents whose symptoms persist through puberty. Anticonvulsants and antihistamines have also been used with limited success in treating this disorder.

Recently, much attention has been paid to diet as a possible aggravating factor in ADD. Sugar, food dyes, milk, chocolate, and artificial additives are among the many things cited as possible contributors to the ADD syndrome. However, elimination of various foods has been found to be helpful in only a minority of cases.

CONDUCT DISORDERS

The category of *conduct disorders* covers a broad range of conditions found among children. They all are characterized by a repetitive and persistent pattern of violating either the basic rights of others or major age-appropriate societal norms or rules. The term "conduct disorder" describes behavior, but says nothing about underlying causes. There is considerable overlap between conduct disorders and ADD; that is, many children with ADD also have a conduct disorder. Also, some children with conduct disorders have "soft" (nonspecific) neurologic signs but do not exhibit behaviors characteristic of ADD.

Conduct disorders are grouped along the dimensions of socialization and aggression. There are four subcategories of this disorder listed in *DSM-III:* undersocialized aggressive, undersocialized nonaggressive, socialized aggressive, and socialized nonaggressive.

Undersocialized children are those who have failed to establish a normal degree of affection for or empathy with others. They lack peer relationships, or these relationships are short-lived and very superficial. They show little concern for the feelings of others, readily manipulate others for their own ends, and appear to lack guilt or remorse. They are likely to blame others and inform on them if it is to their advantage. Socialized children with conduct disorders may show evidence of attachments to others (e.g., gang loyalty), but are callous and manipulative toward people to whom they are not attached and lack guilt when their actions cause such people to suffer.

Aggressive children are characterized in *DSM-III* as engaging in physical violence towards other people (e.g., hitting, biting) or theft outside the home which involves confronting the victim (e.g., purse-snatching, extortion). Nonaggressive children are those who do not engage in violence or physical confrontation, but who persistently violate rules at school or at home. This may take the form of truancy, running away from home overnight, persistent serious lying, vandalism, fire-setting, or theft (e.g., shoplifting).

Children with these disorders typically blame others for their problems and are mistrustful of others. They often hide low self-esteem under a veneer of "toughness." They may be sexually precocious and promiscuous and often become involved in smoking and substance abuse. They are underachievers, and the socialized types often join gangs that engage in antisocial activities. The disorders are much more common in boys than in girls and are more common among the children of adults with antisocial personality disorder and alcoholism.

While a vast number of factors have been proposed as etiologies of conduct disorders, no causal relationships have been demonstrated to date. Poor impulse control, lack of parental care and limit-setting, excessive inborn aggressive drives, cultural norms, and parental role-modeling could all contribute to unusually aggressive behavior. Lack of social bonding appears to be associated with maternal deprivation, harsh or inconsistent treatment by parents (including physical abuse), parental rejection, and ADD. Clearly, children with these disorders stem from a wide variety of biologic and environmental backgrounds.

While habitual antisocial behavior in childhood and adolescence is associated with an elevated risk of serious mental illness in adult life (e.g., depression, schizophrenia, antisocial personality disorder), many children with conduct disorders grow up without such serious disturbances. They often learn through their experience, and many can be helped by various forms of psychological treatment. Moreover, some antisocial acting out in relatively healthy youngsters occurs transiently in response to environmental stresses and disappears when the child's situation changes.

Juvenile delinquency is a widespread and serious problem in our society. More than 40 percent of people arrested for serious crimes are under the age of 18, and adolescents commit half of all rapes and murders reported in this country each year. Delinquent behavior peaks in adolescence, and mental health professionals are commonly called upon to assess and treat delinquent teenagers for emotional disorders that often underlie their antisocial behavior.

Many problems of adolescence contribute to delinquency. Some teenagers who suffer from organic brain damage (e.g., congenitally or as the result of later trauma) have poor impulse control, and the emotional and biological stresses of adolescence push them to the limits of their capacities for socialized behavior. Teenagers who have suffered severe physical and emotional deprivation (e.g., from frequent foster home changes, parental abuse and violence, or parental psychopathology or alcoholism) discharge tension in ways that have been modeled for them by their caretakers. Adolescents who behave violently or promiscuously may do so in an attempt to combat feelings of inadequacy. Delinquent behavior may be a call for help in response to family strife, or it may be the result of parents' encouragement of such behavior (e.g., the father who subtly encourages a son to act out the father's own destructive impulses).

Substance abuse is increasingly common among adolescents (see Chapter 12). In evaluating adolescents who abuse drugs, it is important to consider the possible contributing factors noted above. Moreover, it is particularly important to rule out depression, as some depressed teenagers will attempt to medicate themselves with drugs or alcohol.

Treatment of conduct disorders cannot be outlined in any standard way, because this diagnosis covers behavior problems that have multiple determinants. One child may come from a home in which parents are unconsciously encouraging him to lie and steal, another child may throw tantrums and behave antisocially secondary to ADD, and a third "delinquent" may be attempting to "prove his manhood" in a subculture that prizes and encourages defiance of authority.

Thus, treatment strategies must be based on a careful diagnostic assessment, including consultation with family, school, and any legal or social service agencies involved with the child.

Severely behaviorally disturbed youngsters whose behavior cannot be controlled effectively by parents and teachers may need placement in a residential treatment setting where limits can be enforced, children can be consistently held responsible for their actions, and constructive relationships with peers can be encouraged. In outpatient settings, many children can be helped by therapy that focuses on the consequences of behavior and accepting responsibility for one's actions. Also, many of these children suffer from low self-esteem, and therapy can provide a setting in which these children are valued and respected by the therapist and can in turn learn to appreciate their own strengths. Psychotherapy is often indicated for parents of conduct disordered children when the parents are in some way aggravating or even actively encouraging the antisocial behavior.

SPECIFIC DEVELOPMENTAL DISORDERS

Specific developmental disorders describe impairment in one particular cognitive area of maturation: reading, arithmetic, language, or speech. These disorders are diagnosed in children who may otherwise function well, but who, based on their age and educational backgrounds, have obvious difficulty in one area of learning. Developmental reading, arithmetic, and language disorders correspond to what educators call *learning disabilities*, and these disorders are often not treated in mental health settings at all but are worked with in the educational system. These disorders are quite common; they are estimated to be present in 10 to 20 percent of elementary school children. They are diagnosed twice as commonly in boys as in girls, probably due to a combination of actual increased frequency among boys and greater attention paid in many families and schools to the educational performance of boys.

These disorders are often seen in conjunction with others, particularly with ADD and conduct disorders. In some cases, a child who performs poorly in school secondary to a specific developmental disorder will act out his or her distress by being truant or by engaging in antisocial behavior, and in this way the child warrants the diagnosis of conduct disorder. In most cases, children with specific developmental disorders are not simply lagging behind their peers and do not catch up to them in time. Rather, most children with these problems continue to have signs of these disorders into adolescence and adulthood, although they may compensate quite well for their difficulties.

Developmental reading disorder, often referred to as "dyslexia," involves impaired development of reading skills that cannot be accounted for by the child's mental or chronological age or poor schooling. Assessment of poor performance is based on standardized reading tests (compared with the child's overall intellectual abilities as measured by IQ tests) as well as reading skills observed in the classroom. Examples of the disorder include a 14-year-old eighth grader of normal intelligence from an adequately stimulating home and school environment who reads at the level of a third grader, and an otherwise normally functioning 10-year-old fourth grader who reads at a first grade level.

This disorder often involves some difficulty in integrating and organizing visually derived information. Reading errors include omissions, additions, and distortions of words, and writing errors are often numerous and bizarre. Children with this disorder usually read slowly and comprehend what they read poorly. "Soft" neurologic signs are often present, suggesting some organic basis for the disorder.

Developmental arithmetic disorder is not as common as a reading disorder but is diagnosed by the same means (performance on standardized tests of math skills and performance in class compared with scores on IQ tests). Children with this disorder may also have reading problems.

Developmental language disorder refers to delayed development of language skills, unrelated to hearing impairment or mental retardation. There are two types: expressive and receptive. The expressive disorder involves difficulty with vocal expression ("getting the words out") despite good comprehension. Articulation is generally immature, vocabulary is severely restricted, and sentence construction is poor. The receptive disorder is more serious than the expressive type, in that it involves failure to develop both comprehension and expression. Children with this disorder have reading and spelling difficulties and often show some auditory impairment.

Developmental articulation disorder is a type of speech disorder that is quite common, thought to occur in roughly 6 percent of boys and 3 percent of girls. It involves failure to develop articulation of later-acquired speech sounds such as r, sh, th, f, z, l, or ch. This is a less serious disorder than the language disorders described above, in that the child's abilities to comprehend and express language are normal.

Treatment of specific developmental disorders is largely educational, and many children can make major improvements in their skills with special educational assistance. Learning disabilities are relative discrepancies in skills. Thus, a learning-disabled child may be quite bright and capable of devising strategies to compensate for the disability and thereby function quite well (e.g., the child with a reading disability who learns to remember everything he or she hears in class). However, children with these disorders may lose motivation to learn and give up in the face of repeated failures, so a major part of treatment is to support their self-esteem by putting them in situations (e.g., special classes or special tutoring) in which they can experience some success at their level of ability. When learning disorders are accompanied by coordination difficulties, special physical education programs may be helpful and may enhance the child's self-esteem and ability to interact with peers. Articulation disorders often respond well to speech therapy given in the schools. Psychotherapy for these disorders is not usually necessary, unless the child has developed significant emotional or social problems as a result of teasing by other children or pressure from frustrated adults.

MENTAL RETARDATION

Mental retardation is considered in this chapter because the disorder, although generally life-long, is by definition present before the age of 18. (Similar conditions that begin after age 18 are classified as dementia.) The hallmarks of the disorder are intellectual functioning that is significantly below average (as measured on IQ tests) and resultant deficits or impairment in the person's adaptive behavior (e.g., ability to work, care for self, function socially). Low IQ alone is not sufficient for the diagnosis of mental retardation but must be accompanied by evidence of poor functioning. The prevalence of mental retardation is thought to be about 3 percent among school-age children. Among the rest of the general population in nonacademic settings, the prevalence decreases to roughly 1 percent. Mental retardation may coexist with a wide variety of other psychiatric disorders, such as autism, ADD, and hyperactivity. Also, severe mental retardation is often associated with multiple neurological abnormalities involving neuromuscular function, vision, or hearing. Seizures are common among the severely mentally retarded.

The organic causes of mental retardation are too numerous to list here. The most common (accounting for 25 percent of cases) are inborn chromosomal and metabolic abnormalities, such as Down's syndrome (trisomy 21) and phenylketonuria (PKU). Prenatal infections such as rubella and toxoplasmosis, as well as heavy maternal alcohol consumption, are among the influences that can result in mental retardation. Trauma during delivery (e.g., mechanical injury to the brain or transient loss of oxygen to brain tissue) can also result in mental retardation. Postnatal causes of mental retardation, including infection, hyperbilirubinemia, head trauma (including that resulting from child abuse), brain tumors, and lead poisoning, account for a sizeable proportion of cases.

Psychosocial causes of mental retardation are thought to include deprivation of social, linguistic, and intellectual stimulation. For example, this deprivation may result from parental neglect or from parental deficits in the ability to stimulate children (e.g., when parents are themselves retarded). Mental retardation due to known biologic factors is as likely to occur in upper as in lower socioeconomic groups, but retardation without known organic cause is more commonly found among lower socioeconomic groups.

Subtypes of Mental Retardation

The population of mentally retarded individuals is divided into two large groups, consisting of those with mild and borderline mental retardation (IQ greater than 50) on the one hand, and of the moderately and severely retarded (IQ less than 50) on the other. The vast majority of the mentally retarded fall into the borderline or mild categories.

Those with an IQ of 50 or above tend to live in underprivileged neighborhoods and may have siblings who are mildly retarded. They usually have no obvious neurologic abnormalities or physical handicaps and so appear normal. Usually, the diagnosis of mental retardation is made only after they start school. In this group, psychosocial and hereditary factors seem to be of roughly equal importance in determining intelligence (as they are in determining intelligence in normal individuals).

By contrast, those who have IQs below 50 more commonly show obvious physical and neurological abnormalities and so look "retarded." They are more likely to live in institutional settings, to require special educational programs, or to work in sheltered workshops. Biologic factors generally play a more prominent role than environmental ones in the development of mental retardation in this group. The diagnosis of moderate to severe mental retardation is made earlier than among those with milder impairment—often in the preschool years.

Mental retardation is classified by IQ (the norm is 100), and on this basis the mentally retarded are classified in one of four groups as shown below.

Mild (IQ 50-70). Roughly 2.5 percent of the population have IQs between 50 and 70. These people are termed "educable" and comprise about 80 percent of the population of mentally retarded individuals in this country. They develop social and communication skills before age five and are not distinguishable from normal children until after age five. They can usually learn up to a sixth grade level. As adults, they can usually develop social and vocational skills that allow them to be self-sufficient, but they may need assistance from others in times of stress.

Moderate (IQ 35-49). These people are termed "trainable" and comprise about 12 percent of the population of mentally retarded. They can learn to communicate as preschoolers but are only poorly aware of social conventions. During school age, they do not often progress beyond a second grade level academically but can profit from training in social and occupational skills. As adults they can often care for themselves with moderate supervision and perform unskilled or semiskilled tasks in supervised ("sheltered") workshops.

Severe (IQ 20-34). These people comprise roughly 7 percent of the mentally retarded. During the preschool years, they show poor motor development and little or no communicative speech. They may be able to learn to talk and perform elementary self-care (e.g., personal hygiene) during school age, but they do not profit from vocational training and require a great deal of supervision in living throughout their lives.

Profound (IQ below 20). The profoundly mentally retarded constitute 1 percent of the population of retarded individuals. Throughout life they require a highly structured living environment with constant supervision. Speech and motor development are usually very limited; some people in this category can learn minimal self-care skills (e.g., personal hygiene).

The category of *borderline mental retardation,* also called borderline intellectual functioning in *DSM-III,* has boundaries that are less clear than those of the categories described above. This includes people in the IQ range of 71 to 84. People whose intellectual functioning falls into this range may or may not be classified as retarded, depending on how well they adapt to their life circumstances. For example, a man who has an IQ of 80, who is self-supporting, and who—like his father—functions well at a job requiring semi-skilled manual labor may never come to the attention of an educator or mental health professional. Another man with the same IQ, but who is raised in an upwardly mobile intellectual family, may develop low self-esteem based on an inability to keep up with peers and low status within his family, resulting in behavior problems and an eventual diagnosis. Retardation in this range is highly context-dependent.

Treatment

Treatment of mental retardation begins with identifying and treating somatic causes, such as nutritional deficiencies and seizure disorders. Increased environmental stimulation is sometimes sufficient to assist children with mild or borderline retardation in their intellectual and social development when a deprived home environment has retarded the child's growth. Most treatment is habilitative—that is, it is designed to help the retarded maximize their potential for self-care and social and occupational functioning. Such treatment involves socialization programs to teach speech, hygiene, academic and interpersonal skills, and vocational training with sheltered employment opportunities.

Increasingly, emphasis has been on keeping even the most severely mentally retarded people in the community and out of institutions to maximize their socialization and ability to function in society. Some retarded children may need residential schools to cope with severe behavior problems, and some profoundly handicapped children may need nursing home care. Otherwise, treatment is aimed at family care (in the child's own home or in foster care) and community-based education and training. The mentally retarded are an underserved population in this country. Mental health professionals are often called upon to help the mentally retarded and their families understand the problems the retarded person faces, and to plan for adequate training and assistance. The greater your knowledge about the resources and services available for the mentally retarded in your community, the more effective you will be in providing these clients with the help they deserve.

PERVASIVE DEVELOPMENTAL DISORDERS

Children with *pervasive developmental disorders* show distortions in the development of multiple basic psychological functions, such as attention, perception, reality testing, and movement. Unlike children with specific developmental disorders, who are impaired in one area of cognition but are otherwise normal, these children are globally and severely impaired in their abilities to function intellectually, motorically, and socially.

Infantile autism is a condition in which the child is extremely unresponsive to other people, has gross impairment in communication skills, and shows bizarre responses to various aspects of the environment. The disorder develops before the child is 30 months old.

Autistic children fail to develop normal interest in and attachment to others. Infants do not generally cuddle and are indifferent or averse to physical contact and affection. Older children fail to develop cooperative play and friendships. Some older children gradually develop some awareness of and attachment to parents; however, many autistic children treat human beings as though they were inanimate objects.

Language may be totally absent. Autistic children who can speak usually exhibit immature grammar structure, echolalia (mimicking sounds made by others), reversals of pronouns, difficulty naming objects, and inappropriate nonverbal communications (e.g., bizarre facial expressions and gestures).

Autistic children may respond bizarrely to the environment in a variety of ways. Many of them appear to be "obsessed with sameness" and may react violently to minor changes in their environment, such as new clothes or a change in the child's place at the dinner table. They are often fascinated by motion and stare at fans or other spinning objects, or at water running down the drain. The child may engage in ritualistic behavior (e.g., hand-wringing or hand clapping), and compulsively self-destructive behavior (e.g., head-banging) with apparent imperviousness to pain.

Only 30 percent of autistic children have an IQ above 70. The disorder is chronic. Only one child in six grows up to make an adequate social adjustment and can work regularly, another one in six makes only a fair adjustment, and two-thirds of autistic children remain severaly handicapped and unable to lead independent lives. Many develop seizure disorders in adolescence or early adulthood.

Childhood-onset pervasive developmental disorder is the category that describes children who are grossly impaired in social relationships and show bizarre communication and behavior, but who begin to show signs of the disorder after age 30 months (and before age 12). This disorder, too, occurs more frequently among the mentally retarded, but some children may have "islands" of unusual ability (so-called "idiot savants"). By contrast, children suffering from childhood schizophrenia are usually diagnosed above age 5 and show hallucinations, delusions, or other forms of thought disorder in addition to bizarre speech and behavior. These children are diagnosed by the same criteria used for adults (see Chapter 5).

The etiologies of infantile autism and childhood onset pervasive developmental disorder are not known. However, some factors which are thought to predispose children to the development of infantile autism are maternal rubella (German measles), phenylketonuria (PKU), encephalitis, and meningitis. The prevalence of infantile autism is 50 times as great in siblings of children with the disorder as it is in the general population. Previously, it was thought that "icebox parents" who deprived the child of affection fostered the development of pervasive developmental disorders. However, recent research does not support this notion but instead suggests that genetic and organic factors probably play a prominent role.

Treatment of these disorders is long and difficult. Medication has been of use in treating specific medication-responsive symptoms such as hyperactivity and seizures. Educational and habilitative approaches are most important to help remedy speech and learning disorders and incoordination. Behavior modification programs can help shape some children's behavior along more socially appropriate lines. Children who are severely retarded and behaviorally disturbed may require institutional care, while others can remain at home. Parents need a great deal of support and counseling, both to help them deal with their feelings about their child's difficulties, and to help them preserve time and energy for themselves and other children in the family.

FUNCTIONAL ENURESIS (BEDWETTING)

Enuresis is one of the most common problems of early childhood. It is defined as the involuntary voiding of urine at least twice a month in five- and six-year-olds, and at least once a month in older children. The "accident" most commonly occurs at night in bed during non-REM sleep, so that the child has no memory of wetting the bed. Enuresis occurs in at least 10 percent of four-year-olds, and at age five still affects 7 percent of boys and 3 percent of girls.

Eighty percent of enuretics suffer from primary enuresis—i.e., they have never achieved complete bladder control. Many children in this group lag behind their peers in the development of neurologic and psychological organization of bladder control. In some cases, difficulty over toilet training or conflict between parents is so upsetting to the child that he or she manifests distress through sphincter accidents. Twenty percent of enuretics suffer from secondary enuresis, which occurs after a year or more of being "dry." Psychogenic factors are more commonly implicated in the genesis of secondary enuresis than the primary form, and typical contributing factors include such stressors as the birth of a sibling, parental conflict, starting school, or hospitalization. It is not uncommon for children to develop secondary enuresis temporarily due to regression along the developmental line of sphincter control in response to a specific stressor, and most episodes are so short-lived as to require no treatment. Most enuretics become completely "dry" on their own by age 10.

Whenever a child presents with enuresis, it is always important to rule out an organic problem such as genitourinary tract abnormalities, infection, seizure disorder (with accidents occurring during seizures), and diabetes. The child should always be examined by a physician as part of your evaluation.

When enuresis is the presenting symptom of an underlying emotional disorder, psychotherapy and family therapy can often resolve the symptom by easing emotional stress in the child's life. A variety of behavior modification techniques have been effective with enuretics, including charts and systems of reward with gold stars for dry nights, as well as bladder stretching with fluid forcing and holding of urine during the day for as long as possible. Mechanical devices such as buzzers that wake the child up at the first appearance of moisture on the bed have also been used with good results. Imipramine has been found to be helpful in many cases, although the mechanism by which this antidepressant exerts a therapeutic effect is not understood. The potentially toxic effects of imipramine on the heart make it a treatment to be used with caution. Parents need to be supported by the therapist, so that they can be supportive of their child rather than punitive.

FUNCTIONAL ENCOPRESIS (INCONTINENCE OF FECES)

Encopresis, or incontinence of stool, involves voluntary or involuntary soiling at least once a month after age four that is not the result of an organic cause (e.g., bowel dysfunction). Encopresis is five times as common in boys as in girls and may be either primary (if continence has never been achieved) or secondary (when previously achieved continence is lost). Commonly, soiling results from a cycle of hard, painful stools, which the child holds back as long as possible; leakage around the impacted feces, followed by pain when the child finally defecates; and then holding back of the next stool to avoid further pain. This can be treated with stool softeners and suppositories, which help the dilated rectum resume its normal size, along with a supportive and educative approach to the problem with the child and the parents.

Behavior modification techniques have been used effectively with some encopretic children. Children set goals with the therapist (e.g., learning not to retain feces, or having one bowel movement per day), and when these goals are achieved, the behavior is reinforced with rewards such as gold stars or a special privilege. Behavioral techniques can be particularly helpful in conjunction with psychotherapy, when underlying personality problems play a major role in the etiology of the disorder.

In some instances, encopresis is part of a passive-aggressive, hostile, withholding relationship that the child has formed with the parents. This requires psychotherapeutic treatment of the parents and the child to explore underlying family conflicts, to help parents learn to respect the child's autonomy, and to help the child learn other avenues for the expression of anger and resentment. As with enuresis, encopresis sometimes occurs transiently when the child is under stress, as when a sibling is born or the child starts school. In such cases, the problem often resolves spontaneously when the stressful time is past. In a few instances, encopresis results simply from parental neglect when no one has bothered to toilet train the child.

SEPARATION ANXIETY DISORDER

Separation anxiety is normal in infants and toddlers. Moreover, difficulty separating from parents and anxiety about being away from home are normal for brief periods when children take major developmental steps such as starting preschool, going to camp for the first time, and even leaving home to go to college. However, when separation anxiety is prolonged and severe in older children, it often disrupts the child's life in the way that agoraphobia disrupts an adult's (see Chapter 8). The essential feature of *separation anxiety disorder* is excessive anxiety on separation from primary caretakers or from home or other familiar surroundings, causing major symptoms of physical or emotional distress for at least two weeks.

Children with this disorder have prolonged and unremitting difficulty being away from home to attend school or camp, to sleep over at another child's house, or even to go on errands. Anxiety does not resolve after a few days or a few tries at a new activity, but rather it persists and remains severe. Children may cling to parents and follow them around the house. Often they have physical complaints such as nausea, vomiting, and headaches when separation is about to occur. Adolescents may experience dizziness, faintness, and palpitations at such times.

These children generally fear that some accident or illness will befall them or their parents if they are separated from them. Some children have explicit fantasies of particular dangers, while others experience vague anxiety when separated from parents but do not know what they fear. Concerns about dying and exaggerated fears about robbers, muggers, and monsters are common. Some children do not express fears at all but become intensely homesick to the point of panic when away from home. Difficulty going to sleep, requests to sleep in the parents' bed, and nightmares about separation themes are common among these children. Also, when separated from important people, these children often experience withdrawal, apathy, sadness, and difficulty concentrating.

School Refusal

School refusal is often a symptom of separation anxiety disorder. A child's persistent refusal to attend school and insistence upon staying home with mother or some other primary caretaker (rather than simply wishing to "play hookey" or being kept at home by a parent) is a symptom that you should take very seriously, for it usually indicates distress of major proportions and often reflects a problem in the parent-child bond. In many cases, the child's fear of being separated from mother is related to mother's anxiety about the child's welfare and about being a good mother, with a need for the child's approval. School refusal may be a symptom of other psychiatric illnesses, as well, most notably depression, psychosis, or a severe personality disturbance. Moreover, the child's avoidance of school may be due to a phobia about some element of the school situation rather than difficulty in separating from home. The cause of the child's refusal to attend school will in part determine your treatment strategy.

Treatment of school refusal begins with crisis intervention. When psychological assessment of the child and medical evaluation of the child's physical complaints do not reveal psychosis or some other psychiatric or medical reason to keep the child at home, the child should be returned to school immediately. Family members should be involved in evaluation and treatment. You should make clear to the child and family that there is no reason for the child to stay at home, and that the only way to begin solving the problem is for the child to be back in school. A responsible person in the family needs to be sure that the child gets to school each day and stays there (this often requires the cooperation of teachers as well). The child may cling to mother and cry and throw tantrums in response to the expectation that he or she return to school. Nevertheless, after a few days of firm limits, the child becomes convinced that the parent intends for him or her to be in school, and the protest behavior ceases. When school refusal is due to separation anxiety, the family needs to be offered therapy; in particular, it is often the mother who must have psychotherapy in order to help her uncover her own difficulties in allowing the child to separate and lead an independent life. Systematic desensitization may help children who have developed phobias about particular aspects of the school situation. Antidepressants have been used effectively with some school phobic children, although we do not know the mechanism by which antidepressants alleviate this condition.

School refusal has a relatively good prognosis in younger children, but it is much more serious in the small percentage for whom the disorder recurs in high school. Nearly half of high school children who experience separation anxiety disorder have an underlying psychotic illness and may need hospitalization.

PSYCHOLOGICAL FACTORS IN PHYSICAL ILLNESS

Physical illness is common among children and is always stressful. Children often develop physical symptoms (or consciously feign illness) as a response to emotional distress. Moreover, medical illnesses and their consequences (pain, restrictions, hospitalizations) present children with emotional challenges with which they must cope. Mental health professionals are often called upon to evaluate and treat children who suffer from psychosomatic disorders and emotional reactions to medical illness. Illness may be "faked" deliberately by a child, or emotions may be channeled into physical symptoms when direct expression of distress seems impossible or too threatening. Complaints such as stomachaches and headaches are extremely common in children and adolescents, and these are often reactions to separation anxiety, phobias, and family strife (e.g., in a home where the father physically abuses the mother, a child may develop stomach pain so as not to have to go to school and leave mother alone). Often, chronic stomachaches and headaches run in families, where children who communicate their emotional difficulties through physical symptom formation seem to learn such behavior from their parents. When children are brought to health care professionals complaining of nonspecific symptoms for which no organic basis can be found, it is important to consider depression, anxiety, and family crisis as possible causal factors.

Major medical illnesses are difficult for any child to cope with, and the extent to which illness can be tolerated and adapted to by the child depends on the child's stage of development, on the nature of the illness and the extent to which it interferes with the child's activities, on the child's relationships with parents, and on the parents' reactions to the illness.

Most young children react to illness with regression. They may, for example, revert to bedwetting, thumbsucking, or clinging behavior. This is expectable and usually resolves when the stress of the illness has passed. Younger children often do not understand their condition and interpret illness as a punishment for having been bad. Hospitalization is a major stress for almost any child, particularly for younger children who may have difficulty tolerating separation from parents, frequent encounters with strangers, new routines for dressing and eating, and painful medical procedures.

When illness touches on the special vulnerabilities of a child's developmental struggle at a particular phase of life, the child's anxiety about the illness may be greatly increased. For example, a surgical procedure may greatly exacerbate a five-year-old's castration fears. Similarly, an adolescent immobilized with an injury may have heightened concerns about passivity and loss of self-control. Adolescents may use medical illness as a vehicle for acting out rebellion toward parents and other authorities (e.g., the diabetic teenager who refuses to take his insulin). Some children and adolescents do not express emotional distress during the course of a medical illness, but symptoms such as fears and night terrors may appear after the illness has passed.

Chronic illness poses particular problems for the developing child. Five percent of children and adolescents suffer from some form of chronic illness, with asthma and epilepsy the most common conditions in this age group. Chronic illnesses usually require adherence to some long-term treatment regimen, including special diets, medications, and often restriction of activity. Young children may be confused by their illness and may develop frightening fantasies about it. Children may suffer self-esteem problems if they come to feel significantly different from their peers who do not have such conditions (as is common, for example, among hemophiliacs). Also, children are likely to be influenced by their parents' and siblings' reactions to their illness. Family members may be unduly anxious or depressed or angry about the illness and the stresses it places on the entire household. Parents of children with potentially life-threatening illnesses such as asthma and congenital heart disease often behave overprotectively toward their children, fostering prolonged dependency and a lack of autonomy in the child.

The mental health professional is often called upon to determine the extent to which a physically ill child's emotional stress is due to the child's difficulties, to family tensions, and to the medical condition itself. You can do a great deal to help children and their families cope with illness, by educating them about the illness, by giving parents and children a place to share their fears and frustrations about the condition, by working with families on responsible management of the illness, and by helping to minimize the trauma of medical procedures and hospitalizations. The latter can be done by helping the child to anticipate what he or she is likely to encounter in the hospital, and by promoting frequent visits between parents and child when the child is in the hospital.

DEPRESSION

Depression occurs in children and adolescents as it does in adults, and the depressive disorders are discussed in Chapter 6. However, symptoms of depression in children vary somewhat from those commonly seen in older people, and what follows is a brief discussion of these differences.

There is controversy about what constitute the manifestations of depression in younger children. Many clinicians have advocated the concept of "masked depression"; that is, depression that manifests itself in a variety of symptoms that are not typically associated with a depressed mood. Depressive equivalents in children are thought to include antisocial behavior (such as lying, stealing, running away from home), proneness to accidents, chronic boredom and fatigue, irritability, and escape into fantasy worlds (e.g., preoccupation with fantasy games like "Dungeons and Dragons") to the exclusion of participation in family and school life. Many depressed youngsters will not report depression or sad feelings but will simply look sad most of the time.

Children often become depressed after some loss, such as the death of a parent or friend or pet, parental divorce, or a failing grade at school. In some cases, a child becomes depressed in identification with a depressed parent, or in reaction to the loss of parental care that often results when a parent becomes depressed. Depressive symptoms may be short-lived and self-limited when they occur in reaction to a life event (in which case, the syndrome is diagnosed as an adjustment reaction), or symptoms may persist for many months.

Depression in adolescents often occurs without the unhappy, withdrawn presentation we usually associate with depressive disorders. Teenagers may deliberately hide their depression. Moreover, they may be unaware of feeling depressed, yet manifest their distress in symptoms such as headache, school failure, school refusal, hyperactivity, promiscuity, antisocial behavior, or substance abuse. Vegetative symptoms may or may not be present. While some depressed teenagers lose weight, others gain. They may binge or starve, sleep long or little, be aggressive and boastful or withdrawn and self-deprecating, outgoing or isolative. The depressive picture is complicated by the considerable extent to which adolescents may make use of reaction formation (see Chapter 2). Factors contributing to depression in teenagers are similar to those thought to affect adults: biologic, psychological, and social. The adolescent may be particularly prone to depression when attempts at separation and independence from parents generate feelings of loss and fears of abandonment.

Treatment

Most children and adolescents respond promptly to psychosocial treatment. For younger children, interventions with parents are often more important than direct psychological treatment for the child, particularly when the child needs parental help in weathering a crisis and accepting a loss, or when a parent is depressed. Play therapy is often helpful in allowing younger children to play out and rework problems and conflicts that are troubling them. Older children and adolescents can be greatly helped by psychotherapy, which allows them to verbalize and understand feelings and provides them with experiences that enhance their self-esteem. This may occur individually or in groups.

Some adolescents with vegetative signs who do not respond to psychosocial interventions will respond to antidepressant medication. Younger children have also been shown, in some cases, to benefit from antidepressant therapy. Since prepubertal children are more sensitive to the cardiovascular side effects of tricyclics, these medications should be used with caution by experienced pediatric psychopharmacologists, and always in conjunction with psychosocial treatments.

SUICIDE

In recent years, the news media have given increasing attention to the problem of suicide among adolescents. Suicide is one of the leading causes of death among teenagers and is increasing in this age group. Equally alarming is the dramatic increase in suicides among younger children: the rate of suicide among children ages five through 12 has more than doubled in the last two decades. Suicide is almost certainly underreported in children and adolescents, as it is among adults. Many suspicious deaths are recorded as "accidents."

Factors that prompt children and adolescents to attempt suicide are many and varied. Suicidal behavior commonly occurs around family losses such as separation, divorce, or death of a parent. Suicide by a parent or suicidal behavior and depression in a parent seem to predispose children to suicidal thoughts and behavior. Adolescents and children commonly report making suicide attempts out of anger or desperation at a family or social situation that seems hopeless and intolerable. Very often, suicide attempts represent a call for help, when the child or teenager is in severe emotional distress yet is unable to ask for assistance more directly. Depression can prompt suicidal behavior, as can psychosis (e.g., in response to an hallucination). Younger children may be unable to grasp the concept of death and think only of joining a loved person in heaven, or they may view death as a pleasant place to which they can escape when real life seems unbearable.

Treatment involves taking suicidal thoughts, threats, or gestures very seriously. Even where it appears that suicide threats are clearly manipulative or an expression of anger, the child should be given psychiatric attention immediately, and the extent of the child's distress should be acknowledged clearly. Hospitalization is often necessary when children cannot negotiate a "no suicide" contract, when depression or psychosis require intensive treatment, or where the home situation seems to encourage further suicidal behavior (e.g., when family members give the child the message that he or she is expendable). Psychotherapy is usually indicated for the child and often for parents as well, and the focus is often on dealing with precipitating losses or finding more appropriate ways to express anger. Antidepressants are used less often with suicidal children and teenagers than they are with suicidal adults, but where serious depression is a contributing factor, these medications may be an important part of the treatment plan. As with suicidal adults, antidepressants must be used with great caution in treating suicidal children and adolescents (see Chapters 13 and 16). These medications are potentially lethal in overdose, so access to them must be carefully controlled by the prescribing physician and the child's parents.

CHILD ABUSE

In the past two decades, there has been increasing recognition that child abuse has reached near epidemic proportions in our society. Like suicide, child abuse is underreported, and only a fraction of abused children get professional help. The term "abuse" covers a wide range of maltreatment, including neglect and deprivation of food, clothes, and shelter; emotional neglect; verbal thrashings; actual physical assault; sexual activity; and murder.

Many parents who physically abuse their children were abused themselves as children, although no causal relationship has been demonstrated. Mothers are more likely than fathers to be child batterers, presumably due to the greater responsibility that mothers bear for child-rearing in most households and the resulting greater intensity of the mother-child relationship. In cases of maternal abuse of children, the father often contributes to the problem in important but less obvious ways, through absence from the home or abuse of the mother. Fathers are often the direct cause of abuse as well.

There is a high correlation between a child's premature delivery and low birth weight and subsequent child abuse, presumably because parents have difficulty coping with the child's extra needs and slower development. Also, premature babies are often separated from their mothers for long periods of time immediately after delivery, which may disrupt the normal process of maternal-child bonding. While child abuse occurs in all types of families and cuts across all socioeconomic lines, families in which abuse occurs are typically plagued with unemployment and financial problems, drug and alcohol addiction, divorce, and mental illness. Child batterers are often socially isolated, lacking peers who can suggest ways of handling parenting and disciplinary problems.

Children who are not obviously physically battered, but who show signs of parental neglect and deprivation, are considered to suffer from a maltreatment syndrome. Emotionally and physically deprived infants commonly show signs of failure to thrive (i.e., failure to grow and gain weight at age-appropriate rates), malnutrition, poor hygiene, minor cuts and abrasions, emotional withdrawal, retarded intellectual development, and apathy. These infants often go on to become *psychosocial dwarfs*—children whose physical and intellectual growth has been stunted as a result of chronic parental deprivation.

Physical abuse is often difficult to detect, because children fear retaliation by parents if they report abusive behavior, and because children love and fear the loss of the abusive parent. Battered children are sometimes brought to professionals for medical care with injuries that are the result of "accidents." Physical abuse should be suspected when the parents' history of what happened does not fit with the child's injuries, when families make multiple hospital visits to different hospitals (to avoid discovery of a pattern of injuries), and when parents are reluctant to share information about what happened. Moreover, when physical examination reveals multiple bruises above the waist, and when x-ray studies show multiple old fractures, physical abuse is highly likely.

Sexual abuse is even more difficult to detect than physical abuse. The term "sexual abuse" refers to a variety of situations in which a child under 18 years of age is used for the sexual purposes of another person. This includes any sexual contact with an adult, a significantly older child or adolescent, or involvement of the child in prostitution or pornography. Sexual abuse may occur among children close in age if threats or bribery are used to make a child participate in sexual acts. It most often occurs between fathers or stepfathers and latency age daughters, but it can occur between mothers and sons, fathers and sons, and between adults outside the home and children of either sex. When incest occurs between parent and child, it is usually in the context of a disturbed marital relationship.

Sexually abused children often tell no one of their participation in sexual activities. They usually know that such behavior is wrong even before they have the words to describe it, but they keep silent out of shame, fear, guilt, and a wish to protect the participating adult. No single sign is evidence that a child has been sexually abused. However, the following should lead parents and clinicians to consider the possibility of sexual abuse:

1. Unexplained injuries or pain in the child's genital area, including blood stains in underwear.
2. Sudden changes in behavior, such as fear of a familiar person or place.
3. More general signs of upset, including loss of appetite, nightmares, increased irritability, school difficulties, or abdominal complaints for which no physical cause can be found.

Children often come to the attention of educators and mental health professionals for failing grades or symptoms of depression but with no stated complaints of sexual abuse. A careful and thorough family evaluation, along with the development of a trusting relationship with the child, are essential in uncovering sexual abuse.

Abused children are in great physical and psychological danger, and abuse constitutes an emergency. If the child has any physical complaints, he or she must be given medical attention at once to rule out and treat physical injuries. Physicians and other health care professionals are legally obligated to report instances of abuse and suspected abuse to the relevant child protection agency in the community, and immediate intervention is necessary to ensure that the child comes to no further harm. This often involves removing the child from the home, at least temporarily. Family treatment is essential if the child is to be allowed to return to the home, and foster care is often necessary. Whenever you suspect that a child has been physically or sexually abused, you must be sure that a thorough medical and psychological evaluation is done and that the child's family is involved in exploring the child's current situation. When in doubt, consult a supervisor or someone experienced in working with abused children. Do not leave your suspicions unexplored.

REFERENCES

Achenbach T: The classification of children's psychiatric symptoms: a factor-analytic study. Psychol Monog 80:615, 1966

American Psychiatric Association: Diagnostic and Statistical Manual of Mental Disorders, 3rd ed. Washington, DC, American Psychiatric Association, 1980, pp 35-99

Erickson EH: Childhood and Society. New York, Norton, 1954

Fraiberg S: The Magic Years. New York, Scribner, 1959

Freud A: Normality and Pathology in Childhood: Assessments of Development. New York, International Universities Press, 1965

Johnson AM, Szurek SA: The genesis of antisocial acting out in children and adults. Psychoanal Q 21:323-343, 1952

Lewis M: Clinical Aspects of Child Development, 2nd ed. Philadelphia, Lea and Febiger, 1982

Mahler MS: Symbiosis and individuation: the psychological birth of the human infant. Psychol Study Child 29:89-106, 1974

Mahler MS, Pine F, Bergman A: The Psychological Birth of the Human Infant: Symbiosis and Individuation. New York, Basic Books, 1975

Noshpitz J, Cohen RL (eds): Basic Handbook of Child Psychiatry. New York, Basic Books, 1979

Piaget J: Six Psychological Studies. New York, Vintage, 1967

Rutter M, Hersov L (eds): Child and Adolescent Psychiatry: Modern Approaches, 2nd ed. Oxford, Blackwell Scientific Publications, 1985

Thomas A, Chess S: Genesis and evolution of behavioral disorders: from infancy to early adult life. Am J Psychiatry 141:1-9, 1984

Thomas A, Chess S, Birch H: Temperament and Behavior Disorders in Children. New York, Brunner-Mazel, 1968

Part III

INTRODUCTION

The chapters included in this section cover subjects that every health care professional must understand. They are clinical problems that cross all diagnostic boundaries and often present as manifestations of other medical and psychiatric conditions.

Chapter 11 deals with sexual dysfunctions and deviations—concerns that are often overlooked in diagnostic evaluations. Drug and alcohol abuse is discussed in Chapter 12. Problems of substance abuse have reached epidemic proportions in our society, but they, too, are missed in many medical and mental health assessments. Both of these chapters therefore emphasize diagnosis, with specific techniques for eliciting a history of problems with drugs or sexual functioning.

Suicide and violence are two of the most anxiety-provoking problems you will encounter in your clinical work. Chapters 13 and 14 focus on suicidal and violent clients, respectively, highlighting ways in which you can assess clients' potential for carrying out threats of harming themselves or others and strategies for managing emergency situations.

CHAPTER 11

Human Sexuality: Function and Dysfunction

In our society, mental health professionals are often consulted about sexual problems. Ironically, although they are assumed by many to be experts in this field, they are frequently less knowledgeable about and less comfortable with various aspects of sexual behavior than are some nonprofessionals. As part of your professional training, you must gain some understanding of the broad range of human sexual behaviors, as well as an understanding of your own attitudes toward sex. Such awareness is essential to good clinical work.

TAKING A SEXUAL HISTORY

To learn about the sexual aspects of your clients' lives, you must be comfortable in eliciting such information.

Mental health evaluations and medical histories should routinely include questions that will allow you to establish the client's general attitude toward sex, his or her sexual functioning, and its bearing on important relationships. Sexual functioning should be explored in depth whenever the client's complaints suggest possible sexual difficulties or concerns. Such common complaints as fatigue, headaches, menstrual difficulties, and depression should also alert you to the possibility of underlying sexual dissatisfaction.

When is it best to broach the subject during an interview? Obviously, if the client's chief complaint is of a sexual nature, begin with a sexual history immediately. When this is not the case, it is usually best to wait until you and the client have established some degree of rapport in the interview. A relaxed, matter-of-fact display of interest is most helpful. Ask questions as straightforwardly as possible.

The natural openings for discussion of sexuality are many. People usually talk about romantic relationships or marriages; use this as a point to introduce the topic with a general question, such as, "How has the relationship developed sexually?" or "Can you tell me about your sexual experience with this person?" When a client talks about menstrual functioning, energy level, depression, or other general complaints, you can turn to the subject of sex with a question like, "How does this symptom affect your sexual relationships?" With some clients (e.g., adolescents or severely isolated individuals) who you suspect may have very limited sexual experience, you might begin with a general inquiry, such as, "What have your sexual experiences been like?"

People are commonly concerned that some aspect of their sexuality is abnormal. It will be helpful to frame your questions so that you imply that many people have similar feelings and attitudes. For example, in inquiring about previous homosexual experiences, you might phrase your question as follows: "Many people have sexual experiences with members of the same sex at some point in their lives. Have you had any experiences with other men (or women)?" Or concerning common practices that may be a source of embarrassment, you might word a question as follows, "How old were you when you began masturbating?" rather than "Have you ever masturbated?"

When inquiring about sexuality, take your language cues from the client. This is particularly important in talking with gay and lesbian individuals. If you assume a heterosexual orientation (e.g., asking a man about girlfriends), you may make it more difficult for your client to tell you about homosexual experiences. Thus, when talking about romantic relationships, use neutral terms such as "lover" until your client offers specific names or pronouns that make sexual object choice clear.

Also, be sure to use your client's choice of terms whenever possible to describe sexual experiences and anatomy. Some clients use slang (e.g., "cock" for penis, "screwing" for intercourse), while others would find such terms offensive. Use your judgment, but remember that many words carry different connotations for different people. When in doubt, use the most neutral and widely accepted terms until you develop a common language with your client.

Your Own Attitudes About Sex

Your comfort or discomfort in discussing sexual matters will undoubtedly be communicated to your clients. Many of us were raised in environments in which sex was never discussed, or only mentioned among intimates. It is no small task to learn to speak openly with clients about sexual functioning. You may find that you are embarrassed by or uncomfortable with some of what you encounter as a beginning clinician.

Unresolved conflicts about your own sexual life may hamper your ability to listen and evaluate sensitively. For example, an interviewer who is frightened by his or her own homosexual feelings may have difficulty in evaluating clients' homosexual concerns. Clinicians who believe that sex is "no one else's business" may be reacting to guilt feelings about their own unacknowledged sexual curiosity and may refrain from asking necessary questions. Or such people may overcompensate, asking intrusive and overly detailed questions about matters that are irrelevant to the client's complaints.

Those who are achievement-oriented may tend to think of sex as a performance. Frequency of sexual intercourse, the number of orgasms attained, and the extent of the partner's visible satisfaction during lovemaking are all aspects of sexuality that can come to represent tests of competence. Such notions about sex can greatly distort not only your own sexual experiences, but your understanding of your client's experiences.

Your job is to remain nonjudgmental and professional in your attitude toward your client's sexual life. If you find yourself becoming anxious or imposing your personal values on a client, you must stand back and (with the help of a colleague or supervisor) attempt to understand the source of the problem. Only then will you be able to be effective in helping clients to deal with sexual concerns.

Sample Interview Questions

Proceed from general questions to more specific ones in obtaining a sexual history. The following are suggestions for "openers":

● Tell me about your romantic life.

- How would you describe your sex life at this time?
- Is there anything troubling you about your sex life?
- Have you had any sexual thoughts that concern or disturb you?

The following questions on three more specific areas may help you to focus in on the particular concerns of your client:

Orientation
- Are you primarily attracted to members of the opposite sex? Your own sex? Both men and women?

Current Functioning
- How frequently do you have sexual contact? What does this involve? Are you (or your partner) concerned about the frequency with which you have sex?
- How often do you masturbate?
- What sort of sexual activities have been most satisfying? What sort have been least satisfying?
- Have you had any difficulties in achieving orgasm or in helping your partner to achieve orgasm?
- Are you involved in any sexual activities that worry you or others, or that you must keep secret from others? (See the sexual deviations described later in this chapter.)

History
- What were your parents' attitudes toward sex?
- How would you describe your parents' sexual relationship?
- From whom did you learn about sex?
- Did you have any sexual experiences as a child with older people, such as parents, other adults, siblings, or other children? If so, what were the circumstances?
- Who prepared you for the onset of puberty/menstruation?
- When did you begin masturbating? (Ask about feelings, fantasies.)
- What was your sexual experience like as a teenager? As a young adult?
- How have you felt about yourself as a man/woman?
- Would you say that you are comfortable with yourself as a sexual person?

THE SEXUAL RESPONSE CYCLE

In evaluating your clients' sexual functioning, keep in mind the normal cycle of sexual response. Many texts (e.g., Masters and Johnson

1966) have excellent detailed discussions of this cycle. The brief discussion included here is only meant to provide an introductory overview.

Sexual stimulation produces characteristic responses in men and women that can be conceptualized as a four-phase cycle (Table 11-1). These phases were described by Masters and Johnson in their research on human sexuality and have been useful to clinicians in understanding normal and disturbed sexual functioning.

Table 11-1. The four phases of the sexual response cycle.

Phase I—excitement	Phase III—orgasm
Phase II—plateau	Phase IV—resolution

Phase I: Excitement. Sexual excitement may be brought about by psychological stimulation (through fantasy or by the presence of a desired person), or it may be brought about by physical stimulation (e.g., kissing, caressing). Excitement is characterized by erection of the penis in men and vaginal lubrication in women. Excitement may arise within 10 to 30 seconds after stimulation has begun, and it may last from several minutes to several hours. Another observable physical response in the excitement phase is nipple erection, more common in women than in men. Women also experience thickening of the labia minora and erection of the clitoris due to venous engorgement.

Phase II: Plateau. Continued sexual stimulation brings the individual to the threshold of orgasm, resulting in further physiologic changes and increasing sexual tension in both men and women. In women, the vaginal barrel constricts along the outer third (the orgasmic platform), while the clitoris elevates and retracts behind the symphisis pubis (but may be stimulated indirectly through traction on the labia minora). Breast size increases, and the labia minora become bright or deep red due to venous engorgement. In males, the testes increase in size (up to 50 percent) and are brought up toward the body as the scrotal sac tightens and lifts. Two or three drops of mucoid fluid containing viable sperm are secreted from the penis at this stage, so pregnancy can result from coitus at this stage even if the man withdraws prior to orgasm. In both sexes, heart rate increases, respiration becomes more rapid, elevation of blood pressure is common, and there are voluntary contractions of large skeletal muscle groups. This preorgasmic phase is usually brief, lasting from one-half to three minutes.

Phase III: Orgasm. Increasing sexual tension generally culminates in orgasm, which is experienced as intensely pleasurable. In males, the testes, prostate, and seminal vesicles contract and expel sperm and seminal fluid into the entrance of the urethra. This is followed immediately by three to seven contractions of the urethra and muscles of the penis, ejecting the seminal fluid forcibly through the urethra and out of the penis. In females, orgasms consist of three to 15 involuntary contractions of the lower third of the vagina and strong, sustained contractions of the uterus. Both men and women also have involuntary contractions of the internal and external anal sphincters. In both sexes, muscular contractions during the height of orgasm occur at intervals of 0.8 seconds, and orgasm commonly lasts from three to 15 seconds. Other manifestations of orgasm include voluntary and involuntary movements of large muscle groups (e.g., extension of arms and legs), facial grimacing, and muscular spasm. Blood pressure rises by up to 80 mm systolic and 40 mm diastolic, while heart rate may increase to 180 beats per minute, and respirations up to 40 per minute. Some people also experience a "sex flush," a blotching of the skin in variable patterns on the body that disappears within minutes after orgasm.

Phase IV: Resolution. After orgasm, the resolution phase brings the body back to its resting state by gradual disgorgement of blood from the genitals and a return of these organs to their resting size. If orgasm occurs, resolution is rapid, and may take only 10 to 15 minutes. However, if orgasm does not occur, resolution may take two to six hours (in some cases even up to a day) and may be associated with pelvic discomfort. Resolution after orgasm is characterized by a subjective sense of well-being. For males, there is a refractory period after orgasm in which they cannot be stimulated to another orgasm. This may last from several minutes to several hours. There is no such refractory period in women; they are capable of multiple and successive orgasms.

Female Sexual Response

Most women have certain physical responses in addition to those mentioned above. The female vagina enlarges during sexual excitement and naturally accommodates to the size of the penis (or other object) inserted into it. Lubrication occurs internally, so lubrication of the outer labia must usually be accomplished by manual manipulation or through the thrusting of the penis.

At the moment of orgasm, women have a tendency to increase their pelvic thrusting, while men tend to freeze their thrusting activity. Female orgasm seems to be triggered by stimulation of the clitoris, either directly through masturbation or indirectly, as when the thrusts of the penis cause traction on the labia minora, with resulting stimulation of the attached clitoris. Thus, female orgasm is triggered by clitoral stimulation and manifested by vaginal contractions.

Male Sexual Response

Men tend to show less variation in their sexual response cycles than women do, although there is some variation in the duration of each cycle phase. Men cannot successfully accomplish intercourse without first obtaining an erection that is sufficiently rigid to allow the penis to enter the vagina. Once erection is achieved, it will normally wax and wane if the excitement phase is prolonged; this normal response should not be a cause for concerns about potency.

Men experience two stages of orgasm. The first is a moment of ejaculatory inevitability, when the testes, prostate, and seminal vesicles expel sperm and seminal fluid into the entrance of the urethra. The man "feels the ejaculation coming," and at this point can no longer interrupt the process voluntarily. The second stage is ejaculation, during which the semen is forcibly ejected out of the penis via the urethra. At the moment of orgasm, the man tends to stop his thrusting activity and to hold the ejaculating penis in deep penetration.

Sex and Aging

Some of the most common misconceptions about human sexual response relate to the aging process. As the number of people over age 65 increases in this society, more attention is being focused on all aspects of geriatric life, including sexuality. People vary in their capacity for and interest in an active sexual life beyond middle age. Physical health is important, but—barring major physical illness—other factors seem to loom larger in determining sexual activity in later life— most obviously, the availability of a sexual partner. Also, people who have been sexually active in earlier years are more likely to remain so in later life, as are those who live in an environment that is accepting of their sexuality.

Changes in sexual responsiveness do occur with aging. In aging women, the vasocongestive response is diminished and the elasticity and secretory capacities of the vagina decrease. However, women who continue to have intercourse regularly can minimize these changes and function effectively in spite of them. Aging men take longer to achieve an erection, and erection may be less complete, although adequate for the penis to enter the vagina. The expulsive force of the ejaculation also diminishes, refractory time between orgasms is longer, and greater stimulation is required to achieve erection in the first place. For men, erectile difficulty is the only sexual dysfunction that correlates with advancing age. Some of this erectile failure is psychogenic in origin and can be treated (see below); in other cases, impotence is due to neurologic or vascular disease.

Sexual interest and activity are the rule rather than the exception among people in their fifties and sixties; some people continue to be sexually active even in their eighties. One does not become "used up" sexually; indeed, surveys suggest that a lifelong history of active sexual functioning is a good predictor of sexual activity in old age—"If you use it, you don't lose it."

SEXUAL DISORDERS: DEVIATION VERSUS DYSFUNCTION

Sexual deviations involve a disturbance of sexual *aim*. *Sexual dysfunction* denotes a disturbance of sexual *function*. The difference is thus that deviations are characterized by good and pleasurable sexual functioning, while dysfunctions are not. The sexual deviant's choice of sexual object differs from the norm, and he or she is aroused by stimuli that are not exciting to most people—e.g., a child, an animal, or a shoe. He or she may be excited by bondage or by receiving punishment, by looking at or by exposing the genitals, or by inflicting pain. But arousal and orgasm are physiologically normal and bring the sexual deviant pleasure. Sexual deviations are treated with certain types of behavior and insight-oriented therapy, as discussed below.

Sexual dysfunctions are psychosomatic disorders that make it impossible for the person to enjoy sex or, in some cases, to have sex at all. They involve inhibition of normal physiologic responses—i.e., venous engorgement of the sexual organs, the orgasmic response itself, or both—that makes the experience of sexual activity in some way unpleasurable. Sexual dysfunctions are quite common, and they respond to particular types of sex therapy and to a combination of sex therapy and insight-oriented psychotherapy.

You will encounter clients with sexual dysfunctions in any setting in which you practice, and you are likely to encounter sexual deviations as well. Your receptivity to hearing about such issues, and your awareness of the possibilities for treating these disorders, can be crucial to helping people who are often confused and embarrassed about problems they do not understand.

Table 11–2. Types of female sexual dysfunction.

Type	Definition
General sexual dysfunction	Inability to derive erotic pleasure from sexual stimulation
Orgastic dysfunction	Specific difficulty in reaching orgasm
Primary	Never experienced orgasm by any means of stimulation
Secondary	Experienced orgasm but subsequently developed this difficulty
Vaginismus	Impenetrability of the vagina because of involuntary spasm of the vaginal muscles
Dyspareunia	Pain on intercourse

Female Sexual Dysfunction

The various types of female sexual dysfunction are listed in Table 11-2.

General sexual dysfunction (frigidity). General sexual dysfunction is commonly called *frigidity,* but this is a nonspecific term that carries a pejorative connotation. General sexual dysfunction refers to an inability to derive erotic pleasure from sexual stimulation. Women with this disorder may show little or no physiologic response to sexual stimulation (e.g., no vasocongestion or vaginal lubrication), and they may experience themselves as essentially devoid of sexual feelings. Many of these women consider sexual activity an ordeal that they must endure to preserve a relationship, or sex may be so repugnant to them that any activity is impossible. Some women with this disorder are able to enjoy the nonerotic aspects of sexual contact (e.g., touching, physical closeness), despite their lack of sexual responsiveness. Among the factors that seem to foster general sexual dysfunction are strict parental prohibitions against sexual expression in early life, overwhelming anxiety rooted in childhood conflicts or in current concerns, and hostility directed at, but not directly expressed to, the partner or men in general.

Orgastic dysfunction. Orgastic dysfunction is a more limited disorder that denotes a specific difficulty in reaching orgasm. Women who suffer from this disorder frequently have a strong sexual drive and may reach high levels of sexual arousal. The disorder is termed *primary orgastic dysfunction* if the woman has never experienced orgasm by any means of stimulation, and *secondary orgastic dysfunction* if she previously experienced orgasm and subsequently developed this difficulty. The difficulty in reaching orgasm may be present regardless of the setting, or it may depend on the situation—e.g., some women can have orgasms with masturbation but not during coitus, while for others the situation is reversed. Some women rarely have orgasms with any partner and are surprised when they do, while others only experience difficulty with a particular partner. The diagnosis of a disorder is not always easy, since female response varies greatly. Failure to ever have an orgasm constitutes a disorder in almost all cases. However, not reaching orgasm during coitus (but being able to have orgasms during masturbation) is not necessarily a disorder but may be a normal variation of female functioning.

Women differ greatly in their thresholds for reaching orgasm and require varying amounts of clitoral stimulation, probably due to a combination of physiologic and psychological factors. Coitus actually provides only mild clitoral stimulation (compared with masturbation and other more direct techniques), so only women who can be orgasmic with relatively mild stimulation will have orgasms in this way.

In this and other situation-specific cases, the diagnosis of a disorder depends to a large extent on whether the client (and/or her partner) is disturbed by the problem and feels the need for treatment. If not, there is no reason to label the inability to reach orgasm during coitus "disordered." Many women are satisfied with other means of reaching orgasm and do not seek treatment.

Orgastic dysfunction is the most common complaint among women who do seek treatment for a sexual disorder. When a woman wants to have orgasms and cannot, the cause is often her involuntary inhibition of the response. She may unwittingly do this because the orgasm has acquired some symbolic meaning (e.g., losing control), because its intensity frightens her, because she is in conflict over her erotic feelings, or because she is uncertain about her commitment to her mate or even hostile toward her mate.

Vaginismus. Vaginismus refers to a very specific syndrome in which penetration of the vagina is impossible because of involuntary spasm of the muscles surrounding the vaginal entrance. Whenever penetration is attempted, the vaginal entrance literally snaps shut, so that coitus cannot take place. Even pelvic examinations must often be carried out under anesthesia. In addition to primary spasm of the sphincter vaginae and levator ani muscles, vaginismus may also involve a phobia of coitus and vaginal penetration that prompts avoidance of any situation in which coitus might occur. Some women with this disorder are quite sexually responsive as long as sexual contact does not lead to intercourse.

The diagnosis of vaginismus is made relatively rarely and can only be made definitely when involuntary spasm is noted on pelvic examination. Among the factors that seem to be associated with this disorder are a history of sexual trauma, stern parental prohibitions against sexuality, confusion about choice of sexual object, and a partner's sexual dysfunction (particularly primary impotence).

Dyspareunia. Dyspareunia refers to pain in the genital area during coitus. While it occurs occasionally in men, it is more common in women. Obviously, there are numerous physical causes of pain on intercourse (e.g., in various medical conditions and after surgical procedures), but *functional dyspareunia* refers to pain with no demonstrable physical cause. It is essentially a somatoform disorder (see Chapter 8) and is thought to be due to underlying fears of or conflicts over sexual activity.

Male Sexual Dysfunction

The various types of male sexual dysfunction are listed in Table 11-3.

Impotence (erectile dysfunction). Because a great deal of male self-esteem is invested in the capacity for penile erection, there is probably no other physical condition that is as potentially frustrating or humiliating for a man. Impotence is simply an impairment of penile erection, due to failure of the vascular reflex mechanism to pump

Table 11–3. Types of male sexual dysfunction.

Type	Impairment
Impotence (erectile dysfunction)	Impairment of penile erection that is recurrent and persistent
Primary	Never potent with a partner
Secondary	Potent in the past but subsequently developed erectile dysfunction
Premature ejaculation	Inability to exert voluntary control over the ejaculatory reflex
Retarded ejaculation	Inhibition of the ejaculatory reflex
Primary	Never ejaculated with a partner
Secondary	Ejaculated normally in the past but subsequently developed this difficulty

sufficient blood into the cavernous sinuses of the penis to render it firm. Probably more than half of the male population has experienced occasional transient episodes of impotence, and these episodes are within the limits of normal sexual behavior.

The diagnosis of impotence is made when erectile dysfunction is recurrent and persistent. Men with primary impotence have never been potent with a partner, although they may have full erections when masturbating and may have spontaneous erections. Secondary impotence describes a condition in which a man has functioned well in the past but at some point developed erectile dysfunction. The impotent man may feel aroused and excited in a sexual situation and want to make love, and may even ejaculate, but his penis remains flaccid.

Psychological factors play a crucial role in an overwhelming majority of cases of impotence. Erectile function is impaired in most men when they become anxious. Thus, normal sexual functioning usually occurs only when the man does not feel threatened. There are great variations in the patterns of impotence among men with this complaint, because the precise aspect of the sexual act that arouses anxiety differs. Some men are impotent only upon entering the vagina. Some are impotent with one partner but not another, or are only impotent when they feel the expectation to perform. The source of anxiety may be in the man's current life, or it may stem from early childhood fears and experiences.

Why are some men more prone than others to become impotent when they are anxious? Some clinicians postulate that certain men have a physiologic vulnerability to erectile dysfunction (perhaps because of a highly reactive vasocongestive system) while others do not.

There are numerous medical conditions that can cause impotence. Although these are much less common than psychological factors, they must not be overlooked; any man who complains of impotence should have a medical and neurological work-up in addition to a psychological evaluation. Among the most prevalent somatic causes of impotence are fatigue, early undiagnosed diabetes mellitis, low androgen levels, thyroid disease, kidney disease, liver disease, nonspecific debilitating illness, heart or respiratory illness, and abuse of narcotics, alcohol, or estrogenic and parasympatholytic medications. Neurological diseases that can produce impotence include multiple sclerosis, lower spinal cord damage, and damage to the hypothalamic and temporal lobe regions of the brain.

Premature ejaculation. This is a condition in which the man is unable to exert voluntary control over his ejaculatory reflex, so that when he is sexually aroused, he reaches orgasm more quickly than he and/or his partner would like. Men who suffer from premature ejaculation cannot tolerate high levels of sexual tension and stimulation without ejaculating, and their partners are often left unsatisfied when orgasm occurs too soon and lovemaking ceases. The premature ejaculator may become anxious about reaching orgasm too soon and begin to avoid sexual activity so as not to face the difficulty.

When is ejaculation premature? The definition has been difficult, for no one criterion seems to suffice. The number of thrusts a man can tolerate before ejaculating, the number of seconds of coitus he can endure before ejaculation, and the satisfaction of his partner have all been put forward as criteria for the diagnosis, but all are relative and arbitrary. In fact, the crucial aspect seems to be the man's inability to voluntarily control his ejaculatory reflex, regardless of how many seconds have passed or how many thrusts he has made, and regardless of whether his partner has reached orgasm. The rapidity of orgasm is the primary complaint, but many premature ejaculators also have diminished perceptions of their erotic sensations as they become intensely aroused and therefore are not aware when orgasm is imminent.

Many psychological theories have been put forward to explain the causes of premature ejaculation. Covert hostility toward women has been proposed by traditional psychoanalytic theorists, but it has become clear that the determinants of this disorder are more varied and complex. Many men with this disorder have otherwise good and satisfying relationships with wives or lovers. Other clinicians postulate that early hurried sexual experiences (e.g., with prostitutes, or in the back seats of automobiles) play a role. However, many men with a history of such experiences do not go on to develop this disorder.

Clearly, anxiety plays a role in premature ejaculation, since it does not allow the man to perceive erotic sensations correctly. Also, marital difficulties and underlying psychiatric illness have been implicated in some, but not all, cases of premature ejaculation. Among the factors that do not seem to play a role are masturbatory practices and familial patterns.

Premature ejaculation is very rarely caused by physical factors. Among the physical conditions that may contribute to premature ejaculation are local disease of the posterior urethra (e.g., inflammation of the prostate), spinal cord injuries, multiple sclerosis, and other degenerative neurologic disorders.

Retarded ejaculation. In this disorder (also called *ejaculatory incompetence*), the ejaculatory reflex is inhibited, although erection is usually not impaired. This may be primary, if the man has never ejaculated with a partner, or secondary, if the condition arose after an initial period of adequate functioning. The disorder may be so severe that the man cannot ejaculate when masturbating by himself, but in most cases extravaginal ejaculation is possible. This disorder may prompt the man to prolong intercourse for a very long period (e.g., more than an hour) or to fake orgasms with his partner and then either remain frustrated or achieve release only through masturbation following intercourse.

The causes of this disorder are rarely physical. Among the somatic illnesses that occasionally play a role are depressed androgen levels, undetected diabetes, spinal cord injuries, and drugs that impair the adrenergic mechanism of the sympathetic nervous system, which controls ejaculation (e.g., certain antihypertensive drugs). Thioridazine (Mellaril) can cause retrograde ejaculation, that is, ejaculation which forces semen up the urethra into the bladder rather than out of the penis. As this is painful, physicians must keep this side effect in mind when choosing an antipsychotic drug for males.

The most commonly reported psychological factors that seem to underlie ejaculatory incompetence include a strict upbringing that engenders sexual guilt, strongly suppressed anger, ambivalence toward a partner, fears of abandonment by a lover, or childhood fears of parental retaliation for sexual urges.

TREATMENT OF SEXUAL DYSFUNCTION

Whenever a client presents a sexual complaint, you should proceed with a thorough work-up to determine which type of therapy is indicated. Some people present with complaints of sexual dysfunction but, in the course of giving you a psychiatric history, will reveal serious psychopathology (e.g., depression or psychosis) that requires treatment before sexual concerns can be addressed. In addition to a careful psychological evaluation, be sure that a thorough medical evaluation is carried out, including a medical history and physical examination and, where indicated, a neurologic, urologic, or gynecologic examination and appropriate laboratory studies.

Once you have ruled out organic pathology and serious psychopathology, you have a variety of treatment modalities from which to choose.

Dual-Sex Therapy (Masters and Johnson Techniques)

The new sex therapy originated with the work of William H. Masters and Virginia E. Johnson. This type of therapy relies on behavioral techniques and makes the couple, rather than the dysfunctional individual, the focus of therapy. This is based on the premise that there is no such thing as a partner who is uninvolved in the sexual problem, nor is there one "sick half" in a couple. Both people are expected to participate fully in the therapy and to learn to focus on their own sexual feelings and desires, as well as to learn those of their partner and to improve communication within the dyad.

Treatment is based on the observation that performance anxiety and demands for sexual performance intensify and perpetuate sexual dysfunction. Led by a man-woman team of cotherapists, sessions focus on correcting misinformation or ignorance about sexual functioning, providing support and reassurance, improving communication, and removing the demand to perform sexually.

After a thorough evaluation of the couple, sessions begin with "homework assignments"—exercises that the couple carries out in private. All sexual activity, including intercourse, is prohibited until the therapists feel that the couple is ready. This enforced abstinence is the first step in removing the pressure for sexual performance. The first exercises are *sensate focus* exercises, designed to increase sensory awareness of oneself and one's partner. Each partner takes turns "pleasuring" the other, first touching all areas except breasts and genitals, and later including these areas.

Sessions focus on the couple's experiences in carrying out the exercises—these provide crucial information to the therapists about where there is resistance to sexual activity (e.g., the man who is always too tired to do the exercises or the woman who develops a headache whenever exercises are initiated). Fears and misunderstandings can be clarified in the therapy sessions, and the exercises are repeated until they are pleasurable for both partners. Once this pleasuring is mastered, couples are usually communicating with each other more effectively than when they began treatment, and the sessions move on to specific exercises directed at the particular dysfunction.

General sexual dysfunction is treated with sensate focus experiences to help the woman focus on erotic sensations, followed by genital stimulation by herself and with her partner. Intercourse is initiated when she chooses to do so, and with no pressure to achieve orgasm. As she feels more secure in experiencing sexual feelings with her partner, the woman who suffers from this disorder is likely to be able to achieve considerable pleasure and even orgasm during sexual activity.

Organic dysfunction is treated with exercises that heighten the woman's arousal prior to coitus, to increase her awareness of and pleasure in her vaginal sensations, and to maximize clitoral stimulation. This is done by using masturbatory techniques (and in some cases a vibrator), as well as teaching specific coital positions in which the partner can maximally stimulate the woman. All this is done in situations in which the pressure on the woman to reach orgasm is minimized.

Vaginismus is treated by teaching the woman and her partner to use fingers to gently dilate the vaginal opening, and then to use mechanical dilators to accomplish the same purpose. Once vaginal dilation has been comfortably accomplished by these means, it is usually possible for the male to insert his penis into the vagina easily and without discomfort to his partner.

Premature ejaculation has been very successfully treated by using exercises that repeatedly stimulate the man to the point of near ejaculatory inevitability and then cease stimulation before inevitability occurs, thereby preventing ejaculation (the "stop-and-go" technique). This allows the man to experience intense sexual excitement repeatedly without ejaculating. This technique is accompanied by the forcible prevention of orgasm, when "it is imminent," by using the "squeeze" technique, which involves squeezing the head of the penis with the thumb and the first and second fingers. The squeeze technique has had almost universal success in treating premature ejaculation.

Ejaculatory incompetence is dealt with in the opposite manner. Exercises are aimed at achieving intravaginal ejaculation, since in most cases ejaculation during masturbation is not impaired. The woman stimulates the man manually to orgasm in her presence, with the penis in gradually closer proximity to the vaginal opening. Eventually, she stimulates her partner to the point of ejaculatory inevitability and inserts the penis into her vagina without interrupting the ejaculation process. A single episode of intravaginal ejaculation often breaks the male's block against intravaginal ejaculation.

Impotence has been alleviated by creating nondemanding sexual situations in which the man can experience erections without the pressure to have intercourse. Exercises include masturbation, stimulation of the penis to erection by the partner, and gradual introduction of the penis into the vagina by the partner in the woman-on-top position. Even when the penis is inserted into the vagina, no thrusting is allowed at first, or only minimal movements to maintain the penis in a stimulated state. Thrusting is allowed in subsequent exercises, and orgasm naturally ensues. Relieved of the demand to perform, the man who can gradually achieve erections and achieve vaginal penetration usually proceeds at his own pace to have effective coitus.

Masters and Johnson have reported high rates of success for these treatment approaches, with an overall rate of 80 percent success for all dysfunctions combined. They report the greatest success with premature ejaculation (97 percent) and the most limited success with primary impotence (59 percent). Although some critics argue that results are temporary, these behavioral techniques have proved valuable in the treatment of sexual dysfunction.

Psychodynamically Oriented Sex Therapy

Combining psychodynamic psychotherapy and sex therapy enables clinicians to treat people whose sexual complaints are associated with other mental disorders. This therapy may continue for longer than the usual 10-15 sessions involved in sex therapy alone, and it may involve individual work with each partner as well as work with the couple. This approach is particularly useful for couples who have difficulties in their relationship that clearly extend beyond the realm of sex. Couples are given "homework assignments" as described above, but sessions also focus more intensively on the psychological conflicts and distortions that hamper the relationship—often problems that originated for each partner in early childhood relationships.

When one partner is more obviously in need of psychological support and help than the other, individual sessions can be tailored to that person's needs and carried out in addition to the couple's therapy sessions. For example, if a woman who complains of general sexual dysfunction discovers in couples therapy that she harbors deeply rooted hostility toward men, she may want to work with the therapist individually to understand more about the origins of this anger, while continuing in joint meetings to explore the ways in which she unwittingly distances her husband.

The combination of psychodynamic and sex therapy is commonly used in general mental health facilities, while sex therapy alone is often used in clinics that limit their work to the treatment of sexual dysfunctions.

Hypnotherapy

Some clinicians have found hypnotic suggestions useful in alleviating anxiety (e.g., in a man with secondary impotence) and in removing psychological impediments to vaginal lubrication, erections, and orgasm. This is not a couple's approach, and is aimed at specific symptoms rather than an individual's general ability to experience and communicate his or her sexual feelings in a relationship.

Behavior Therapy

Behavior therapy was initially developed to treat phobias, but the technique of systematic desensitization has also been applied to sexual situations that arouse anxiety (see Chapter 15). The client identifies situations that arouse anxiety and foster symptoms (e.g., when vaginal penetration results in impotence), and the therapist gradually desensitizes the client to these anxiety-provoking situations. Like hypnotherapy, this approach is generally for individuals rather than couples.

Group Therapy

Groups have been useful in treating people with sexual dysfunction, since they can impart sexual information, provide reassurance, and offer mutual support to people who suffer from similar difficulties. Some groups consist of people of one sex who have the same disorder; others are composed of couples. Groups are particularly useful for people who need to explore interpersonal difficulties, as well as specific sexual problems.

Individual Psychotherapy

Classical psychodynamic theory holds that sexual dysfunctions have their roots in early childhood experiences and conflicts that therapy can help to elucidate. When irrational fears and fantasies are brought to light and understood, the symptoms of sexual dysfunction often lessen. However, the psychodynamic approach is less effective than the behavioral approach of Masters and Johnson in rapidly removing specific sexual symptoms. Individual psychotherapy is most useful for people whose sexual dysfunction is part of a larger constellation of psychological difficulties and who have other symptoms for which psychotherapy is indicated.

SEXUAL DEVIATIONS

Sexual deviations (also called *perversions* and *paraphilias*) are disorders that involve unusual sexual-object choices or sexual acts (Table 11-4). The person who suffers from a perversion generally requires these specific acts or objects or images in order to be sexually aroused and to achieve orgasm. He or she must repeatedly recreate the needed situation or fantasy. Perversions most often involve one of the following: the use of a nonhuman object for sexual arousal (excluding vibrators and other objects designed for that purpose), the experience

Table 11–4. Types of sexual deviations.

Type	Definition
Transsexualism	Persistent sense of discomfort about one's anatomic sex and strong desire to change one's genitals and secondary sex characteristics
Transvestitism	Dressing in clothes appropriate to the opposite sex for purposes of arousal
Fetishism	Use of a nonhuman object as the preferred method of achieving sexual excitement
Zoophilia	Repeated sexual arousal through contact with an animal
Pedophilia	Sexual contact with prepubertal children as the preferred means to sexual excitement
Exhibitionism	Exposure of the genitals in public to unsuspecting strangers to achieve sexual excitement
Voyeurism	Repeatedly looking at unsuspecting people who are disrobing or engaging in sexual activity
Sexual masochism	Obtaining sexual gratification through mental suffering or bodily pain
Sexual sadism	Inflicting physical or psychological pain on another to achieve sexual excitement

of suffering on the part of the individual or of his or her partner, or sexual activity with a nonconsenting partner.

Many people with perversions do not regard themselves as ill and only come to mental health facilities for help when their behavior has brought them into conflict with society (e.g., with their families or with the law). People with sexual perversions are grossly impaired in their ability to participate in mutually gratifying sexual relations with consenting adults, and marital difficulties are common.

Perversions are much more common in men than in women, but the reasons for this are not clear. Environmental factors (particularly early childhood experiences) appear to play a major role in the genesis of sexual perversions, and sons often develop the specific perversions of their fathers. Since these disorders are relatively uncommon, they will be discussed only briefly.

Transsexualism

This disorder involves a persistent sense of discomfort and inappropriateness about one's anatomic sex and a wish to change one's genitals and secondary sex characteristics in order to live as a member of the opposite sex. Transsexualism must be distinguished from transvestism and homosexuality (see below), neither of which necessarily involves a desire to change one's sexual anatomy. Cross-dressing and homosexual behavior are common among transsexuals, but the eventual goal for these people is often surgical and hormonal treatment leading to reassignment of gender. Surgical procedures to change external anatomy from male to female are more common than the reverse procedure.

Transsexualism is often associated with moderate to severe personality disturbance. Surgical correction does not bring about a satisfactory sexual adjustment for some transsexuals, and depression and suicide attempts are frequent complications of this disorder. Thus, careful and detailed psychiatric evaluation must be a prerequisite to surgical procedures for anyone wishing to change his or her sex.

Transvestism

Transvestism involves dressing in clothing appropriate to members of the opposite sex for purposes of arousal and as an adjunct to masturbation or coitus. This generally occurs among *heterosexual* males and may range from occasional cross-dressing to intense involvement in an elaborate transvestite subculture. When not cross-dressed, the transvestite usually appears and acts masculine. Homosexual experiences are reported in this population, but sexual preference is generally for members of the opposite sex. Cross-dressing often begins in adolescence, but may start earlier, and it is often used to alleviate anxiety in addition to providing erotic stimulation. Transvestism must be distinguished from cross-dressing by homosexuals, which is often carried out in order to attract homosexual partners, and from transsexualism, which involves a conscious desire to change one's anatomy in order to become a member of the opposite sex.

Fetishism

Fetishism involves the use of a nonhuman object as the preferred (or only) method of achieving sexual excitement. These objects tend to be shoes, undergarments, gloves, or other items of apparel closely associated with the human body. Fetishes may also involve body parts (e.g., feet, hair) rather than inanimate objects. The object may be the sole focus of sexual activity (e.g., masturbation into a shoe) or may be integrated into sexual activity with a partner (e.g., the demand that the partner wear high-heeled shoes).

The fetish differs from simple experimentation to achieve sexual arousal, since people with true fetishes require the presence of a specific object (at least in fantasy) for arousal to occur, and the object is preferred over human beings. The desired object is usually linked to someone important from the individual's childhood and serves to help maintain some special relationship in fantasy with that person.

Zoophilia

Zoophilia involves repeated sexual arousal through contact with an animal. Sexual contact with animals (masturbation or coitus) is not uncommon among adolescents, particularly those raised in rural settings. However, true zoophilia involves preference for sexual contact with an animal even when other sexual outlets are possible.

Pedophilia

Pedophilia involves sexual contact with prepubertal children as the preferred or only means of achieving sexual excitement. Pedophiles tend to fall into two distinct groups: those who choose children of the opposite sex (heterosexual pedophiles) and those who choose children of the same sex (homosexual pedophiles). Virtually all pedophiles who come to the attention of mental health professionals are men.

Heterosexual pedophiles tend to be socially maladjusted men, often alcoholics with troubled marriages. The incidence of heterosexual pedophilia peaks among late adolescent boys and among men in their forties and sixties. They generally prefer to engage in sexual activity with eight- to 10-year-old girls.

Homosexual pedophiles tend to be men who have never married, and they tend to prefer prepubertal or pubescent boys as the objects of sexual activity. Many of these men were themselves sexually abused by older men when they were children.

There are few reliable statistics on the relative incidences of homosexual and heterosexual pedophilia, but a great majority of incidents (some estimates are as high as 90 percent) are perpetrated by heterosexual men. Especially common is sexual activity between fathers (or stepfathers) and their preadolescent or early adolescent daughters. Thus, contrary to popular myth, homosexual men do not pose the most significant sexual threat to children in our society.

Exhibitionism

Exhibitionism involves exposure of the genitals in public to unsuspecting strangers as a means of achieving sexual excitement, with no attempt at further sexual activity with these strangers. The exhibitionist is usually aware of the desire to shock observers. Exhibitionists are exclusively men, and they generally expose themselves to women and girls. They may begin this practice at any time after the onset of puberty, but the disorder most commonly begins in the mid-twenties. These men are frequently arrested for their behavior, but they generally do not constitute a danger to those to whom they expose themselves.

Voyeurism

Voyeurism involves repeatedly looking at unsuspecting people (usually strangers) who are disrobing or engaging in sexual activity. This activity is the voyeur's preferred means of achieving sexual excitement. No sexual activity with the person is sought, but the voyeur often achieves orgasm through masturbation during the voyeuristic activity or afterwards, while recalling the activity. Such people (usually men) are usually isolated, withdrawn individuals who prowl neighborhoods looking for opportunities to "peep." This behavior often gets the voyeur into minor legal difficulties.

Voyeurism differs from sexual excitement achieved by watching a partner undress, or by viewing pornography, in that sexual partners and pornographic entertainers are willing participants and are aware of being watched.

Sexual Masochism

Masochism consists of sexual gratification obtained through mental suffering or bodily pain. The individual prefers to be excited or can only be excited by being bound, beaten, humiliated, or tortured. The diagnosis is made on the basis of one or more episodes in which an individual achieves excitement through suffering. Masochistic sexual behavior occurs among heterosexuals and homosexuals. It may begin at any time but most commonly begins in early adulthood. It may be quite dangerous, particularly if the individual must engage in increasingly harmful activities in order to be aroused. Permanent bodily injury, castration, and even death may result from such activity. Masochistic individuals often engage in sadistic sexual practices as well. Sexual masochism is distinct from masochistic personality in that masochistic personality traits are not associated with conscious sexual excitement.

Sexual Sadism

Sexual sadism involves inflicting physical or psychological pain on another person as a means of achieving sexual excitement. The partner may be consenting or nonconsenting, and this mode of sexual arousal is both repeated and preferred over others. Sexual sadism occurs among both heterosexuals and homosexuals and most commonly begins in early adulthood. The harm inflicted on a partner may be mild and may not escalate over time, or harm may be quite severe and result in death or permanent disability or disfigurement of the victim. Severe sadistic practices can result in legal action and imprisonment. Sexual sadists sometimes engage in masochistic activities as well.

Treatment of Sexual Deviations

Sexual deviations are thought to be psychologically based and rooted in early childhood experiences. Thus, many clinicians have found psychotherapy to be the treatment of choice in these disorders. Psychoanalysis attempts to elicit and resolve early childhood conflicts that are responsible for the perversion, but many disturbed people (e.g., those with severe personality disorders or psychoses) cannot tolerate such intense treatment. Individual psychotherapy can be useful to help clients identify the feelings and fantasies that prompt deviant sexual behavior, to help them find more acceptable means of obtaining sexual gratification, and to help them diminish the extent to which perverse behaviors interfere with other aspects of their lives.

Antiandrogen agents such as medroxyprogesterone (Depo-provera) have been used in men with sexually hyperactive perversions (e.g., in those who are involved in compulsive sexual assaults) to decrease sexual activity and thereby decrease dangerousness to self and others.

HOMOSEXUALITY

Imagine a textbook discussion of heterosexuality as a clinical entity. Most of us take heterosexuality for granted in our dealings with other people; it is considered the norm. Yet a large portion of the population consists of men and women who prefer same-sex partners for sexual activity. You undoubtedly have encountered and will continue to encounter gay people in your personal and professional life. Whether your gay friends, colleagues, and clients feel they can tell you about their sexual orientation will depend in large part on your sensitivity and receptivity to nonheterosexual orientation and life-styles.

It has been said that the world's population of gay people have about as much in common as do the world's population of coffee drinkers. There is tremendous diversity in personality traits, life-styles, and sexual practices among people whose primary orientation is homosexual. It is difficult even to define the gay population. How would one classify the many people who are heterosexual in practice and homosexual in fantasy, or those who are sexually active with both men and women, or others who make abrupt mid-life changes in their sexual-object choices?

Prevalence

Homosexual behavior occurs in virtually all societies. The prevalence of homosexuality is difficult to determine, in part because of problems in defining what constitutes homosexuality and in part because much homosexuality goes unreported owing to societal prejudices and pressures against open disclosure of a homosexual orientation. The best data probably remain those of Kinsey and his coworkers, who in their 1948 and 1953 studies of sexual behavior in men and women interviewed more than 11,000 men and nearly 8,000 women. Kinsey found that 4 percent of men were exclusively homosexual throughout their adult lives, while another 13 percent were predominantly homosexual for at least three years between the ages of 16 and 55. Most surprising to the American public was the disclosure that 37 percent of the men in Kinsey's sample reported at least one sexual experience with another man leading to orgasm during their postpubertal years. His findings showed the prevalence of homosexuality among women to be roughly one-third that found among men. About 28 percent of the women in his sample reported some homosexual experience or arousal at some time from the onset of puberty, with 13 percent experiencing associated orgasm. He estimated the prevalence of exclusive homosexuality among women in his sample to be between one-half and one-third of that among men.

Causes

Why do some people grow up with a heterosexual orientation and others with a homosexual one? There are no clear-cut answers. In attempting to elucidate the causes of homosexuality, researchers have explored a variety of psychological and biological hypotheses.

Traditional psychoanalytic theory views homosexuality as an arrest of psychosexual development. For men, the disturbance is thought to result from early childhood experiences with a close-binding, intimate mother and a passive, hostile, or absent father. For women, no such clear-cut family pattern has been hypothesized, but traditional theorists believe that female homosexuality involves unresolved developmental difficulties. These psychoanalytic hypotheses have not been consistently validated in clinical studies of gay men and women. And this research is significantly flawed, for most of it has been conducted by using populations of gays who have consulted a psychiatrist for emotional difficulties, thus biasing the sample toward those who are psychologically troubled.

Genetic theories of the origins of homosexuality have been supported by twin studies that show a substantially higher rate of concordance for homosexuality among monozygotic (identical) than among dizygotic (fraternal) pairs of twins. However, some cases of discordance among identical twins have been reported, and studies of twins reared together versus those reared apart (which would better separate genetic from environmental factors) have yet to be carried out. Thus far, it has been impossible to prove or disprove that genetic factors play a role in homosexual orientation.

Neuroendocrine studies of possible causes of homosexuality have focused on the hypothalamus and the pituitary gland. Studies of serum testosterone levels have not consistently shown differences between homosexual and heterosexual populations. However, new research is focused on the hypothesis that variations in sex hormone levels in the uterus may program the developing fetus for a heterosexual or homosexual orientation. To date, no conclusive data have emerged from this research.

In summary, the numerous theories about psychological and biological causes of homosexuality remain unproven. It is likely that both developmental and biological factors play a role in the genesis of homosexuality, as they do in the genesis of heterosexuality.

Life-Style

Much publicity has been given to the gay life-style, which stereotypically involves frequent anonymous sexual contacts and little sustained emotional attachment. The subculture of gay bars and baths that facilitates such impersonal contacts has come increasingly into the public eye in recent years, as homosexuality has been more openly discussed. To be sure, such stereotypes do hold for some gay people, more commonly for men than for women. However, the pattern of frequent anonymous sexual contacts is typical of only one subset of the gay population; those who are involved in stable, intimate relationships are often less visible.

Some clinicians cite fleeting relationships as evidence that gay men in particular cannot sustain intimate emotional ties; others argue that our society provides no social supports that encourage gay people to form lasting relationships in the way that the institution of marriage is socially sanctioned. It is also true that, as the divorce rate climbs to nearly 50 percent and singles bars become a more prominent part of heterosexual culture, heterosexuals and homosexuals come to look increasingly similar with respect to the frequency with which they sustain intimate relationships. In dealing with either heterosexual or homosexual clients, you must never make assumptions about life-style or sexual behavior; wait until your client shares that information with you.

Psychopathology

There continues to be considerable controversy within our society and within the mental health profession about whether homosexuality per se is a mental disorder. Although Freud did not believe it to be so, many later psychiatrists have adhered to the notion that homosexuality is pathological. Recent studies of large nonpatient populations of heterosexuals and homosexuals do not support the thesis that homosexuality is associated with pathological personality traits or increased emotional distress or social dysfunction. Thus, the American Psychiatric Association has removed homosexuality from its *Diagnostic and Statistical Manual of Mental Disorders* as of the third edition (*DSM-III*).

Obviously, the range of psychopathology found among homosexuals is as broad as that found among heterosexuals. But homosexuality per se is only cited as a disorder in *DSM-III* when it is ego-dystonic—i.e., when an individual strongly desires to change his or her homosexual orientation to a heterosexual one in order to lead a heterosexual life-style.

Treatment

Many different treatments have been employed to help people who want to change their homosexual orientation. Psychotherapy, psychoanalysis, and behavior therapy have been the modalities most commonly employed, and all have met with limited success. Some clinicians estimate that one-third of gay men who enter treatment with this goal in mind achieve a heterosexual orientation through therapy. However, others are more pessimistic about the possibility of achieving a lasting reorientation of sexual preference through any form of treatment. For men, factors reported to weigh in favor of achieving a heterosexual reorientation include youthfulness (under 35), some experience of heterosexual arousal, and high motivation. Few data are available for homosexual women.

Many gay people who are troubled by their sexual orientation have been treated at counseling centers that do not aim to change one's sexual perference, but instead direct treatment interventions toward enabling the person to be more comfortable with a gay life-style—decreasing the shame, guilt, and anxiety that are too often associated with homosexuality.

Advice to Mental Health Professionals

Unfortunately, many health care professionals are either insensitive or openly hostile to the concerns of those with a bisexual or homosexual orientation. You can do a great service to all of your clients by paying attention to some simple interviewing techniques:

- Do not assume that you know your client's sexual orientation until you are told.
- Do not assume that you understand your client's sexual practices or life-style until he or she tells you.
- Do not assume that a client who is homosexual is troubled by his or her sexual orientation.
- When you are taking a sexual history, use neutral terms like "lover" and "relationship" until your client tells you whether sexual relationships have been with men or women or both.
- Use your client's words for his or her sexual behavior—some people call themselves "homosexual," but for others this term carries negative connotations and "gay" is more comfortable.

REFERENCES

American Psychiatric Association: Diagnostic and Statistical Manual of Mental Disorders, 3rd ed. Washington, DC, American Psychiatric Association, 1980

Freund K: Should homosexuality arouse therapeutic concern? J Homosexuality 2:235-240, 1977

Group for the Advancement of Psychiatry: Assessment of Sexual Function: A Guide to Interviewing [Vol 8, Report 88]. New York, GAP Publications, 1973

Hetrick ES, Stein TS (eds): Innovations in Psychotherapy with Homosexuals. Washington, DC, American Psychiatric Press, 1984

Kaplan HS: Disorders of Sexual Desire and Other New Concepts and Techniques in Sex Therapy. New York, Brunner/Mazel, 1979

Kaplan HS: The New Sex Therapy. New York, Brunner/Mazel, 1974

Kaplan HS (ed): Comprehensive Evaluation of Disorders of Sexual Desire. Washington, DC, American Psychiatric Press, 1985

Kinsey AC, Pomeroy WB, Martin CE: Sexual Behavior in the Human Male. Philadelphia, WB Saunders, 1948

Kinsey AC, Pomeroy WB, Martin CE, et al: Sexual Behavior in the Human Female. Philadelphia, WB Saunders, 1953

Masters WH, Johnson VE: Human Sexual Response. Boston, Little, Brown, 1966

Meyer JK: Paraphilias, in Comprehensive Textbook of Psychiatry, 3rd ed. Edited by Kaplan HI, Freedman AM, Sadock BJ. Baltimore, Williams and Wilkins, 1980, pp 1770-1783

Sadock VA (ed): The psychiatric aspects of sexuality [Part 1], in Psychiatry Update: The American Psychiatric Association Annual Review. Edited by Grinspoon L. Washington, DC, American Psychiatric Press, 1982, pp 7-73

Saghir M, Robbins E: Male and Female Homosexuality. Baltimore, Williams and Wilkins, 1973

Chapter 12

Alcohol and Drug Abuse

Drug abuse and drug dependence are major social problems in our culture, yet it is difficult to define exactly what sort of behavior constitutes abuse. The use of mind-altering substances is sanctioned in amost every group in Western society. Which substances, then, are not permissible? And among sanctioned substances, how much is too much? It may be useful to begin with some definitions.

The World Health Organization defines *drug abuse* as excessive drug use that is inconsistent with acceptable medical practice. Some drug abuse results in *tolerance*, which is an altered physiologic state caused by continuous use of a drug, resulting in a diminished response to the same dose of the drug over time, so that progressively larger doses are required to produce the same drug effect.

Drug dependence refers to the psychological or physical compulsion to take a drug on a continuous or periodic basis in order to experience its psychic effects or to avoid the discomfort of its absence. Clinicians often speak of two types of drug dependence: *physical dependence* involves an altered somatic state due to continued drug use that results in physiologic symptoms (abstinence syndrome) when the drug is abruptly discontinued; *psychic dependence* is a less specific term used to refer to drug dependence without any apparent physical component. Psychic and physical dependence often occur together, so that treatment must address *both* somatic and psychological crav-

Table 12–1. Effects of some commonly abused substances.

Drug	Tolerance	Psychic dependence	Physical dependence
Alcohol	+	+ +	+ +
Amphetamines	+ +	+ +	0?
Barbiturates	+ +	+ +	+ +
Caffeine	+	+	0
Chlordiazepoxide (Librium)	+ +	+ +	+
Cocaine	+	+ +	0
LSD	+ +	+	0
Marijuana	+	+	0
Nicotine	+	+ +	+
Opiates	+ +	+ +	+ +

Key: 0 = no effects, + = mild effects, + + = marked effects.
Source: Vaillant GE: Alcoholism and drug dependence, in *The Harvard Guide to Modern Psychiatry*. Edited by Nicholi AM Jr. Cambridge, MA, Harvard University Press, 1978, p 568.

ings. Table 12-1 lists some of the more commonly abused substances and their effects.

Obviously, not all drug abuse results in drug dependence, nor does every instance of drug abuse imply the presence of an illness. When does the use of mind-altering substances constitute a disorder that requires treatment? *Drug use is pathological when it in any way impairs an individual's family and social relationships, health, job efficiency, or ability to avoid legal difficulties.* This definition is deliberately broad, in order to include the almost infinite variety of ways in which drugs can hamper people's lives.

ALCOHOLICS AND POLYDRUG ABUSERS

What sorts of people use particular drugs? Although drug abusers are often classified by clinicians according to the substances they abuse, such categorization actually tells us very little about the people involved. One common myth is that alcoholics tend to remain "faithful" to alcohol and do not generally go on to abuse other substances, while those who abuse opiates or barbiturates or hallucinogens are likely to abuse other drugs, including alcohol, during the course of their lives. In fact, many people—whether primarily categorized as alcoholics or as polydrug abusers—use whatever substances are available to alter their psychic state.

What Causes People to Abuse Drugs and Alcohol?

Obviously, there is no single factor that accounts for why some people develop these disorders and others do not. The following variables seem to be important in determining patterns of drug abuse:

Availability of drugs. People who live and work in situations where drugs are readily accessible are more prone to abuse them (e.g., bartenders). While availability is a necessary condition for drug abuse, it does not, in and of itself, cause people to abuse drugs.

Onset of action of the drug. Drugs that act quickly (e.g., alcohol, fast-acting barbiturates) are more prone to be abused than those that exert their effects more slowly.

Development of tolerance and physical dependence. Withdrawal symptoms are unpleasant and may be life-threatening. The avoidance of these symptoms is a powerful factor in the continued use of drugs that create physiologic dependence (e.g., alcohol, heroin).

Genetic background. The child of an alcoholic, adopted at birth into a nonalcoholic family, is at a greater risk of developing alcoholism than the child of a nonalcoholic who is adopted into a nonalcoholic family. There thus appears to be some genetic predisposition to alcoholism, although the importance of this factor has yet to be fully elucidated. No comparable studies have been done of polydrug abusers.

Childhood environment. In addition to the genetic factors mentioned above, alcoholics (particularly men) are more likely than nonalcoholics to have alcoholic parents and siblings. The process by which drinking habits are "handed down" from one generation to another is thought to be based on the mechanism of *identification*, whereby children unconsciously adopt characteristics of important caretakers and others who are role models as they grow up. No general statements can be made with certainty about the childhood experiences of polydrug abusers. Some writers claim that polydrug abusers tend to come from noncohesive home environments where one or both parents were neglectful of or abusive toward the children, but this hypothesis has yet to be well substantiated empirically.

Culture. Drug abuse is less likely where drug use is prohibited on religious grounds, or where there are clear guidelines for nonabusive drug use. Thus, rates of alcoholism are very low among Moslem and Mormon communities, where alcohol is prohibited, and among Italians and Jews, who allow children to drink in socially sanctioned ways but prohibit drunkenness.

Socioeconomic status. Drug abusers often fail to conform to popular stereotypes. To be sure, there are sociopathic addicts who live on the street and steal to finance a heroin habit. But other "hard-core" addicts and alcoholics include physicians, teachers, housewives, and students—people from all backgrounds and socioeconomic groups.

Mental illness. Many people who abuse drugs and alcohol suffer from mental disorders. It is often difficult to distinguish between psychiatric symptoms that result from substance abuse and those that prompt it. However, it is clear that many patients begin to abuse drugs to "medicate" preexisting emotional disorders such as depression, anxiety, and psychosis (e.g., the depressed student who becomes addicted to cocaine). Disorders that commonly underlie drug abuse include affective disorders, anxiety disorders, somatoform disorders, and personality disorders (e.g., borderline, narcissistic, and antisocial personality disorders). No one personality type has been found among substance abusers. People who become alcoholics have often been stereotyped as passive, dependent, and depressed; polydrug abusers are thought to be primarily sociopathic. But these generalizations are not valid. Alcoholics and polydrug abusers vary greatly with respect to personality type and underlying psychopathology.

Mental health professionals are often consulted for treatment of emotional problems by people who minimize the extent to which their drug use affects their mental health. It is virtually impossible to get an accurate picture of a substance abuser's baseline state of mental health while he or she continues to use drugs. Thus, accurate assessment and effective treatment of mental illness are not possible until substance abuse has ceased.

ALCOHOLISM

It is estimated that 5 to 10 percent of the adult population in the United States is afflicted with alcoholism. It is more prevalent among men than women, but the incidence among women is increasing. Not surprisingly, it is also more prevalent among the urban poor and deprived minority groups, although it cuts across all class, ethnic, and geographical lines. A public health problem of major proportions, alcoholism is also significantly underdiagnosed—perhaps as many as half of the alcoholics seen by health care professionals go entirely undiagnosed. This occurs in part because alcoholics tend to strongly deny that they have a problem; in many cases, only family and friends can supply accurate information about drinking habits and resulting impairment of functioning. The alcoholic is likely to rationalize job difficulties and interpersonal problems as the *causes* rather than the *results* of drinking. And clinicians do not generally suspect alcohol abuse among people who do not conform to the stereotype of the skid-row bum.

Alcoholics commonly do not seek treatment until they are forced to by others. This often involves some sort of confrontation or coercion. For example, an exasperated spouse may threaten to leave if the alcoholic does not stop drinking. Or an irate employer may give the alcoholic one last chance to sober up or be fired. Unless the alcoholic's way of life seems significantly threatened, he or she is not likely to view drinking as a problem that requires treatment.

You will most often deal with alcoholics who want to hide the severity of their drinking problem from you, from friends and family, and from themselves. They will tend to minimize the extent to which they abuse alcohol and see their current physical or psychological symptoms as unrelated to drinking.

You will not diagnose alcoholism if you do not look for it. A drug and alcohol history must be part of every mental health evaluation. You must be particularly diligent about pursuing any clues or intuitions you have about the presence of alcohol abuse, or you may miss a problem that is primary to your client's complaints.

Diagnosis

Ask every client about the amount and frequency of alcohol use. *Assume* alcohol use and begin with such questions as, "How much do you drink?" "In what situations?" "How often do you take a drink?"

Give clients who are vague about amounts and frequency some suggestions that are more likely to *overestimate* drinking than to underestimate, for example, "Do you have several drinks each day?" When you suspect a problem, the following questions may help you clarify the situation. They are grouped roughly according to the severity of the symptoms they are designed to elicit.

- Do you sometimes feel a little guilty about your drinking?
- Do you often find that you want to continue drinking after your friends say they have had enough?

- Are you irritated when your family or friends comment on your drinking?
- Have you ever argued with someone close to you about your drinking?

- When drinking with others, do you try to have a few extra drinks when others will not know it?
- Did you ever wake up "the morning after" and discover that you could not remember part of the evening before, even though your friends tell you that you did not pass out?
- When you are sober, do you ever regret things you have done or said while drinking?
- Do you try to avoid family or close friends when you are drinking?

- Are you having more financial or work problems lately?
- Do you eat little or irregularly when you are drinking?
- Have you ever been in a car accident after you have been drinking, or have you ever been arrested for drunk driving?
- Do you sometimes have "the shakes" in the morning and find that it helps to have a little drink?
- Do you sometimes drink steadily for several days at a time?
- After periods of drinking, do you sometimes see or hear things that aren't really there?

Positive answers to any of the questions at the beginning of this list should make you think seriously about alcoholism and explore the matter further. If you suspect that your client is denying the seriousness of the problem, ask to speak with family members, and do so with the client present in the room. This should help you assess the extent to which alcohol has impaired work, home life, or health, and whether it constitutes an illness requiring treatment. In particular, be alert to a history of withdrawal symptoms ("the shakes," delirium tremens) or "blackouts" (memory loss while intoxicated), for these are clear signals that the problem is significant and may result in serious withdrawal reactions in the future.

Treatment

Once alcohol abuse has been diagnosed, the decision must be made as to what forms of treatment are indicated, keeping in mind the client's motivation for treatment. Obviously, emergency situations must be treated first. Anyone presenting with severe intoxication that threatens to compromise respiratory functioning, or with severe withdrawal symptoms like delirium tremens or seizures, should be admitted immediately to a medical ward or intensive care unit. For information on the management of these situations, consult a general medical textbook.

Clients who present for mental health evaluation are generally those for whom there is no medical emergency, but they may nevertheless require careful medical and psychiatric treatment in order to avert consequences of alcohol abuse or withdrawal.

Detoxification. Detoxification is the first step in the treatment of those who are addicted to alcohol and have experienced significant withdrawal symptoms when they have stopped drinking in the past. Detoxification is generally carried out on a medical or psychiatric inpatient unit, in order to allow careful monitoring of physical status and to prevent potentially lethal withdrawal reactions. Inpatient treatment also allows the alcoholic to begin other types of therapy (discussed below), which can be continued on an outpatient basis.

Table 12–2. Early manifestations of alcohol withdrawal.

Signs	Symptoms
Tachycardia (increasing pulse rate)	Irritability
Elevation of systolic blood pressure	Agitation
Sweating	Difficulty concentrating
Fever	Insomnia
Hyperventilation (rapid breathing)	Abdominal pain
Hyperreflexia (more pronounced	Nausea, vomiting
deep tendon reflexes)	Diarrhea
	Tremulousness ("shakes")

Physiologic withdrawal from alcohol usually begins six to 24 hours after the person has stopped a period of heavy drinking and may begin as late as 36 hours after the alcoholic's last drink. The early signs and symptoms of alcohol withdrawal are shown in Table 12-2.

Later complications of alcohol withdrawal include the following:

1. Worsening of early symptoms noted in Table 12-2, especially
   - rapid pulse,
   - sweating,
   - agitation, and
   - tremor.
2. Seizures:
   - Most likely in the first 24-48 hours after the last drink;

- Usually nonfocal and generalized;
- Self-limiting; and
- Generally preceding agitation, delirium, and hallucinations.
3. Alcoholic hallucinosis:
   - Most common in the first 24-48 hours after the last drink; and
   - May involve visual or auditory hallucinations, or both.
4. Delirium tremens (DTs):
   - Usually occur 50-100 hours after the last drink;
   - May last up to two weeks;
   - Involve hallucinations, delusions, or both;
   - Includes a hypermetabolic state: elevated body temperature, dehydration, blood chemistry imbalance; and
   - Associated with mortality as high as 15 percent.

Major withdrawal syndromes can usually be prevented by treating earlier manifestations before they become severe. The key is early and aggressive treatment, for it is much more difficult to "catch up" once withdrawal has progressed beyond the preliminary stages.

Treatment of early signs of alcohol withdrawal. Chlordiazepoxide (Librium) is an effective pharmacologic substitute for alcohol that has a wide margin of safety, little respiratory depression, low addiction potential, anticonvulsant effects, and a long half-life (24-30 hours). It both alleviates the signs and symptoms of early withdrawal and prevents progression to more severe syndromes (DTs, seizures).

Treatment should be begun as soon as clients show any of the early signs of withdrawal: evaluated pulse rate (over 110 beats per minute), elevated systolic blood pressure, sweating, or elevated temperature. These signs are more reliable indicators than subjective symptoms like anxiety and agitation, which may be present for many reasons other than withdrawal. The therapeutic procedure that a physician would likely follow is outlined below:

1. Administer 50-100 mg of chlordiazepoxide orally at the first signs of withdrawal (the dose will depend on the person's physical size and extent of recent alcohol abuse). For persistent symptoms, the dose may be repeated in an hour.
2. People experiencing withdrawal can then be put on an ongoing regimen of 25-100 mg of chlordiazepoxide orally every four hours as needed to keep vital signs stable during the first day. The average person will require 300-400 mg/day on the first day; the total daily dosage should not exceed 600 mg.
3. Further doses should be given as needed for agitation, high blood

pressure, or rapid pulse. A useful guideline is to medicate so as to keep the pulse rate below 110, provided the person is alert.

4. After the first 24 hours, if symptoms are controlled, the dosage of chlordiazepoxide may be cut in half each day until it is tapered off within four to five days.

5. If more than 400 mg/day of chlordazepoxide is required to control symptoms in the first day of withdrawal, 50 mg of chlorpromazine (Thorazine) can be added orally to each 100-mg dose of chlordiazepoxide, but this may complicate the treatment, since chlorpromazine may increase the likelihood of having a seizure.

Once withdrawal symptoms have been controlled, other forms of treatment may be initiated.

You may be surprised by the onset of alcohol withdrawal among people who are admitted to the hospital for seemingly unrelated medical or psychiatric reasons but who have a history of recent heavy drinking. These people may only admit to the full extent of their alcohol abuse when, in a setting where alcohol is suddenly unavailable, withdrawal symptoms set in. You must therefore consider the possibility of alcohol withdrawal whenever you see a hospitalized patient who has a history of alcohol abuse.

Wernicke's encephalopathy and Korsakoff's syndrome. The medical consequences of chronic alcohol addiction, such as cirrhosis of the liver and nerve damage, are well outlined in general medical texts. One neuropsychiatric syndrome deserves special mention here because it is characterized by dramatic psychological symptoms. Chronic alcoholics develop the syndrome, presumably because of a prolonged inadequate diet that results in thiamine deficiency.

Wernicke's encephalopathy is an acute, life-threatening condition characterized by clouding of consciousness, ophthalmoplegia (weakness of the muscles controlling movement of the eyes), and ataxia (a wide-based gait, falling, or inability to walk or stand).

At autopsy, people who develop this condition are found to have brainstem hemorrhages, particularly in the area of the mamillary bodies. The condition comes on rapidly and requires emergency treatment with thiamine to prevent death and minimize residual brain damage. *Anyone* with a history of chronic alcohol abuse who manifests acute psychiatric or neurologic symptoms should be given 100 mg of thiamine intramuscularly. Symptoms often respond dramatically to treatment, but residual impairment is common.

Korsakoff's syndrome is a chronic condition that remains when Wernicke's encephalopathy is treated. It may also occur after one or more episodes of delirium tremens. The most prominent feature of Korsakoff's syndrome is *recent memory impairment,* although peripheral nerve damage, ataxia, and oculomotor difficulties may also be present. Classically, these people have been described as using confabulation—i.e,. fabricating answers to questions in an attempt to fill in details they do not recall. However, confabulation is actually infrequent and is not necessary to establish the diagnosis. The most common memory impairment involves difficulty in learning new information (e.g., your name). Korsakoff's syndrome improves in about 75 percent of people who stop alcohol abuse and are maintained on an adequate diet for six months to two years, but only about 25 percent of those with this syndrome achieve full recovery. The only prevention against Wernicke's encephalopathy and Korsakoff's syndrome is an adequate diet; after emergency treatment with thiamine, an adequate diet is the only necessary treatment for those recovering from the syndrome.

Long-Term Treatment of Alcoholism

Most clinicians consider alcoholism a disease rather than a moral failing. This viewpoint is useful in helping to alleviate the heavy burden of guilt carried by many alcoholics. However, the disease concept does not absolve alcoholics from responsibility for their drinking, nor does it imply that other people can bail them out of their difficulties. The treatment of alcoholism is long and difficult for alcoholics, families, and treaters alike. Alcoholics are asked to give up forever a substance they truly (if ambivalently) love.

Effective treatment involves giving clients a nonchemical substitute for the lost addiction, reminding them continuously that even one drink can lead to relapse, repairing the social and medical damage that has occurred, and restoring their self-esteem. A variety of treatment modalities have been employed to achieve these goals, the most effective of which are listed below.

Alcoholics Anonymous (AA). This is the most effective treatment known for alcoholics. It provides continuously available group support by individuals who have themselves suffered from alcoholism. Meetings are held in many cities at every hour of the day and night, so that support is available as frequently as the alcoholic wishes it. These meetings involve peer support and gentle confrontation of the ways in which alcoholics deny their illness. AA techniques also help the alcoholic understand the conditioned and impulsive aspects of drinking. AA replaces drinking companions with a new group of peers with whom the alcoholic can identify. It allows members not only to receive help from other alcoholics, but also to give help to others, thereby enhancing self-esteem.

Many alcoholics are initially reluctant to participate in AA. In recommending this treatment, you should be consistently supportive and, if possible, find a way for other AA members to personally introduce the client to these meetings. Because alcoholism often takes a devastating toll on the families of alcoholics, you may want to refer them to *Al-Anon*, a self-help group that helps family members to deal with their own emotional difficulties, as well as teaching them about alcoholism and how to avoid interfering with the alcoholic's recovery. *Alateen* is a similar organization that offers support to adolescents who are coping with alcoholic parents.

Psychotherapy. This is not the primary treatment of choice for alcoholism, for it cannot provide the continuous support that is often required. However, when used adjunctively with other modalities like AA, it can be extremely useful—e.g., in helping to uncover family problems that perpetuate the client's drinking, and in helping the client to see ways in which drinking is motivated by certain benefits (*secondary gains*). In most cases, psychotherapy cannot be effective until the client stops drinking, for only then can the therapy address the uncomfortable feelings and symptoms that the alcoholic habitually "medicates" away with ethanol.

Disulfiram (Antabuse). This medication blocks the normal oxidation of alcohol so that acetaldehyde accumulates in the bloodstream and causes unpleasant symptoms, such as rapid pulse and vomiting. Obviously, the use of this medication is voluntary (usually in oral doses of 125 or 250 mg/day), and clients must be made aware of its adverse interactions with alcohol. Although Antabuse provides a deterrent to drinking, it does not help with such factors as low self-esteem and the loss of the addicting substance. By itself, therefore, it is of limited use in the treatment of alcoholism. However, many clinicians use it in conjunction with AA or psychotherapy.

Behavior modification. Hypnosis, desensitization, relaxation training, and aversion therapy (coupling alcohol use with noxious stimuli like shocks or nausea) have been somewhat successful in treating alcoholism. In particular, aversion therapy that couples alcoholism with vomiting has shown some promise.

Adjunctive services. Halfway houses, vocational rehabilitation programs, and other social institutions that give alcoholics support and help them recover lost skills have been useful as part of a treatment plan that includes other modalities like AA.

OPIATES

Opium is an ancient drug around which entire cultures and economies have revolved. Today, many opium-related compounds are used illegally in this country. In addition to the natural alkaloids of opium—morphine and codeine—there are important synthetic derivatives—such as heroin, dihydromorphinone (Dilaudid), and oxymorphone (Numorphan)—as well as purely synthetic opioids, such as meperidine (Demerol), methadone (Dolophine), phenazocine (Prinadol), pentazocine (Talwin), and dextropropoxyphene (Darvon).

All of these drugs are sedating; more importantly, they are the strongest pain-killers known. Thus, they are highly useful for medical purposes. However, they have strong potential for the development of tolerance, as well as psychological and physiologic dependence. Although the majority of narcotics addicts live in the slums of large cities and obtain drugs on the street, addiction cuts across all class and social lines. Some health care professionals who have ready access to narcotics become addicted to them. Men outnumber women by almost four to one among narcotics addicts.

Many addicts seek treatment for their addiction in outpatient settings, but you may also encounter them in hospital emergency rooms where they are experiencing acute symptoms of overdose or withdrawal.

Overdose

Overdose with narcotics often occurs because the user is unaware of the strength of the illicit supply he or she has purchased. Also, one's tolerance to a given dose of narcotic varies according to how much one has used recently; addicts may overdose even on their usual "fix" if their tolerance has been lowered by short supply of the drug.

The signs of acute overdose are the following: constricted pupils, diminished pulse rate, diminished respiratory rate, pulmonary edema (the lungs fill with fluid), and stupor or coma. Acute overdose requires emergency medical treatment, as outlined below. First, the person's vital functions must be supported and glucose must be administered intravenously. Then, an *opioid antagonist* must be given to block the effects of the drug. Although there are several drugs that block the action of opiates, naloxone (Narcan) is the drug of choice, since it has no physical effects in the absence of opiates and therefore will not complicate the situation if it turns out that the person has not been abusing opiates but suffers from some other medical problem. The usual initial adult dose is 0.4 mg intravenously, although up to 1.2 mg may be required to reverse coma and respiratory depression. Comatose people should be put into physical restraints before Narcan is given, since they may be combative as they emerge rapidly from coma. Narcan will reverse the signs of acute overdose within minutes, but its effect may wear off within 30 to 120 minutes, at which time the narcotic will again produce symptoms of overdose. Thus, people who emerge from coma must not be allowed to leave the hospital but must be monitored carefully for up to 48 hours, repeating the administration of Narcan as needed.

Withdrawal

Withdrawal from opiates has been given much publicity in films and on television, and the abstinence syndrome associated with narcotics is very unpleasant. However, abrupt withdrawal is *not* life-threatening in otherwise healthy people, as it may be from severe alcohol or barbiturate addiction. In fact, in terms of discomfort and medical danger, opiate withdrawal has been compared to a one-week bout with influenza. The symptoms are listed in Table 12-3.

Table 12–3. Symptoms of opiate withdrawal.

Early (12–36 hours after last dose)	Late (48–72 hours after last dose)
Yawning	Abdominal cramps
Sweating	Diarrhea
Gooseflesh (piloerection)	Vomiting
Insomnia	Elevated blood pressure
Dilated pupils	Increased respiratory rate
Loss of appetite	Increased heart rate
Muscle cramps	Fever
Tremor	

Treatment of Opiate Withdrawal

Methadone substitution. Methadone is a synthetic opiate that has proved to be effective in treating withdrawal from narcotics because it is long-acting and produces little euphoria (even so, it is commonly abused by recovering addicts). It is used for withdrawal primarily on an inpatient basis and in certain specialized outpatient clinics. It is given orally, beginning with 10 mg every four to six hours as needed for signs of withdrawal, and generally no more than 40 mg in a 24-hour period. The dose is adjusted to the minimum level that will suppress symptoms and is then decreased by 5 mg (or 20 percent) every day until it is discontinued. It is important to use objective signs (blood pressure, temperature, heart rate) to assess the person's condition, rather than relying on subjective complaints.

Clonidine. Recent studies have demonstrated that clonidine is very effective in alleviating the signs and symptoms of withdrawal from opiates, presumably by suppressing the activity of norepinephrine, a neurotransmitter in the central nervous system that appears to mediate the withdrawal process. Clonidine is nonaddicting and produces no euphoria, so it is not likely to be abused. New research suggests that it may be the most effective treatment available for withdrawal from methadone, heroin, and other opiates.

Outpatient methadone maintenance. This is a controversial treatment designed to provide addicts with methadone as a long-term substitute for street drugs, in order to reduce the craving for these drugs. Methadone is given in doses of up to 120 mg orally per day, and addicts are monitored carefully with urinalyses and other control measures. However, abuse of methadone and its illicit sale on the street have been complications of such programs. Methadone maintenance must be carried out in conjunction with other support services that address the social aspects of addiction.

Long-acting opioid antagonists. These agents, such as naltrexone, prevent addicts from experiencing the effects of narcotics, and thus are thought to act as deterrents to drug abuse. The long-term use of opioid antagonists is still an experimental form of treatment, but some clinicians have achieved promising results with low rates of relapse.

CENTRAL NERVOUS SYSTEM DEPRESSANTS

Sedatives, hypnotics, and antianxiety agents all depress the central nervous system (CNS). They are often referred to as *downers.* Most are prescription drugs that are either obtained illegally or obtained legally from physicians but misused. The pharmacologic properties of these drugs are described in Chapter 16. Downers are commonly abused along with alcohol and opiates, and both abuse and overdose frequently involve combinations of drugs. Individuals who use barbiturates and other sedative-hypnotics are very prone to develop psychological dependence, followed by increasing tolerance and physical dependence.

Overdose

The symptoms of intoxication and overdose with CNS depressants resemble those of drunkenness—drowsiness (coma in severe overdoses), slurred speech, lack of coordination, memory impairment, confusion, nystagmus (rhythmical oscillation of the eyeballs), tremor, decreased muscle tone, agitation, paranoia, and inappropriate affect.

Management of overdose. If the person is *awake,* induce vomiting or perform gastric lavage to clear the stomach of any unabsorbed substance. Send blood and urine samples and gastric contents for toxicologic analysis. Monitor and support respiratory and cardiac functions for at least 24 hours.

If the person is *comatose* or *semicomatose,* attempt gastric lavage if the drug was taken less than 12 hours before. Alkalinize the urine to increase excretion. Support basic life functions through intubation, administration of oxygen, plasma expanders, and vasopressors.

Obviously, severe overdose with CNS depressants requires immediate medical attention and necessitates admission to a facility where intensive care can be provided.

Withdrawal

Withdrawal from CNS depressants can be quite dangerous if it occurs abruptly. In particular, withdrawal can result in seizures and cardiovascular collapse, and it carries a significant risk of death. The possibility of withdrawal must be considered for every person who presents with a history of abuse of or dependence on CNS depressants. The withdrawal symptoms are listed in Table 12-4.

Treatment of Withdrawal

Treatment is conducted on an inpatient basis and relies on substitution of pentobarbital for the abused CNS depressant. Pentobarbital is a short-acting barbiturate that is used to alleviate withdrawal symptoms and subsequently tapered over many days. Treatment begins with a pentobarbital tolerance test on day 1, to determine how much pentobarbital must be given initially to prevent severe withdrawal.

Table 12–4. Symptoms of withdrawal from CNS depressants.

Mild	Severe
Agitation	Seizures
Anxiety	Delirium
Loss of appetite	Lowered body temperature
Vomiting	Cardiac arrest
Increased heart rate	
Postural hypotension (drop in blood pressure)	
Hyperreflexia (increased deep tendon reflexes)	
Tremor	

Pentobarbital tolerance test. First, a 200-mg test dose of pentobarbital is given orally. If intoxication results (with nystagmus and/or ataxia), then tolerance is not presumed to be great, and the person is maintained on 150-200 mg of pentobarbital orally every six hours for the first day of treatment.

If no intoxication results from the 200-mg test dose, 100 mg is given orally every 2 hours until intoxication develops. The total dose required to produce intoxication is then given every six hours for the first 24 hours of treatment. That is, if intoxication develops after 400 mg has been given, the dose for day 1 is 400 mg orally every six hours.

After the first 24 hours, the dose of pentobarbital is reduced by 10 percent each day and withdrawn gradually over a period of about three weeks. Subjects are monitored carefully for signs of intoxication or withdrawal, with subsequent adjustments in dosage.

Some clinicians use phenobarbital instead of pentobarbital in the treatment of withdrawal, because there is less fluctuation in blood levels of phenobarbital and because it has antiseizure activity. In this procedure, 30 mg of phenobarbital is substituted for each 100 mg of pentobarbital, in three divided doses, and the dose is decreased 30 mg/day.

If someone is dependent on both opiates and barbiturates, barbiturate withdrawal is carried out first.

CENTRAL NERVOUS SYSTEM STIMULANTS

Amphetamines

Amphetamines are prone to abuse by a wide variety of people, including students who want to be able to stay up for many hours preparing for examinations or writing papers. However, amphetamine use in large doses can produce acute delirium and psychosis.

Table 12–5. Symptoms of amphetamine intoxication and overdose.

Mild	Severe
Restlessness	Confusion
Irritability	Delirium
Weakness	Hallucinations
Confusion	Paranoia
Talkativeness	
Anxiety	
Tremor	
Increased deep tendon reflexes	
Insomnia	
Euphoria, with lability of mood	

Overdose is potentially lethal. The symptoms of amphetamine intoxication and overdose are listed in Table 12-5.

Treatment of acute intoxication involves decreasing CNS irritability and controlling psychotic symptoms. Toward this end, support and reassurance in a quiet setting may suffice in cases of mild intoxication. In more severe cases, 25-50 mg of chlorpromazine (Thorazine) administered orally every six hours will ease agitation and diminish psychosis.

Amphetamine psychosis occurs in a more chronic form after prolonged use of the drug. The psychotic symptoms can be difficult to distinguish from schizophrenia. Symptoms include talkativeness, hyperactivity, stereotyped or repetitive behavior, bruxism (grinding the teeth), picking movements, suspiciousness, and (in more severe cases) persecutory delusions, hallucinations, ideas of reference, and hypersexuality. Management of amphetamine psychosis is also carried out with antipsychotic medication (e.g., chlorpromazine in the doses noted above) to decrease agitation and diminish psychotic symptoms.

Although physical addiction to amphetamines does not develop, a sudden withdrawal of the stimulant after prolonged use or administration of high doses results in a marked decrease in CNS activity known as "crashing," which is characterized by drowsiness, fatigue, apathy, and severe depression that may lead to suicidal ideation. People who "crash" need sleep, as well as physical and emotional support, until CNS activity returns to normal.

Cocaine

Cocaine use has increased dramatically in the United States in recent years. It enjoys a special status as the recreational drug of the affluent. Its use results in an initial stimulation of the CNS like that seen in amphetamine use, followed by CNS depression. The drug is commonly absorbed via the nasal lining after "snorting," but smoking and intravenous use are also common and are more likely to be the routes in severe overdoses. Overdose may result in psychosis and even cardiac arrest.

Antipsychotic drugs help to diminish psychosis in cases of cocaine overdose, and propranolol is used to decrease cardiac excitation. Although cocaine does not create physical dependence, it can create a psychological dependence resulting in chronic use.

HALLUCINOGENS

Hallucinogens include a wide variety of substances grouped together somewhat arbitrarily based on their ability to induce altered states of awareness that resemble those of natural psychoses. Some hallucinogens, like psilocybin (mushroom) and mescaline (peyote cactus), come from natural sources, while drugs like D-lysergic acid diethylamide (LSD) and dimethyltryptamine (DMT) are synthetic.

Signs and symptoms of hallucinogen intoxication include alteration of mood (often euphoria), vividness of real or fantasized sensory illusions and hallucinations, synthesia ("overflow" from one sensory modality to another), and confusion. Many other psychological manifestations may be present, including a sense of time slowing, a loss of body boundaries, and feelings of grandiosity or omnipotence.

Although each hallucinogen has slightly different characteristics and produces somewhat different signs and symptoms, they all produce adverse reactions in some people. These reactions include acute panic attacks, psychosis, flashbacks, and precipitation of underlying psychosis (e.g., in people with latent schizophrenia). Whether a person has an adverse reaction to a hallucinogen (a "bad trip") depends on such factors as the dose of the drug, the setting in which it is used, and the personality characteristics of the user. LSD intoxication is particularly common and is manifested by such physical signs as dilation of pupils, increased deep tendon reflexes, muscle weakness, increased blood pressure, increased heart rate, and fever.

Treatment of hallucinogen intoxication generally involves support, reassurance, and diminishing stimulation around the person until the drug wears off. In many cases, putting the person in a quiet, dimly lit room and talking to help him or her distinguish psychotic symptoms from reality will suffice to weather the crisis. However, severe panic may be treated effectively with oral diazepam (Valium). Unless psychosis is unusually severe and prolonged, it is best to avoid using antipsychotic medication because of possible adverse anticholinergic reactions resulting from the combination of a hallucinogen and an antipsychotic.

Phencyclidine (PCP) is unique in action compared with other psychedelic drugs, and it is not a true hallucinogen. A synthetic drug initially developed as a possible anesthetic agent for humans, it is now licensed only for use as an immobilizing agent for nonhuman primates. Often called "angel dust," it is a common drug of abuse. Its psychological effects include changes in body image (e.g., "My head is growing larger"), depersonalization, anxiety, disorganization of thought, depression, and hostility. PCP abusers sometimes behave with great violence under the influence of the drug. Physical signs of intoxication include elevated blood pressure, rapid respiration, and neurologic signs such as nystagmus, muscle spasm and rigidity, and ataxia. PCP intoxication can result in coma and death.

Treatment of mild to moderate intoxication is different from that for hallucinogens in that "talking people down" is not usually helpful and may even increase the person's anxiety. Instead, placing the subject in a quiet, dimly lit room with a minimum of stimulation is successful in most cases. Diazepam (Valium) is used intravenously if severe muscle spasm or seizures result. Antipsychotics are not generally helpful. Most cases of intoxication resolve after several hours of reduced stimulation (e.g., in a secluded room in an emergency ward), but some result in prolonged and severe behavioral disturbances, exaggeration of preexisting thought disorders, and serious medical complications that require hospital admission.

CANNABINOIDS

Cannabinoids, such as marijuana and hashish, are mild euphoriants with some sedative effects. Many people use these drugs as others use alcohol socially. It is estimated that as many as 30 million Americans have had some experience with marijuana, but only a fraction of that number use the drug heavily on a continuous basis. Signs and symptoms of acute intoxication include disconnected speech, recent memory impairment, emotional lability, depersonalization, and confusion, as well as increased heart rate, conjunctival injection (redness of the eyes), and decreased body temperature. While adverse reactions such as panic, psychosis, and depression do occur as a result of cannabis intoxication, these reactions are rare.

The effects of chronic use of cannabinoids are the subject of some debate. Chronic psychotic states secondary to cannabis use have been reported in Eastern cultures where doses are presumably much higher, but such reactions have been rare in the West. Some clinicians have identified an *amotivational syndrome* of low drive, poor judgment, introversion, loss of insight, poor communication skills, and depersonalization. This syndrome occurs in people who use marijuana heavily on a regular basis for many months or years. At this time, however, it is not clear whether heavy cannabis use causes or results from this condition of low motivation, and adverse effects of intermittent cannabis use have not been clearly identified.

TREATMENT OF POLYDRUG ABUSE

Your first task in dealing with people who abuse drugs is to avoid stereotyping them. As was noted above, polydrug abusers come from all backgrounds—including highly educated professionals and "sweet little old ladies." If you only look for people who come in covered with tattoos and needle marks, you will fail to notice the many cases in which substance abuse is a major problem.

Your second task is to take a nonjudgmental approach to the evaluation and treatment of drug abusers. Health professionals often see addicts as hopeless cases. Your first impulse in dealing with such people may be to try to usher them out as quickly as possible. *Every drug abuser you see deserves a thorough medical and mental health evaluation*, with particular attention to possible underlying mental illness (e.g., affective illness, anxiety disorders, personality disorders). You should either do the evaluation yourself under the supervision of a physician, or you should refer the client to a physician who is experienced in the treatment of drug abuse or to a drug treatment center.

Treatment of drug abuse is difficult. Detoxification and crisis management are only the beginning of a long and difficult course to recovery. Like alcoholism, polydrug abuse involves substituting a substance for human contact. Many addicts' lives revolve around the process of obtaining drugs, and this provides a daily structure and a set of personal contacts that must be replaced even after physical addiction is eliminated. Also, polydrug abusers often "medicate" unpleasant feelings (anxiety, depression) that are likely to persist or worsen when the drug is taken away.

Reformed drug abusers who come from lower socioeconomic groups often find little support among peers who are likely to be antisocial and to encourage drug abuse. Thus, an important part of treatment for many people consists of helping them to establish new support systems. This may take the form of self-help groups like *Narcotics Anonymous* or *Pills Anonymous* (similar to Alcoholics Anonymous), vocational rehabilitation programs, day care centers, or drug-free residential communities (e.g., Synanon).

Psychotherapy cannot, in and of itself, provide the continuous support and peer group encouragement many recovering substance abusers require. However, as an adjunct to other treatment programs, psychotherapy can help some drug abusers to cope more effectively with feelings and problems that may have promoted drug use in the first place. Family therapy can also be useful in pointing out the family's pathological patterns of coping with stress. Group therapy can be especially useful in providing support, as well as in confronting drug abusers with the consequences of their self-destructive and antisocial behaviors, especially when other group members are themselves recovering or recovered drug abusers. No one treatment modality is as useful as a combination that provides the client with support, daily structure, and vocational skills that help to increase self-esteem.

REFERENCES

Cohen SE: Cannabis: impact on motivation, part I. Drug Abuse and Alcoholism Newsletter 9(10), 1980

Gold MS, Redmond DE Jr, Kleber HD: Noradrenergic hyperactivity in opiate withdrawal. Am J Psychiatry 136:100-102, 1979

Mendelson JH, Mello NK: Biologic concomitants of alcoholism. N Engl J med 301:912-921, 1979

Mirin SM, Weiss R: Substance abuse, in The Practitioner's Guide to Psychoactive Drugs. Edited by Bassuk E, Schoonover S, Gelenberg A. New York, Plenum Press, 1983, pp 221-290

Showalter CV, Thornton WE: Clinical pharmacology of phencyclidine toxicity. Am J Psychiatry 134: 1234-1237, 1977

Vaillant GE: Alcoholism and drug dependence, in The Harvard Guide to Modern Psychiatry. Edited by Nicholi AM Jr. Cambridge, Mass, Harvard University Press, 1978, pp 567-577

CHAPTER 13

Suicide

The intentional destruction of one's own life is an act of enormous power. Suicidal intent and suicidal behavior constitute one of the most emotionally charged of medical emergencies—for clients, for their families, and for clinicians.

Approximately three-quarters of those who commit suicide consult a physician (most often with medical complaints) within six months before their death. Each year, the average psychotherapist encounters more than a dozen clients who are seriously contemplating suicide. Suicide is ubiquitous and confronts practitioners in every branch of health care.

The pathways to suicide are many, but virtually all suicidal people have reached a state·of intolerable emotion. The rage, defiance, despair, and helplessness that you will encounter in such people is often frightening and confusing.

Suicidal people invariably arouse intense emotions in those close to them. Families and friends may react to suicide threats with sympathy, anxiety, or hostility. They may feel impotent and overwhelmed; they often blame themselves for the crisis; and they usually feel responsible for its outcome.

You, too, are likely to find your equanimity challenged by the suicidal client. As a human service professional, you are charged with helping people to improve the quality of life—yet people who are intent on killing themselves often go to great lengths to thwart those aims. They may reject every offer of aid, thereby making you feel what they feel—helpless and angry. Or they may attribute to you unrealistic powers over life and death, and make you believe that you alone will be responsible if they carry out their self-destructive plans. Suicidal clients force you to confront the limitations of how much responsibility you or anyone else can take for another's life. If you are to deliver effective care in such situations, you must learn to tolerate your own fear and anger and frustration without retaliating against the client.

Often, in the midst of emotional turmoil, you will be called on to make a considered judgment about the lethality of the client's intentions and actions. You must use that judgment to intervene in a quick and decisive manner. There are no foolproof formulas for the prediction of suicide risk, and lethality remains a matter of clinical judgment. But the study of suicide has yielded valuable guidelines for emergency assessment, and these guidelines, along with a heightened sensitivity to your own reactions, can make the care of the suicidal client safer and more efficient.

MYTHS ABOUT SUICIDE

A great many misconceptions about suicide have flourished, even among mental health professionals, and these can hinder clinical work:

Suicidal people are fully intent on self-destruction and have the right to die. Nearly all suicidal people are ambivalent about dying— they want to die and at the same time wish to be saved from death. For many, the fact that they have reached the mental health care setting in which you work is evidence of these mixed feelings.

Once decided upon, suicide is inevitable. Strong suicidal intent usually represents an acute condition, and intent generally falls sharply after the immediate circumstances compelling the event are survived.

People who talk about killing themselves are not the ones who actually do it. In more than 80 percent of cases, people who succeed at suicide have given definite warnings of their intent to die.

Improvement following a suicidal crisis means that the period of risk is over. Most completed suicides occur within three months after an acute crisis, when "improvement" affords the suicidal person more energy with which to put his or her intentions into effect.

Discussing suicidal thoughts and plans with the client will fix ideas of suicide more firmly in his or her mind. In fact, the careful eliciting of such thoughts and plans can be enormously relieving to people who have been unable to share their feelings of desperation. Sensitive and open discussion may well ease the crisis, and will rarely if ever exacerbate it.

EPIDEMIOLOGY OF SUICIDE

- Suicide is among the 10 leading causes of death in the United States (ninth as of 1978).
- Roughly 1 out of every 10,000 people kill themselves each year in the United States (in 1980, 12.7 per 100,000 population).
- Estimates of the total number of suicides in the United States each year range from 25,000 to 55,000. (Many suspected suicides are never proved.)
- One out of every 10 people in the general population have at some time had suicidal feelings that *they* would label "serious."
- For every completed suicide, there are between 10 and 40 attempts. (Many attempts are never reported.)

RISK FACTORS

Suicidologists have long searched for "suicide profiles." They have looked at everything from the phases of the moon to birth order in the family in an effort to solve the mystery of why certain people resort to suicide. The following is a list of the risk factors that are most consistently identified in recent studies:

Age. The risk of suicide increases with age and peaks among people in their late seventies. However, over the last 25 years there has been a more than threefold increase in the rate of suicide among adolescents and young adults.

Sex. Men commit suicide three times more frequently than do women. However, women *attempt* suicide two to three times as often as men. Men tend to use knives, firearms, and other violent methods of suicide, while women show a preference for self-poisoning (such as taking a drug overdose).

Race. The suicide rate is higher for whites than for nonwhites. However, the rate among young black adults in ghetto areas has recently increased sharply.

Marital status. Suicide rates are lowest for married people and higher for those who are separated, divorced, or widowed.

Living situation. People who live alone are at a higher risk of suicide than people who live with others.

Employment status. People who are unemployed are at higher risk of suicide than those who are working in or out of the home. Professionals (especially male physicians) are also at a disproportionately high risk.

Physical health. Physical illness, or the perception that one is ill, is more frequent among those who commit suicide. In particular, there is a high correlation between completed suicide and visits to a physician for medical complaints during the preceding six months.

Mental health. Among the mental illnesses that have been correlated with a high risk of suicide are depression, manic-depressive illness, schizophrenia, and personality disorders. In general, the presence of major mental illness should alert the clinician to the possibility of suicide.

Alcohol abuse or addiction. Alcoholism markedly increases the risk of suicide.

Previous suicide attempts. A history of suicide attempts has been estimated to increase the risk of completed suicide by as much as 64 times that of the general population.

The following factors, while less easily quantifiable, have also been associated with completed suicides:

Hopelessness. Several studies have concluded that the specific symptom of hopelessness about one's life situation is more highly correlated with suicide than is the more general category of depression.

Interpersonal loss. There is a high correlation between interpersonal loss and suicide. *Loss* is defined as the separation from, divorce from, or death of a significant other, and may include relatives, friends, lovers, and therapists. The risk of suicide is particularly high among alcoholics who have suffered interpersonal losses within the previous six weeks.

Life stresses. A high frequency of major life events in the previous six months has been found among those who commit suicide. Such events include job changes, moves, births, graduations, financial reversals, marriage, retirement, and menopause. Such changes are important to identify in assessing both the precipitants of a suicidal crisis and the possibilities for therapeutic intervention.

Interpersonal conflict. Longstanding intense interpersonal conflict with family members or other important people is associated with a high risk of suicide and has led some observers to characterize suicide as a fundamentally dyadic event. Such conflict, if unremitting, may continue to jeopardize the life of the client after a particular crisis has passed.

ASSESSING THE SUICIDAL CLIENT

When to Assess

Like many other potentially lethal conditions, suicidal intent can present itself to health care professionals in a variety of subtle and obscure ways. Many suicidal people express their desperation covertly, and the danger to their lives may go unnoticed.

You must ask about suicide *whenever* it crosses your mind, and you must address this question to *every* new client who presents with an emotional complaint. Even this will not be sufficient unless you are attuned to the types of verbal and nonverbal clues that desperate people often give.

Verbal clues. Direct statements about suicide are easy to identify, but people may couch these in an off-hand or joking manner. *Statements about killing oneself are to be taken seriously until proven otherwise.*

Suicidal people will often speak indirectly about their desire to die. They commonly express frustration with particular aspects of their lives ("My job is too much—I can't handle it any more") or they describe a general state of unhappiness ("I can't take it—nothing is going right"). Hopelessness is particularly evident among people who are suicidal. Statements such as, "I might as well give up because I can't make things better for myself" or "I don't expect to get what I want," may allude to a client's deep-rooted sense that the future is intolerable. Such declarations often sound like everyday "garden variety" complaints, but it is here that careful inquiry may elicit profoundly self-destructive ideas and plans.

Behavioral clues. People who are unable to verbalize their wish to die may act it out in a number of ways. The client who abruptly decides to make a will, buy a casket, or give away prized possessions may be putting affairs in order prior to suicide. Nonlethal experimentation with potentially lethal agents (drugs, weapons) may be a prelude to a serious attempt. A new interest in life insurance policies, cemetery plots, or gravestones may seem like prudent planning and may only in retrospect appear to reflect suicidal intent. Accidents and accident-proneness are very common among suicidal people, who may be genuinely unaware of the ways in which they put themselves in danger so as not to have to acknowledge the existence of suicidal impulses. All of these behaviors should alert you to the possibility of suicide and should prompt the sort of examination described below.

How to Assess

People on the verge of suicide are desperate. Their usual methods of coping with life have failed, and they may feel very ashamed of their condition. A nonjudgmental, objective concern on the part of the clinician may do much to alleviate these clients' burdens of humiliation, enabling them to be more open about their feelings and plans.

Whenever possible, the suicidal client should be interviewed in a quiet and relatively private setting. When the client has made a suicide attempt, it is essential that the interview be conducted only *after* the client has had a full medical evaluation and is medically stable. Initially, you will usually want to speak to the client alone, and at some later point speak with friends or family in person or by telephone. You should make it clear to everyone involved how the evaluation will proceed. A calm and organized approach will help to ease the extreme tension that suicide threats inevitably generate in clients and family members or friends. Avoid premature reassurance, for the client may interpret this to mean that you do not understand the seriousness of the situation.

Obviously, this sort of assessment requires time and thoughtful attention to emotional nuances—and both of these factors are usually in short supply in such places as a busy outpatient clinic. Nevertheless, you must take care to establish a setting in which you can gather the data you need.

What to Assess

Assessment of suicide risk must focus on suicidal intentions, suicide attempts (if any have been made), general psychiatric condition, and potential resources for correcting the situation. An outline is provided in Table 13-1.

Suicidal Ideation

You must entertain the possibility of suicide with every new client you see in a mental health care facility. You need to ask about suicidal ideation, even when no attempts have been made and the client has not spoken of feeling suicidal.

The exploration of suicidal thoughts can usually be done most tactfully and yield the most useful information when the interviewer

Table 13–1. Outline for suicide assessment.

Assessing suicidal ideation
   Pervasiveness of suicidal thoughts
   Extent to which plans have been formulated
   Lethality and availability of proposed method
   Likelihood of rescue from proposed attempt

Assessing a suicide attempt
   Damage done
      Agent used
      Impairment of consciousness
      Extent of physical harm
      Reversibility of physical harm (recovery time)
      Treatment required
   Likelihood of rescue
      Location of attempt
      Person who acted as rescuer
      Probability of rescue
      Patient's participation in rescue
      Delay until discovery

General psychiatric evaluation
   Social situation—important relationships and recent changes in these
   Occupation—change in status or performance
   Psychiatric history—previous suicide attempts, depression, psychosis,
      current treatment
   Drug and alcohol history
   Medical history—recent change in physical health
   Mental status examination
   Availability of community resources (family, friends, etc.)

begins with general questions and proceeds to specifics. A sequence
of inquiries might go as follows:

- How is your life going?
- How are you feeling in general?
- How bad does it get?
- Do you sometimes feel like giving up?
- Do you ever think you would be better off dead?
- Have you thought of ending your life?
- Do you ever feel close to harming yourself?
- How would you do it?
- Where would you get the means to do it?
- At what time and in what place would you do it?
- How close have you come to killing yourself?
- Do you feel that you will kill yourself in the near future?
- What has kept you from killing yourself until now?
- Does anyone else know of these feelings?

Each question narrows the focus of the discussion. In some cases,
you will find that your client's responses to general inquiries do not
point toward suicidal thoughts; more detailed questioning about suicide plans will then be unnecessary. In other cases, the client will
gradually divulge carefully worked-out schemes for self-destruction.

In discussing suicide plans, the *key factors* are the *lethality* of the
method, the *availability* of the method, and the *likelihood of rescue.*
Tactful questioning does not increase a client's desire or ability to plan
for suicide.

Direct denials of suicidal intent are usually truthful. People often
admit to seriously considering suicide, but insist that they would not
actually harm themselves, citing children, spouses, jobs, or other
factors in their lives that keep them from killing themselves. Such
reassurances are usually reliable, at least temporarily. Of course, one
can be misled; you must be especially wary of clients who act self-
destructively and at the same time deny any suicidal intent. In such
cases, judge clients by their actions rather than their words.

Attempted Suicide

Mental health professionals are often called upon to treat people
who have survived a suicide attempt. In such a situation, you must
make a judgment about the risk of another attempt in the immediate
future. This involves a careful evaluation of the suicide attempt itself,
since the lethality of an attempt has considerable prognostic significance for later self-destructive behavior. *No one* who has made a

suicide attempt should be sent home from a treatment facility without a mental health evaluation.

Below are a number of questions you can ask to quickly estimate the lethality of a particular self-destructive act. These questions evaluate the damage caused by the attempt and the degree to which rescue from this attempt was likely. The possible answers are listed in order of increasing dangerousness.

Physical harm done in the suicide attempt. The following questions can help you evaluate the physical damage done in an unsuccessful suicide attempt. Since superficial wrist scratches will inspire less alarm than a gunshot wound, the management of two such cases would differ greatly.

1. What agent was used?
   a. Least lethal: ingestion, cutting, stabbing.
   b. Intermediate: drowning, asphyxiation, strangulation.
   c. Most lethal: jumping, shooting.
2. Was consciousness impaired?
   a. Alert.
   b. Semicomatose, with confusion.
   c. Comatose.
3. How much physical harm did the person do?
   a. Mild: superficial, self-limited (e.g., scratching without significant blood loss).
   b. Moderate: requires a physician's attention, but not life-threatening (e.g., wound that requires sutures, fractures of small bones, damage to small arteries).
   c. Severe: penetration of vital organs or large blood vessels, skull or large bone fractures, neurologic changes.
4. How quickly can the person recover from the physical effects of the attempt?
   a. Within 24 hours.
   b. Within one to six days.
   c. Questionable, possible residual damage.
5. What medical treatment is required?
   a. First aid.
   b. Hospital admission.
   c. Intensive care.

The likelihood of rescue from the suicide attempt. A person who has attempted but not completed suicide has obviously been rescued, and it is useful to determine how likely that rescue was. For example, taking an overdose at home in the living room with others nearby is quite different from taking the same dose while alone in a hotel room in a strange city. The likelihood of rescue provides one measure of the lethality of any given suicide attempt, as well as data for judgment about continued suicide risk.

The following five questions will give you some idea about how far the client went to conceal or publicize the attempt.

1. What was the setting in which the attempt was made?
   a. Familiar: where the subject would be recognized (e.g., home, office, school).
   b. Nonfamiliar but not remote: where the subject would not be recognized, but could be observed to be in trouble by a passerby (e.g., bridges, subways, public buildings).
   c. Remote: where discovery could not be counted on (e.g., deserted areas, alleys, rural roads).

2. Who initiated the rescue?
   a. Key person: someone who knows the subject (friend, relative, therapist).
   b. Professional: someone whose job is such that he or she would initiate rescue (e.g., physician, police officer, taxi driver, telephone operator).
   c. Passerby: someone with no obligation to initiate rescue, who happened on the scene by chance (e.g., hotel staff member, pedestrian, washroom attendant).

3. What was the probability that someone would rescue the client?
   a. High, almost certain: rescuers were nearby or were faced with the attempt immediately (e.g., spouse was expected home).
   b. Moderate, uncertain (e.g., a rescuer was nearby but would not know of the attempt).
   c. Low, accidental: rescue was by chance (e.g., subject took precautions to avoid discovery).

4. To what extent did the client participate in the rescue?
   a. Asked for help.
   b. Left clues (e.g., staggered, left notes or empty bottles in conspicuous places).
   c. Did not ask for help.

5. How much time elapsed before the attempt was discovered?
   a. Less than one hour.
   b. One to four hours.
   c. More than four hours.

General Psychiatric Evaluation

Suicidal ideation and attempts only make sense in the larger context of a person's life. A careful general history will help you to identify risk factors for suicide, as well as problems that might be amenable to change. One question to keep in mind is, "Why now?"—what prompted this person to choose suicide at this particular point in life? Another question to ponder as you hear about the client's current life is, "What would this suicide accomplish for the client?" Explore the following areas:

Social situation. Current living situation, family, recent changes in or losses of love relationships or important friendships.

Occupation. Job, home responsibilities, school; recent changes in status or performance.

Psychiatric history. Previous suicide attempts (method, severity), depressive episodes (depressed mood, sleep or appetite disturbance, diurnal variation in mood), psychotic symptoms (hallucinations, delusions), psychotropic medications, psychiatric hospitalizations, current therapy.

Drug and alcohol history. Patterns of use or abuse; consider psychosis or depression secondary to drug use or drug withdrawal.

Medical history. Ongoing conditions and treatment, recent changes in physical health.

Mental status examination. Focus on presence or absence of depression, psychosis, and homicidal ideation. The wish to kill others is commonly associated with the wish to kill oneself. Also, hallucinations or delusional beliefs may dictate suicide (e.g., a voice commands the person to leap from a window), and the client is at serious risk as long as this form of psychosis persists.

Availability of Resources

You must listen to the client's story with an ear for possible interventions. Hospitalization is indicated for many who are at risk of suicide, but others can be treated as outpatients if they have adequate resources in the community.

Family and friends. The attitude of those closest to the client provides important information about treatment possibilities. Significant others who are concerned but not panicked, and who recognize both the seriousness of the situation and the need for treatment, are likely to promote the client's safety and recovery. Such people, if available to stay with the client, can be instrumental in helping the client to weather the suicidal crisis. At the other end of the spectrum, a person who has no one to whom he or she is close would leave the mental health facility facing the prospect of returning to an impoverished world.

Often, those closest to the client are overwhelmed with panic and confusion, or with anger. They may be incapable of assisting in follow-up care. It is even more lethal if friends and family are indifferent to the crisis. They may minimize the dangerousness of the situation and discourage the client from seeking professional help.

Most lethal is the setting in which significant others covertly encourage the client to commit suicide. The husband who ignores his depressed wife's suicide threats, or who leaves a bottle of tranquilizers lying about, may consciously or unconsciously wish for his wife's death. If the history demonstrates such collusion, you must arrange to get the client out of this environment until some intervention can be made.

Other resources. "Significant others" whose help can be enlisted in follow-up care include psychotherapists, family physicians, and clergy. Important people in the client's life should be identified and considered as possible resources, particularly if you contemplate outpatient treatment. As a rule, any ongoing caretakers (physicians, therapists) should be contacted while the evaluation is taking place.

TREATMENT

Use your judgment about continued risk and available resources to arrive at a plan of action. Do this with the help of the client, the client's family and friends, and any ongoing caretakers who are available to collaborate in the process. The options are essentially the three described below.

Send the client home. The client who has not made a suicide attempt, and who expresses vague ideas but denies any clear self-destructive plan or intent, is probably a candidate for outpatient treatment, consisting of follow-up by you, the family physician, or a clinician at a mental health facility. The choice will depend on the client's preferences and the cooperation of those to whom the referral is made. A definite appointment within the following day should always be confirmed before the client is allowed to leave.

For the person who *has* attempted suicide, hospital admission is often the treatment of choice. However, if the client denies further suicidal intent, the attempt itself indicates low risk, the client is not locked into a hopeless or frightened position by depression or psychosis, and concerned relatives or friends can stay with the client, you may consider sending the client home. Follow-up care by a mental health professional should take place *the next day.* This may be through a community mental health center or other local facility, or with a private therapist. It is essential that a definite follow-up plan be formulated, that the relevant agencies be contacted, and that the client have an appointed time and place for follow-up care before he or she is allowed to go home.

Outpatient treatment will be based on the client's needs and diagnosis and may range from a few sessions of crisis intervention work to long-term psychotherapy and pharmacotherapy. Possibilities include individual treatment, couples or family therapy, or group therapy. For a description of various treatment modalities, see Chapters 15 and 16.

Voluntary admission to a hospital. Many people who have definite plans for suicide, and most who have actually made serious attempts, will need hospital admission. Hospitalization affords a safe place in which to weather the crisis, as well as the chance for intensive evaluation and prompt initiation of treatment. Desperate suicidal people will often agree to hospitalization, especially if family or friends support such a move. If you suspect that the client may attempt suicide again even in the hospital, admission to a locked psychiatric unit where the client will be under careful observation may be indicated.

Forced hospitalization. Unlike most other conditions, suicidal intent carries with it a legal mandate for treatment. A person you judge to be at immediate risk of suffering serious bodily harm *must* be hospitalized, according to the law in most states. Thus, the client who is bent on self-destruction and refuses voluntary admission must be committed to a psychiatric unit. Commitment is generally done by a licensed physician, who must explain this course of action clearly and decisively and, if necessary, use ancillary personnel to detain the client against his or her will.

Because suicidal people often have enormous conflicts about

their wishes, present your plan of treatment as clearly and firmly as possible. Decisions about suicide risk should be clearly documented in the client's chart.

HAZARDS IN TREATING THE SUICIDAL CLIENT

The mirage of health. Some people may look healthiest immediately *after* a suicide attempt, if the attempt has mobilized support from family, friends, and caretakers. People who give perfectly rational explanations for their attempts (eliciting sympathy, getting attention) may convince you that they are out of danger. However, do not let such a person leave your care without a thorough mental health evaluation and without making arrangements for follow-up care. The probability of a subsequent, more serious attempt is extremely high if the person's condition and life circumstances remain unchanged.

Debating the wisdom of suicide. You may find yourself drawn into an argument over the pros and cons of suicide. Remember that almost all suicidal people are ambivalent about dying, and they may well opt to live once the crisis has passed. Impromptu existential debates are rarely helpful.

Monitoring your own reactions. You may be quite disturbed by a suicidal client's despair, or by what you see as the client's manipulativeness. Some health care professionals find themselves furious or frightened by talk of suicide. Others find their clients to be "kindred spirits" and may unwittingly ignore distress signals in an effort to see them as healthier than they really are.

You must be attuned to your own reactions to suicide, so that your "blind spots" and personal prejudices do not obscure the nature and severity of the illness. When you sense that your feelings are in some way interfering in your work with a suicidal client, do not hesitate to seek help from a colleague or supervisor. No one needs to manage a difficult crisis alone, and knowing when to ask for support is an essential aspect of good clinical care.

REFERENCES

Havens LL: The anatomy of suicide. N Engl J Med 272:401-406, 1965

Miles CP: Conditions predisposing to suicide: a review. J Nerv Ment Dis 164:231-246, 1977

Murphy GE, Wetzel RD: Suicide risk by birth cohort in the United States, 1949 to 1974. Arch Gen Psychiatry 37:519-523, 1980

Paykel ES, Myers JK, Lindenthal JJ, et al: Suicidal feelings in the general population: a prevalence study. Br J Psychiatry 124:460-469, 1974

Schneidman ES, Farberow NL, Litman RE: The Psychology of Suicide, 2nd ed. New York, Jason Aronson, 1976

Sletten IW, Barton JL: Suicidal patients in the emergency room: a guide for evaluation and disposition. Hosp Community Psychiatry 30:407-411, 1979

Tefft BM, Pederson AM, Babigian HM: Patterns of death among suicide attempters, a psychiatric population, and a general population. Arch Gen Psychiatry 34:1155-1161, 1977

Weisman AD, Worden JW: Risk-rescue rating in suicide assessment. Arch Gen Psychiatry 26:553-560, 1972

CHAPTER 14

Violence

Threatened and actual violence are ever more pervasive in our culture. Mental health professionals have long been prominent among those who work with "dangerous" individuals, but the issue of which violent acts to attribute to mental illness continues to cause heated debate in both courtrooms and emergency rooms.

Popular wisdom holds that insane people are dangerous people. Yet this notion does not hold up under scrutiny. Although some investigators report slightly higher rates of violent crime committed by released psychiatric inpatients than by the general population, this difference can be accounted for by patients who have a record of criminal activity prior to hospitalization. Psychiatric patients who do not have prior criminal records are, if anything, less prone to violent behavior than the general populace. The President's Commission on Mental Health addressed this issue in its 1978 report:

> The sporadic violence of so-called "mentally ill killers" as depicted in stories and drama is more a device of fiction than a fact of life. Patients with serious psychological disorders are more likely to be withdrawn, apathetic, and fearful. We do not deny that some mentally ill people are violent, but the image of the mentally ill person as essentially a violent person is erroneous. (p. 56)

Our understanding of violence is sadly limited. The literature abounds with studies that show the mental health profession's poor

341

record in the prediction of dangerousness. Yet mental health professionals continue to be called upon for expertise in evaluating violent individuals and forecasting their future behavior. Psychiatric assessment of "dangerousness" remains central to the decision to commit a potentially violent person to a psychiatric hospital against his or her will. Such opinions are often influential in distinguishing "patients" from "prisoners," and in determining whether a violent person is to be treated or punished. Although the complex relationship between mental illness and criminal justice is beyond the scope of this discussion, it is of critical importance in modern mental health care.

This chapter deals with violence on a personal level—how it affects you in your work as a health care professional. Although most mentally ill people are not violent, threatening behavior does occur in mental health settings—and indeed in all health care facilities—for we regularly deal with people who are under severe emotional stress. You may be faced with violence where you least expect it (e.g., from an enraged father who cannot accept the death of his hospitalized child), so it is essential that you become familiar with some basic principles of management. As an informed professional, you can make critical judgments that prevent injury, diminish fear, and deliver much-needed care to people who are on the verge of losing control, or who have already lost it.

SOME BASIC PRINCIPLES

Violence generally denotes an assault on objects or people. Where people are involved, it implies an intrusion that threatens another person's sense of safety or well-being. We often speak of verbal violence as well as physical violence, but "violence" will be used here to denote physical harm done by one human being to another.

Violence is a behavior, not a diagnosis. Violent behavior cuts across all diagnostic categories, and it is common among people who have no diagnosable mental disorder. It is not an illness, but in some cases, it is a symptom of an underlying illness.

Violence or the threat of violence preempts all efforts at treatment. It demands immediate management, for you cannot care for someone competently when you feel that you are in danger. Much like a cardiac arrest, the violent act in a mental health care setting is an emergency that must be responded to and effectively controlled before you can step back and think about underlying causes and possible remedies.

Minimizing or denying your own fear is the most dangerous thing you can do in dealing with people who may act violently. It is also the most common error made by inexperienced mental health profes sionals. Your own reaction to a client constitutes important data about how safe you are and how close the client is to losing control. It may be your only clue to an imminent attack. If you do not pay attention to your own responses, you put yourself, your client, and other people in real danger of being harmed, even killed. If this sounds overly dramatic, remember that mental health care professionals are at times the unfortunate victims of those they treat.

Why are we so prone to deny our fears in working with poten- tially violent people? As professionals, many of us harbor the unre- alistic belief that we should be able to cope with any problem under any and all circumstances. Admitting that we are afraid, or that we need help, is not consonant with that belief. You are not omnipotent if you summon security guards, or if you end an interview and leave the room after acknowledging to your client that you are concerned about his or her threatening behavior. You may be accustomed to putting your personal feelings aside until a crisis is over. But in fact, failing to attend to your own fears as you sit with a threatening client is like a nurse or physician failing to monitor someone's pulse and blood pressure during a cardiac arrest—you ignore critical data and thereby risk making the situation worse.

CLUES TO VIOLENCE

Potential violence may be easy to ignore, and it often goes unrecog- nized. Health care professionals who are hurried, emotionally with- drawn, or overly sympathetic may screen out clues to dangerousness and allow their clients' warnings to go unnoticed. You must be atten- tive to a variety of verbal and behavioral clues if you are to help people who cannot keep their violent impulses in check.

Threats. Roughly 5 percent of homicidal threats culminate in murder. Even when made in an offhand manner, threats of harm to others must be taken seriously and actively explored. A client may make casual threats to test your receptivity to the problem, and a concerned response allows the client to make a more explicit request for help.

Body space. The individual who remains constantly vigilant may be ready to lash out violently in self-defense. Such people reveal their inner terror in a variety of ways:

- *Shrinking from physical contact* (such as when approached for a handshake);
- *Feeling crowded* (paranoid people require roughly four times as much space as others do to maintain comfortable conversational distance);
- *Retreating when approached suddenly;* and
- *Protecting the rear* (a fear of being approached from behind and surprised by an assailant).

Physical findings. Unusual numbers of scars, lacerations, bruises, old fractures, and missing teeth may indicate that a client is habitually involved in violent activities.

Your gut response to the client. This is often the only clue to dangerousness. It is better to be overcautious and to overestimate possible danger than to underestimate it and be sorry.

EMERGENCY MANAGEMENT OF THE VIOLENT CLIENT

When people become violent or threaten violence in mental health care facilities, your first priority is to *ensure safety*—the client's, the staff's, and your own. No effective treatment can begin until care givers and client feel that the threat of danger has been removed.

Your second task is to *quiet the client and develop an alliance.* Many violent people assume a hostile and aggressive posture to defend themselves against intense feelings of helplessness and fragility. They are often fearful of losing control over their violent impulses. The following measures will help maintain a safe environment in which some collaboration between you and the client can take place (Table 14-1).

When a Client Is Potentially Violent But Danger Is Not Imminent

If you are interviewing someone who has a history of violent behavior, or who you sense might become agitated and lose control, you must structure your interview so as to maximize everyone's safety.

Show available force. Before you begin, or at any point when you sense danger, bring security guards and other personnel into the interview room or station them outside the room within the client's view. People who fear losing control of their impulses will find out-

Table 14–1. General guidelines for managing a violent client.

When there is a possibility of violence	When violence is present or imminent
Show available force	Summon help
Establish a nonthreatening setting for the interview	One staff member should assume leadership
Establish a collaborative tone in the interview	Remove all weapons from the client
Set verbal limits on threatening behavior	Seclude the client
Monitor your own reactions	Set physical limits on violent behavior when verbal limits do not suffice
Know when to stop the interview	Administer medication (antipsychotics, benzodiazepines) if needed to ease agitation and combativeness

side controls reassuring, and you will feel more comfortable with help nearby.

Establish a nonthreatening setting for the interview. Remain at least at arm's length from the client. Leave the client and yourself clear access to an exit, so that either one of you has the freedom to leave at any time (e.g., do not sit between your client and the door). The door to the interviewing room should remain open at all times. *Never approach the client from behind.*

Establish a collaborative tone in the interview. The most helpful interviewing style is a straightforward and respectful manner that honors the client's reasonable requests. You should show empathic concern but avoid appearing too warm or too friendly at the outset—this may frighten a paranoid client. Openly inquire about any veiled threats made against you or others, and encourage the paranoid client to see you as an ally against perceived enemies.

Set verbal limits on threatening behavior. When dealing with someone who is obviously agitated, try to help him or her *verbalize* feelings rather than acting on them. You may want to reassure the client that you will not allow anyone to be harmed—neither the client nor others. (Many paranoid people lash out because they are frightened that they will be attacked.)

Monitor your own reactions. Your gut responses to the client throughout the evaluation and treatment process may be your only clue to the client's level of hostility and degree of self-control. If you begin to feel unsafe, address this openly with the client and then remedy it; otherwise, the client will sense your uneasiness, and his or her own fears of losing control may intensify. You could, for example, ask security personnel stationed outside the interviewing room to come in, so that both you and the client feel safer to proceed.

Know when to stop. If you have taken precautions as noted above, but the client continues to be agitated and threatening, do not continue the interview. Instead, let the client know that you sense his or her difficulty in maintaining self-control, and that you are going to continue the interview at another time, when both of you can feel safer. Remember, you have nothing to lose by stopping an interview when you sense danger, and everything to lose by continuing.

When a Client Behaves Violently or Is on Verge of Losing Control

Summon help. Call for help at the first sign that a client may become violent (or before a violent person arrives, if advance warning is given). This help may include security guards, police (where necessary), or anyone capable of helping to restrain an assaultive individual.

Assume leadership. Both staff and client must feel that you can take charge and direct a team effort. Give your directions clearly and tell the client what to expect at each step. *No surprises.* Keep your distance from the client and do not block the doorway.

Remove all weapons. No treatment can be delivered to an armed client. This includes pills and liquor as well as knives, guns, and other instruments of force. Do not take a weapon directly from the client, but ask that it be placed on a table; then remove it. Explain that it will be held for safekeeping. Police help must be enlisted if an armed client refuses to cooperate with staff, and the client may need to be searched for weapons.

Seclude the client. Take the client away from large, populated areas (e.g., a waiting room) to a more secluded setting. This will limit the potential targets of any violent outbursts and quiet the client, especially when hostility and hypervigilance are due to fear of others. Seclusion is a common technique for decreasing agitation, since a seclusion room diminishes sights, sounds, and voices when the client's normal ability to screen out such environmental stimuli is impaired.

Set physical limits on violent behavior when verbal limits do not suffice. Remember that severe agitation is very frightening for the client as well as for others, and physical restraint is often relieving. Physical restraint involves using belts, straps, or other devices to restrict the client's movements, often by strapping the person's arms and legs to a bedframe as he or she lies on a mattress. Physical restraints provide concrete external controls when the client has lost his or her internal controls. Wrist and ankle restraints must not be used punitively, but only when physical harm to self or others appears imminent. The primary clinician should generally not take part in restraining the client for two reasons: 1) others are usually more skilled in this procedure, and 2) physical struggles between therapist and client may make later work impossible. One person should generally be assigned to restrain each of the person's extremities; this should be done with a minimum of struggling and as humanely as possible. The use of restraints does not replace personal contact and empathy.

Medication. The use of medication against the client's will as a *chemical restraint* is warranted only when there is immediate danger of injury to the client or to others. Of course, the medication must be prescribed and administered by qualified personnel. However, a client or patient who is acutely anxious will often willingly accept medication if the reasons for treatment and the effects of the medicine are carefully discussed in advance, and if the plan of treatment is presented in a firm and confident manner.

Antipsychotics may be given orally or intramuscularly to control agitation and combative behavior. A physician responsible for a violent patient's medication may, for example, prescribe 2-5 mg of haloperidol (Haldol) orally or intramuscularly every 30 minutes until agitation subsides. This is a drug of choice in many cases, since it does not cause the rapid drop in blood pressure that commonly results from certain other major tranquilizers. Another likely choice would be chlorpromazine (Thorazine), with 25-50 mg given intramuscularly or 50-100 mg given orally every 30 minutes until agitation subsides. Chlorpromazine is more likely than the higher-potency neuroleptics (e.g., haloperidol) to cause hypotensive reactions (sudden drops in blood pressure) and must therefore be used intramuscularly with caution.

Benzodiazepines (minor tranquilizers) are particularly useful for those who are agitated but not actively violent and for the elderly, who are more sensitive to hypotensive reactions. A physician might call for 5-20 mg of diazepam (Valium) to be administered orally or intramuscularly every four to six hours, or 50-100 mg of chlordiazepoxide (Librium) every six to eight hours.

For severe alcohol withdrawal, a physician might prescribe 10-30 cc of paraldehyde orally every four hours.

Amobarbital sodium (sodium amytal) is another powerful sedative, which may be used in oral doses of 100-200 mg as needed to produce sedation.

PROFILES IN VIOLENCE

There is enormous diversity among those who resort to violence, but certain personal characteristics are common. If you are alert to these correlates of violence, you can use them to put your client's threats or behavior into perspective and to judge his or her potential to act violently in the future.

Previous violent behavior. Previous violent behavior is the most valid predictor of violent behavior in the future. The probability of future violence increases with each violent act. This includes a history of arrests, assaults on people or property, and a history of accidental or intentional involvement in another person's death.

Age. Violent behavior peaks among teenagers and those in their early twenties. Juvenile violence is increasing at nearly twice the rate of violence among adults. The earlier one is violent, the greater the likelihood that one will continue to be violent.

Sex. Ninety percent of those arrested for violent crimes are male. But much domestic violence (e.g., child abuse) perpetrated by women goes unreported.

Race. Blacks account for 12 percent of the population but 48 percent of all arrests for violent crime in the United States each year. The reasons for this disproportionate representation of blacks among violent criminals are not entirely clear, but social injustices and economic discrimination against blacks in this country are obvious contributing factors.

Drug and alcohol abuse. Substance abuse is highly correlated with violent behavior and predisposes one to violence through a variety of mechanisms (see below).

Socioeconomic status and employment stability. Violence is markedly increased among members of lower socioeconomic groups and among those with a history of unemployment or irregular employment.

Self-destructive behavior. This factor is often overlooked. Self-mutilation and suicide are disproportionately common among people who act violently toward others.

Other factors that correlate with violent behavior include increased residential mobility ("absent roots"), being single, lower IQ, and lower level of educational attainment.

Childhood Correlates of Violence in Adults

Which children grow up to be violent? We do not know, but the following factors have been found to be particularly prevalent in the childhood experiences of people who behave violently as adults:

- *Parental deprivation and abuse.* Violent people frequently give histories of parental neglect or abandonment, as well as parental abuse (verbal, physical, or both). Those who were victims as children commonly become victimizers as adults.
- *Early exposure to violence.* Parental and sibling brutality witnessed in the home provides a model for conflict resolution through violence.
- *Frequent disruptions in family life.* This includes parental separation or divorce, frequent moves, and school changes.
- *Bedwetting, firesetting, and cruelty to animals.* This "triad" is encountered frequently among children who have poor impulse control, but what was once thought to be a clear relationship between this triad and subsequent violent behavior has been challenged in recent studies.
- *Temper tantrums and frequent fights.*
- *Authority problems.* These include truancy, school problems, and difficulties in the military or in other employment situations.

ETIOLOGIES OF VIOLENCE

In evaluating a client who has acted violently, you must consider the possible causes of this behavior. Many mental disorders underlie violence; some of the most important ones are listed below. But since most violence is perpetrated by people who do not suffer from a major mental disorder, your first task is to determine whether the problem is psychiatric.

You may find it helpful to try to fit your client's behavior into a broader conceptual scheme of the etiology of violence. Most of us keep our violent impulses in check most of the time. What, then, has prompted this person to act on his or her violent impulses in this setting at this time?

Does the person suffer from an impaired ability to test reality? People who are hallucinating may hear voices commanding them to act violently—for example, a man may hear his dead mother's voice commanding him to kill his father. Someone who is having visual hallucinations might see you as a vampire who is about to attack.

Paranoid thinking plays a prominent role in many acts of violence. People who resort to the use of violence frequently believe that they are being persecuted, harassed, or unfairly treated; they view the world as hostile and threatening; and they often lash out in "self-defense." Paranoid ideas generally begin with the misinterpretation of real events. The paranoid person who acts violently often does so because of a distorted view of his or her situation.

Does the client suffer from an impaired ability to control his or her impulses? We all have violent impulses. On a daily basis, we hear ourselves and others make such statements as, "I wanted to wring his neck!" Yet we control these urges, sometimes so rigidly that we push them out of our awareness entirely. We do not attack others whenever we feel like it. People who do not control themselves may not have developed a normal capacity for self-control as children, because of poor parental control, neurologic impairment, a severely disturbed home environment, or other factors we have yet to elucidate. Such people often give histories of impulsivity in many areas of their lives, including sexual behavior, employment, drug abuse, and reckless driving. Other people lose the ability to control their impulses only temporarily—e.g., under the influence of disinhibiting substances such as opiates or alcohol.

Does the client show impaired judgment? Judgment is a complex mental function involving a variety of cognitive skills. Obviously, psychosis or drug use can impair one's ability to judge how to behave in a given situation. Other factors that may impair judgment include anxiety, depression, and neurologic impairment (e.g., as a result of head trauma).

Does the client use violence explicitly to manipulate others? Many people suffer from no impairment in mental functioning but simply use physical force deliberately and in a calculated fashion to intimidate or to achieve what they want at others' expense. Such people do not require mental health care, but rather disciplinary action.

Mental Disorders and Violence

Some of the more common mental disorders may foster violent behavior. They are listed in Table 14-2 and described briefly below.

Table 14–2. Some disorders that may underlie violent behavior.

Psychotic illnesses
  Schizophrenia
  Mania
  Psychotic depression
  Brief reactive psychosis
 	
Personality disorders, especially:
  Paranoid personality disorder
  Borderline personality disorder
  Obsessive-compulsive personality
    disorder
  Antisocial personality disorder
 	
Sexual disorders
	Drug intoxication or withdrawal
	  Alcohol
	  Opiates
	  Amphetamines
	  Barbiturates
	  Cannabis
	  Cocaine
	  LSD
	  Phencyclidine (PCP)
	
	Organic conditions
	  Temporal lobe epilepsy
	  Brain damage
	  Dementia
	  Adult minimal brain dysfunction
	  Altered androgen levels
	  Delirium

Psychotic Illnesses

Schizophrenia. Delusional beliefs and hallucinations become the "motives" for violence.

Mania. Delusions and hallucinations, coupled with uncontrolled rage and hyperactivity, predispose the client to violence.

Psychotic depression. The hopeless person may kill family members or a lover in the delusional belief that this "spares them grief" and may go on to commit suicide. Elderly people with agitated depression can be surprisingly combative.

Postpartum depression. This is a special category of depression. Typically, the mother becomes anxious prior to delivery, develops delusions about her husband's infidelity, and becomes depressed after delivery. She is at risk of harming her newborn child.

Personality Disorders
Any of the personality disorders may be accompanied by violence, particularly those listed below.

Paranoid personality disorder. Constant, pervasive paranoia may erupt into violence when the paranoid person feels that he or she is under attack.

Borderline personality disorder. Poor impulse control and persistent anger may prompt borderline individuals to behave violently toward those who are important to them, but anger turned against the self is more common.

Obsessive-compulsive personality disorder. The highly controlled, obsessional individual may "explode" under severe stress.

Antisocial personality disorder. This disorder is characterized by failure to accept social norms, recklessness, impulsivity, and unstable relationships. Often labeled "sociopaths," people who have this disorder characteristically feel no remorse for antisocial behavior.

Sexual disorders
Sexual dysfunction. Threats to sexual identity, particularly impotence from any cause, may prompt a show of force in an attempt to demonstrate virility.

Homosexual panic. Men whose unconscious homosexual strivings come to the surface (e.g., in the military or other situations of forced intimacy) may become acutely anxious and paranoid. The individual who is in the midst of homosexual panic believes others are accusing him of "forbidden" homosexual wishes and practices, and he may pick fights in an attempt to prove his manhood. Such men frequently brawl in barrooms with "drinking buddies."

Drug-Related Violence
Drugs may precipitate violence in three basic ways:

- Substances with disinhibiting effects can take away an individual's self-control, particularly when that control was tenuous in the first place.
- Intoxication may result in delirium or toxic psychosis, in which confusion, delusions, and hallucinations prompt violent behavior.
- Drug withdrawal syndromes may include agitation, confusion, and psychosis.

Some drugs commonly implicated in acts of violence are alcohol and opiates (43 percent of all violent crimes are committed by people who are under the influence of opiates or alcohol), amphetamines, barbiturates, cannabis (marijuana, hashish, synthetic tetrahydrocannabinol), cocaine, LSD, and phencyclidine (PCP).

Less common causes of violent behavior, but sometimes encountered among medical and psychiatric patients, are L-dopa, benzodiazepines, and tricyclic antidepressants.

Organic Conditions
Some organic conditions may produce violent behavior, such as those listed below.

Temporal lobe epilepsy. People who experience psychomotor seizures are at risk for developing impulsive and irritable behavior patterns, characterized by angry outbursts. These outbursts do not occur at random but are often provoked. They do not occur during seizures, do not commonly result in serious injuries, and alternate with prolonged periods of "good behavior." Families often note that the person seems to have undergone a gradual personality change.

Brain damage. Traumatic lesions most often associated with violence are those involving the frontal or temporal lobes, particularly the limbic system and the area of the amygdala and hippocampus. Brain damage that prompts subsequent violent behavior may occur at birth, or later in life as the result of falls, motor vehicle accidents, etc.

Dementia. Alzheimer's disease and senile dementia diminish integrative capacity and produce confusion, which often results in combative states, even among seemingly frail elderly people.

Adult minimal brain dysfunction. This syndrome of aggressiveness, impulsivity, and mood disorder is often found in people with a history of minimal brain dysfunction in childhood.

Altered androgen levels. An uncommon cause of violent behavior, it is found in some cases where violence is associated with sexual activity.

Delirium. Delirium may result from a variety of causes, including metabolic encephalopathies (see Chapter 9).

ASSESSMENT

Clinical evaluation of people who behave violently must include a detailed exploration of violent acts and impulses, along with thorough psychiatric and medical histories. People rarely exhibit random violence but become dangerous to others only under specific circumstances. You must therefore pay close attention to the particular social, biologic, and psychological stressors that trigger violent impulses in each person. Only by constructing individual "profiles" of violence can you tailor treatment to individual clients' needs. Also, if you can identify specific settings, events, and other factors that trigger violence in your client, you will improve your ability to predict when he or she may act violently in the future.

Evaluating Violence

The following questions may help you assess a client's current status after a recent episode of violent behavior or violent threats.

Current Crisis
- What happened?
- Who decided that you needed help? (You? A relative? A friend?)
- Do you think your behavior is a problem? Do others think so? If so, in what way?
- What prompted this crisis? (Fears of others, threats from others, etc.)
- Where did it happen? (In a bar, at home, at work)
- Who was involved? (Spouse, policeman, passerby)

In as much detail as possible, reconstruct exactly what was said, what was done, and who was involved. Also note whether drugs or alcohol were involved. What were the client's thoughts and feelings throughout the episode?

Potential Victims
- Who do you feel angry at now?
- Is there anyone you would like to hurt/kill?
- Is there anyone you feel wants to hurt you?
- Are you likely to see these people soon?

Available Weapons
- How would you carry out your threat/protect yourself?
- Do you have a gun, knife, etc.?

History of Violent Behavior
- How far back does your trouble with violence (getting into fights) go?
- What is the most violent thing you have ever done?
- How badly have you hurt someone in the past?
- What is the closest you have come to killing someone?
- Where do fights usually occur? With whom? What do you usually fight about?
- Do you get into fights (in general or with a specific individual) more or less often than you used to?
- Are the fights getting worse?
- Have you ever been arrested? (Document dates)
- Have you been convicted of any crimes? (Document crimes, sentences)
- Have you ever been hospitalized because of your violent behavior?
- What weapons have you used in the past? Against whom?
- Do you ever hit your spouse/child?

Try to get a detailed picture of previous situations in which the client has acted violently—e.g., when intoxicated, upon ending a relationship, when fired from a job, when manic.

Environment
Assess the client's family situation, along with any unusual peer pressures.

- Has anything recently changed at home or with friends? Has an important relationship recently or suddenly been threatened? (Note that 75 percent of all emergency commitments occur when family members are attacked or threatened. Half of all homicides are committed by family members or lovers.)

- Are you the only one at home/at work/among your friends who gets into fights?
- Have you had trouble at work lately?

Judgment

Can the client accurately appraise situations and anticipate the consequences of his or her actions?

- Do you think you will need to behave violently again?
- What do you think will happen to you if you do what you have in mind?

Psychiatric Evaluation

A general psychiatric evaluation is part of every assessment of the violent client. Special attention should be paid to the following areas:

- History of drug and alcohol use,
- Childhood history (abuse or neglect, violence in the home, tantrums, frequent fights, school difficulty, delinquency, problems with authority),
- Sexual concerns, and
- The mental status examination, particularly delusions (e.g., thought control, thought broadcasting), hallucinations (commands or threats from imaginary beings), depersonalization, paranoia, suicidal ideation, and impulsivity.

TREATMENT

When a client comes to you in an outpatient clinic or emergency room with a history of recent violent or threatening behavior, you must judge whether it is safe to allow that person to return to the community. Obviously, your decision will be based on many factors, including the client's mental status, the presence of underlying medical or psychiatric illness, and your assessment of the likelihood that the client will harm someone if released.

If you are concerned that a client will be violent if allowed to go home, it is safest to hospitalize him or her so that you have more time to thoroughly evaluate the situation. Again, it is better to be safe than sorry.

Hospitalization

Indications for hospitalization include 1) specific homicidal intent with a definite, workable plan and the availability of weapons and intended victims; 2) lack of internal controls—impulsivity, poor judgment, faulty reality testing; 3) lack of social supports—family and friends are unavailable or are themselves in danger; 4) acute psychosis; and 5) toxic states that do not clear rapidly.

People who fear their own violent impulses may willingly agree to hospitalization. Involuntary commitment is justified in most states only when there is a substantial risk of physical harm to others or evidence that the client has placed others in a reasonable fear of harm.

When involuntary commitment is indicated. Involuntary commitment must be presented to the client in a firm and nonpunitive manner. Staff must remain with the client at all times to prevent escape, and transportation must be carried out by ambulance and/or by security forces. Hospitalization should not mean rejection—whenever possible, if you do the initial assessment, you should make a follow-up visit once the client is admitted to the hospital.

When involuntary commitment is not indicated. You face a dilemma when the client does not fit the criteria for commitment and refuses voluntary hospitalization, but there is concern that a specific intended victim might be harmed. Recent court rulings (e.g., *Tarasoff v. Regents of University of California*) have upheld the idea that clinicians are obligated to warn intended victims when clients express homicidal intentions toward specific people. Since it constitutes a breach of confidentiality in the therapist-client relationship, this concept is under heated debate. Also, given mental health professionals' demonstrated inability to reliably predict their clients' future violent behavior, many feel that the profession has become legally bound to perform a task of which it is incapable. Nevertheless, the clinician must contact and warn intended victims if clients are sent home with persistent thoughts of violence focused on particular individuals. A useful therapeutic stance is to inform the client that the rules of confidentiality do not hold in cases where the client's or someone else's life is in danger.

When you make judgments about a client's dangerousness, it is essential that the basis for these judgments and subsequent interventions be carefully documented in the client's record.

Outpatient Treatment

Clients who reveal no clear violent intention or plan, and who have no history of violence, may be followed up in outpatient treatment if they appear capable of allying themselves with you and seeking help before they act on violent impulses. Before the client is sent home, it is essential that precise arrangements for follow-up be made, ideally involving you if you performed the initial assessment.

Psychotherapy. Psychotherapy can be helpful to clients who want and can use an ongoing relationship. The therapist should assume an interested but nonintrusive attitude, avoiding all physical contact and initially avoiding the use of humor, which may be misunderstood by a suspicious client. The focus of work is on helping the client recognize violent urges and behavior patterns, and on finding verbal or other means of ventilating these urges without acting them out. Clients must learn to predict the times and situations when they are likely to act violently, and to develop means of preventing such acts.

Clinicians disagree about the best treatment regimen for violent or potentially violent people. Some consider regular outpatient appointments with one therapist the treatment of choice. Others recommend treatment on an "as needed" basis at one facility by a variety of health care providers, in order to dilute the intense and potentially overwhelming feelings that might develop in a therapy relationship and that could actually promote violence toward the therapist. Most clinicians agree that violent people need access to one institution on an ongoing basis for crisis intervention.

Pharmacologic treatment. There are no specific medications for the long-term management of violent behavior. Medication should be used only when it is likely to alleviate an underlying mental disorder, and only after a thorough discussion with the client (Table 14-3).

In rare cases of intractable violence, psychosurgery has been effective. In violence associated with sexual activity, antiandrogen therapy which reduces blood levels of male sex hormones with drugs like medroxyprogesterone (Depo-provera) has proved useful. However, both treatments raise particular ethical problems for the clinician.

YOUR REACTIONS TO VIOLENCE

Anxiety in dealing with violent people is real and must be used as data rather than ignored. In the struggle to remain in control of the

Table 14–3. Some medications that may be indicated in the management of violent behavior.

Medication	Indication
Antipsychotics	Psychosis and overwhelming anxiety
Lithium	Affective disorders and disorders of impulse control (e.g., episodic dyscontrol)
Antidepressants	Depression
Benzodiazepines	Anxiety
Anticonvulsants	Underlying seizure disorders, including psychomotor seizures
Disulfiram (Antabuse)	Alcohol addiction

situation, you may defend against your own uneasiness in a variety of unproductive ways:

Denial. You may overlook important evidence of the client's dangerousness (e.g., not hearing veiled threats, forgetting to ask about weapons) and see only the client's nonthreatening qualities.

Reaction formation. "I'm afraid of you" may become "I'm not afraid of you," and your fear may be transformed into an overly warm and solicitous manner that can raise a paranoid client's level of anxiety.

Withdrawal. If you feel helpless in treating a violent individual, you may avoid or openly reject the client without being aware of your own emotional withdrawal.

Retaliation. Anger at the client can be expressed through punitive treatment (e.g., the unnecessary use of restraints). You may find yourself enraged at someone who threatens you, and you may actually find pleasure in the "revenge" involved in restraining a violent person with medication or by physical force. If this happens, simply step back from the situation and allow others to take over for you. Anger and fear are normal reactions to violence—you need not be ashamed of them. However, you are obliged as a professional to remove yourself (at least temporarily) from the treatment situation if such feelings begin to influence your clinical decisions.

Treatment for the Treaters

Working with people who resort to violence is extremely stressful. Witnessing violent behavior, and fearing for your own safety, are experiences that arouse some of our most primitive emotions. You must have support in doing such work, as outlined below.

Group support. Staff members who have been involved in a crisis with a violent client commonly meet when the crisis has passed to "decompress" and discuss their reactions to what has happened.

Supervision. Supervisors who have experience in working with violent people can help you understand your reactions to threatening clients and improve your therapeutic skills.

Review of security procedures in the facility where you work. This may allay some anxiety and will improve your future efficiency in managing crises with violent clients. Review in detail plans for summoning help and procedures for carrying out physical restraint.

Visit a maximum security psychiatric facility. This is likely to broaden your perspective on how violent behavior can be controlled and treatment facilitated.

Peer support. The most helpful support usually comes from your colleagues, who best understand your reactions as a trainee in a stressful situation.

Violence, perhaps more than any other clinical situation, highlights the fact that you cannot care effectively for others if you do not take care of yourself.

REFERENCES

Benson DF, Blumer D: Temporal lobe epilepsy and its psychiatric significance, in Psychiatric Aspects of Neurological Disease. New York, Grune and Stratton, 1975, pp 119-217

Drugs that cause psychiatric symptoms. The Medical Letter 23:9-12, Feb 6, 1981

Lion JR: Evaluation and Management of the Violent Patient. Springfield, Ill, Charles C Thomas, 1972

Monahan J: The Clinical Prediction of Violent Behavior. Washington, DC, National Institute of Mental Health, 1981

President's Commission on Mental Health: Report to the President. Washington, DC, President's Commission on Mental Health, 1978, p 56

Rada RT: The violent patient: rapid assessment and management. Psychosomatics 22:101-109, 1981

Rockwell DA: Can you spot potential violence in a patient? Hospital Physician 10:52-56, 1972

Tupin JP: Management of violent patients, in Manual of Psychiatric Therapeutics. Edited by Shader RI. Boston, Little, Brown, 1975, pp 125-136

Part IV

INTRODUCTION

The two major forms of treatment in modern psychiatry are the psychotherapies and the somatic therapies. Chapter 15 is a discussion of several different types of psychotherapy. The array of psychosocial treatments now used in mental health care is vast. This chapter could not begin to teach you about all of them, and no attempt is made to do so. Instead, the chapter includes an extensive discussion of traditional psychodynamic psychotherapy and a much more cursory description of some other important treatment modalities.

Why the emphasis on psychodynamics? First, as a mental health practitioner, you will need to have more than a superficial understanding of this approach to treating mental illness, since it continues to be the major form of psychotherapy used in the mental health field. Second, Freudian psychodynamic theory is the foundation upon which many subsequent theories of the mind were constructed, and it is the school of thought to which many psychological theorists have reacted. Your understanding of the "basics" will greatly enhance your ability to think critically about the many ways in which these principles have been modified in later efforts to understand and treat psychiatric disorders.

Chapter 16 covers the somatic therapies, beginning with a general discussion of the principles of psychotropic medications. You should read this section in its entirety. The subsequent sections on specific classes of medication are for you to refer to as questions about particular medications arise in the course of your clinical work. Electroconvulsive therapy (ECT) is discussed at the end of the chapter.

Chapter 15

Psychotherapies

Contact with other human beings can relieve distress, change behavior patterns, and alter our views of ourselves and the world. All psychological therapies rely on this fundamental premise. From the infinitely complex ways in which people interact, psychosocial theorists attempt to tease out the factors that promote emotional well-being and those that foster ill health. These studies have yielded a variety of schemes for understanding emotional life and treating psychological impairment.

The term *psychotherapy* includes the means by which a therapist attempts to provide new interpersonal experiences for another human being. These experiences are designed to enhance one's ability to manage subjective distress and to participate in loving relationships and satisfying work.

To be sure, these are ambitious goals. They are, in essence, no different from the goals any health care professional brings to work with people, for the aim of all therapeutics is to improve the quality of life. Most medical practitioners rely heavily on the use of concrete aids in their therapeutic interventions: medications, surgical procedures, and an ever-increasing array of tools and machines. Psychosocial therapists, by contrast, rely on themselves as the primary agents of treatment. Yet the medical and psychosocial models of therapy are much closer than they at first appear. Regardless of specialty, experienced practitioners invariably attest to the therapeutic power inherent in human relationships.

HOW CAN A HUMAN RELATIONSHIP BE THERAPEUTIC?

Each type of therapy discussed in this text emphasizes a particular view of mental illness and particular treatment techniques. Yet all therapeutic situations share certain important factors that promote recovery.

The client brings to therapy an expectation that help is possible. Psychotherapy prescribes that the therapist and the client work together in specific ways that they both believe will be a means of restoring health. The therapist offers a sincere, interested, attentive, and reliable presence; the client generally comes to view the therapist as a benign and powerful force. Most clients come to treatment with the hope that the therapist has benevolent powers.

Where does this hope come from? Human beings spend many years in a dependent relationship with their parents and other caretakers. As children, we learn that needs can be satisfied, fears allayed, and pains eased by the care and attention of adults. This learned expectation of help becomes activated in many situations in our adult lives, such as when we consult health care professionals.

These hopes serve as the cornerstone for successful treatment. In psychoanalytic terms, this phenomenon is referred to as positive transference, since we transfer positive expectations we had for early caretakers to people we expect to play similar roles in our adult lives. As a rule, people who have not learned to trust in this manner were deprived of care during early infancy. Such people may bring to therapy ingrained attitudes of suspicion and hate that take months or even years to overcome, or their mistrust may be so pervasive that it is impossible to establish a therapeutic relationship.

Psychotherapy gives the client a conceptual scheme for making sense of bewildering mental phenomena. Each type of psychotherapy provides a set of concepts that people can use to label and explain confusing subjective states and seemingly inexplicable behaviors. This enhances the person's sense of control over problems.

The therapist offers the expectation that the client can make positive life changes. Although this may appear obvious, many people come to therapy believing that they are incapable of self-improvement. Relatives and friends may share this pessimism, and everyone in the client's life may be quite comfortable with the view that the client is "disturbed" or "a mental case" or "the one with problems." In such situations, the therapist offers a different perspective and an unwillingness to share these stereotyped views.

The client adopts certain of the therapist's positive attitudes. This happens through identification, a process that occurs in all of us from early childhood onward, as we consciously and unconsciously take on the characteristics of important others (e.g., parents, teachers) we want to be like. The client in psychotherapy identifies with the therapist's attitude that problems can be faced squarely, and that seemingly unbearable thoughts and feelings can be tolerated and managed. For example, a client who is brutally self-critical can identify with the therapist's more tolerant and realistic view, thus gaining the ability to be more flexible and less demanding of perfection.

Therapy offers a safe place for taking risks. The client learns that it is possible to discuss "forbidden" feelings, attitudes, and experiences with another person without being judged or reprimanded. Developing a trusting, confiding, emotional relationship with the therapist is, in and of itself, a considerable achievement for many isolated and inhibited people, and this relationship serves as a model for developing more satisfying relations with others. The client can also use therapy to experiment with new behaviors, in a situation that carries no real threat of punishment.

The safety of therapy lies in its structure: the sessions have clear boundaries of time and space; the therapist is restrained, professional, and nonjudgmental; and the activities that go on between client and therapist are strictly limited. These limitations are at times frustrating, but also reassuring. For example, a client who is frightened by sexual impulses can learn that it is possible to talk about such feelings without having to act on them.

Therapy expands one's horizons and increases one's options. This occurs in innumerable ways. Many forms of therapy help the client arrive at a fuller awareness of self, particularly those aspects of the self that were previously disavowed or distorted. Therapy also helps clients see the ways in which they repeatedly distort their perceptions of others. This opens up the possibility of dealing with people in more productive and satisfying ways. Some therapists explicitly teach new behaviors; others attempt to teach new cognitive styles. All therapies offer new possibilities for viewing oneself and dealing with the world—i.e., they reopen the future by facilitating growth.

Psychotherapy cannot alter the problems of the world in which clients live. It cannot, for example, eliminate stress or poverty. But therapy can enhance self-acceptance and help clients cope more effectively with their environment.

MODELS OF PSYCHOTHERAPY

There are two basic models of psychotherapy. Psychodynamic therapies are based on the idea that people can achieve greater understanding of the psychological forces that motivate their actions, and that insight achieved through psychological exploration opens up possibilities for change in personality and behavior. The classic insight-oriented therapy is psychoanalysis, which will serve as a prototype for our discussion of psychodynamic change.

A second model is that of the behavior therapies. Behavior therapies do not aim to develop insight or bring about personality change, but they instead use directive techniques to remove specific symptoms. Persuasion and learning theories provide the theoretical bases for these therapies.

Behavior therapy and psychoanalysis may be seen as two ends of a very broad spectrum of psychological treatments. In fact, most therapies involve some admixture of supportive-directive work and self-exploration.

THE PSYCHODYNAMIC MODEL OF CHANGE

Psychodynamic therapy encompasses a vast array of treatment modalities, including individual, group, couples, and family therapy. Sigmund Freud (1856-1939) is generally acknowledged to be the major figure in the genesis of this approach, for he was the first person to systematize a method of understanding seemingly unintelligible behavior in adult life by relating such behavior to childhood experiences.

All psychodynamic therapies share the assumption that the present is shaped and governed by the past—i.e., that our present attitudes and styles of reacting to the world are, to some extent, carryovers from our attitudes and reactions to people and events earlier in life. Psychodynamic theorists focus on childhood—particularly on infantile experience—in attempting to understand mental health and mental illness. This is not to say that childhood trauma is invariably the cause of psychological difficulties in adult life. Indeed, human behavior cannot be reduced to simple causal explanations. Nonetheless, how children experience pleasure and pain, reward and punishment, in the context of family and social life prompts the gradual development of personality traits, ideas about oneself, and expectations of others.

Each of us develops along different lines. We have different caretakers as children and different family constellations; we play different roles within those constellations; and we bring different inborn characteristics to our dealings with the world. Each person's "take" on the world is unique, and the psychological traits and forces that develop early in our lives are highly individual, like fingerprints. These forces are modified as life proceeds, but the extent to which early roles and attitudes persist into adulthood and rule our adult lives is considerable.

Many of these psychological forces operate without our being aware of them. They are *unconscious*. The unconscious consists of fantasies, feelings, expectations, memories, attitudes—virtually all types of mental phenomena (see Chapter 2).

Why do some things lie outside our awareness? Material is pushed into the unconscious because it reflects experiences that are unacceptable at the time and in the circumstances in which they first occur. For example, a small boy may be totally unaware that he feels murderous rage toward his abusive mother. The child *represses* his anger—i.e., banishes it from his consciousness—because he cannot resolve the conflict between his wishes to murder his mother and his very real need for mother's care and protection.

The idea of *conflict* is central to the psychodynamic model of mental illness. Conflict refers to the opposition between seemingly irreconcilable forces. Examples include a wish to excel and a wish not to defeat others, or a wish to please someone that can only be achieved by doing something that is considered wrong.

Many of those who seek psychological treatment are enmeshed in conflict and are in some way hampered by it. Battles between opposing psychological forces can consume a tremendous amount of energy and leave the individual exhausted and incapable of effective functioning, as seen in the following example:

A young man who had unconsciously adopted his parents' strong prohibitions against sexuality found himself caught in a desperate struggle between his own sexual longings and the dictates of a stern conscience. Sexually frustrated and incapable of forming a satisfying sexual relationship, he sought gratification in other, less intimate activities. He turned to auto racing, which, although objectively more dangerous, was emotionally safe. Despite his considerable success in this endeavor, he remained unsatisfied with his life and preoccupied. Moreover, he began to have difficulty completing projects at work and was increasingly unable to concentrate on even the simplest of tasks.

In many cases, such as this one, people who are caught between conflicting intrapsychic demands or desires find themselves unable to derive satisfaction from work or play. They may feel anxious or depressed, or they may develop discrete symptoms such as phobias or compulsive rituals; however, because the conflict is unconscious, they are not aware of the cause of their distress.

Psychoanalytic theory holds that conflict fosters the development of symptoms in three stages:

1. The presence of an unresolvable conflict,
2. An attempt to repress the conflict, and
3. The return of the repressed conflict to conscious life in a disguised form: as a symptom (e.g., anxiety or compulsive behaviors) or as a pathological character trait (e.g. passive-aggressive characteristics).

Life events and the process of growing up can ease internal conflicts, and many people find their way out of such dilemmas without psychotherapeutic intervention. However, some people become "stuck" and cannot find satisfactory solutions on their own.

Psychological conflict often manifests itself in disturbed relationships with others—a phenomenon that is especially prominent in many personality disorders. People with these disorders characteristically transpose their intrapsychic dilemmas onto a larger interpersonal stage and rely on distorted perceptions of others to ease their internal distress. For example, a man who cannot accept his feelings of murderous rage toward his family may develop the belief that other people are "out to get him." What starts out as danger from within—the threat that he may act on unacceptable impulses—is transformed into a danger from without, and the patient is able to assume the role of victim instead of victimizer. Not surprisingly, such distortions can upset family, friends, and even entire social institutions. A person enmeshed in such struggles with the world is likely to be brought to treatment when those around him or her become exasperated.

The notion of conflict provides a framework for understanding many symptoms of mental illness. However, some people—particularly those who are more severely impaired—seem to have an absence of certain emotional and intellectual capacities that are normally acquired in the process of growing up. They are thought to have psychological *deficits* that make them incapable of certain activities most of us take for granted. Examples of psychological deficits include a lack of the capacity to control violent or sexual impulses, the inability to anticipate the consequences of one's acts, and the inability to understand the difference between one's own and another person's feelings.

In pursuing the nature of mental illness, psychodynamic theorists and clinicians continue to debate whether certain symptoms and character traits result from conflicts or from deficits. This controversy has important implications for treatment.

Sources of Data in Psychotherapy

People come to psychotherapy because they have problems and need help. Their presenting complaints usually involve immediate life events and specific symptoms, but they are generally unaware of the deeper issues that underlie their complaints as in the following case:

> A 23-year-old woman sought therapy after breaking up with her 45-year-old boyfriend. She reported that she became inexplicably anxious and had to flee the relationship as it became more intimate. She was aware that other relationships, also with older men, had ended in a similar fashion but she did not understand why. In the treatment that followed, the client and her therapist explored the origins of her need to flee from intimacy, particularly when it involved older men. Eventually she recalled a childhood experience in which an uncle's physical affection had frightened and excited her. She was also able to recall the shame she felt not only because her uncle had caressed her body but also because, from time to time, she wished that he would do it again. In her adult life she found herself pursuing older men but, at the same time, she unconsciously equated sexual intimacy with her fear of sexual exploitation and with her forbidden interest.

As a therapist, how would you work with a client to understand the presenting problem? The therapist has several sources of data about how clients' minds work. First, they offer information about their past experiences: their relationships with important people and how they felt and behaved in a variety of situations. Second, as sessions proceed, clients generally bring information about their current lives and relationships. Third, the client forms a relationship with the therapist. This relationship is a powerful tool, because clients bring the same set of unconscious conflicts and motives to therapy that they bring to their dealings with other people in their lives. Thus, they are bound to recreate in therapy many of the pathological patterns that brought them into treatment in the first place. The therapist can then help the client step back from the relationship and attempt to understand its unsatisfying and destructive aspects.

This brings us to two of the most important concepts that psychoanalytic theory has contributed to our understanding of the human mind: *transference* and *resistance*.

Transference

We are not born knowing how to relate to other people. From the first moment of life, the infant begins to form relationships and, in doing so, learns patterns of dealing with others that are not arbitrary but are determined both by the infant's inherent temperament and by the environment into which he or she is born. The way we learn to form relationships is strongly influenced by the particular people who are important to us early in life—most often, parents, other primary caretakers, and siblings. We carry our feelings for these people with us into adult life, and they serve as templates on which we form later relationships.

Thus, our reactions to new people in our lives are not only based on how we experience them in reality. We also tend to displace onto new people the feelings and attitudes we had toward early significant figures (parents, siblings, etc.)—transferring feelings from old relationships to new ones. This happens with particular intensity when someone in the present resembles someone important from the past. The resemblance may be in very particular details (appearance or tone of voice) or it may simply be in the nature of the relationship itself (e.g., that of an authority figure). An individual may thus stir up intense feelings of worship or hatred, longing or fear, that are totally inappropriate to one's real knowledge or experience of that person. This is *transference*, and it is, for the most part, unconscious.

Transference feelings are present to some extent in all of our relationships, and they help determine our choices of friends, lovers, and colleagues. But transference reactions are likely to occur with particular strength toward people who perform functions that were originally carried out by parents—including teachers, lovers, celebrities, bosses, and, of course, therapists.

Clients instinctively reenact their earliest interpersonal patterns and conflicts in the relationship with the psychotherapist. They do this by attempting to coerce the therapist into being something other than a therapist—a lover, a protector, or a competitor.

> A client complained that throughout his adult life he had always established highly idealized relationships with women, but the women he went out with always fell short of his expectations. Similarly, in the therapeutic situation, his therapist (who happened to be a woman) always disappointed him in that she "never quite understood what I was driving at," she sometimes had to change his appointment time, and she occasionally had the temerity to interrupt treatment in order to go on a family vacation. Eventually the client began to realize that what he really wanted in a relationship was the nurturance he believed his mother had provided. Further exploration, however, revealed that in fact his mother had been somewhat cold and ungiving. Thus, what he expected from other people (especially women) was the perfect "idealized" mother of his fantasy life. Anger at others for continually disappointing him and anger at himself for feeling so dependent colored all his relationships and eventually caused others to become angry at him and to leave, proving that they were in fact as undependable as his mother had been.

Because psychotherapy sessions are unstructured and the therapist remains a relatively neutral, nondisclosing figure, the psychotherapeutic situation encourages transference feelings to blossom. When these feelings become sufficiently intense, the therapist can help clients to discover their distortions of the therapy relationship and to discover how they misperceive and misjudge other relationships in their lives. Such revelations can have major therapeutic impact, because they are based on clients' actual experiences in the therapy sessions.

Countertransference

Countertransference is, in essence, the therapist's transference to the client. Like transference, countertransference feelings are inappropriate to the therapy situation, because they are actually the result of a relationship in the therapist's past. For example, a male social work intern may find in talking with an older female patient that he is reluctant to explore the sexual concerns for which the client has come to him for help. At the root of the difficulty lies the fact that the client reminds the intern of his mother, and he reacts to her in subtle ways as if she were his mother. In this case, the intern must recognize his distortions (e.g., with the help of a supervisor) in order to provide assistance to his client. Countertransference is, for the most part, unconscious. Thus, it is imperative that therapists-in-training have supervision and, if possible, be in psychotherapy themselves, so that they become well enough acquainted with their own countertransference responses to be able to deliver effective treatment without imposing their own distortions onto therapeutic relationships.

Resistance

People come to therapy for help, and they usually express a desire to cooperate in the hope of getting better. Toward this end, they try to form an alliance with the therapist. Paradoxically, they also try to keep the therapist and themselves at a distance from the sources of their emotional pain. Indeed, people in emotional distress have often spent much of their time and psychic energy warding off pain, and many have achieved a tenuous, if unsatisfactory, emotional balance. The therapeutic relationship offers the prospect of psychological insight and change, but any change threatens to upset this hard-won emotional balance.

Even clients who suffer distressing symptoms will feel safer holding on to familiar ways of coping with the world than venturing into unknown territory. And they may have "good" reasons for not getting better—increased attention from others, decreased responsibility, a desire to make others feel guilty for their suffering, or an unconscious need to punish themselves. Thus, clients may be aware of wanting to get better, but at the same time they are largely unaware of their fears about change. They are also likely to be unaware of how they attempt to keep themselves and others away from their real feelings and concerns. This distancing process is known as *resistance*.

Resistance can assume innumerable forms, and examples are easy to find in daily clinical work. Clients may arrive late for appointments, thus leaving less time for therapeutic work, or, once in the therapist's office, they find that they have nothing to say. Others discover that they are suddenly well after one visit and need no more help (a phenomenon that has been called "flight into health"). Some deliberately withhold information, while others "forget" important data because of conflict over whether to disclose it. Any means of distracting attention from the task of therapy can be seen as resistance—e.g., when the client is seductive or amusing, when the client tries to divert the discussion to talk about the therapist's private life, or when the client rejects the therapist's efforts to engage in conversation. The client's use of psychiatric jargon is also a resistance when it is used to ward off genuine understanding.

Resistance may be so strong as to completely undermine the therapy, but such sabotage can often be avoided if the therapist addresses the problem, along with the feelings that prompt resistances. However, resistance is more than just an obstacle that needs to be overcome. Like everything else in therapy, resistance constitutes important data about how the client's mind works. The ways in which clients keep their true feelings out of the interviews are likely to be the ways in which they avoid them in other areas of their lives. In therapy, people can learn to recognize these defensive maneuvers and understand how they get in the way of forming satisfying relationships.

To facilitate the clear emergence of transference distortions and resistances in the therapy hours, particular therapeutic techniques— *free association* and *dream analysis*—are especially helpful. They are used most often in psychoanalysis but also, to a lesser extent, in other types of dynamic therapy.

Free Association

Free association is a process by which clients say whatever comes to mind as they talk with the therapist. They are instructed not to change the sequence of undirected thoughts and not to withhold feelings or thoughts that seem irrelevant, illogical, or distressing. This sort of uncensored, uninhibited verbalization is not easy to achieve, for the flow of thoughts is interrupted by the client's various resistances to the work of therapy. Over time, patterns of resistance can be understood and clarified as they emerge to obstruct the free flow of material.

Free association is facilitated in psychoanalysis by the use of the couch, so that the supine client does not look at the therapist and is at more liberty to pursue his or her own thoughts. Also, the psychoanalyst says relatively little, so that the flow of associations can continue uninterrupted. In face-to-face psychotherapy, free association is not used per se, but the client's associations and the order in which they occur provide critical information about unconscious mental content.

The reluctance to associate about some matters can be instructive of the unconscious wish to avoid certain feelings or material, and changes from one subject to another can signal an unconscious linkage that can then be illuminated, as in the following case example.

A client, informed of her therapist's upcoming vacation, suddenly became silent. When asked what was on her mind, she recalled a series of memories about the unexpected death of her father. Subsequently she related this memory to her now acknowledged dread of the forthcoming interruption in her treatment. What remained unspoken, however, was the considerable rage she felt toward the therapist for "leaving her," unconscious fear that her rage might be destructive enough to harm the therapist.

Dream Analysis

Dream analysis is another means of discovering unconscious material. Dreams differ from most mental content in that they lack some of the careful censorship the mind exerts over unconscious ideas during waking life. Thus, dreams often reveal underlying motives and yearnings more clearly than consciously directed thoughts. Freud called dreams a "royal road to the unconscious." Carl Jung was among the first to study the symbolic meanings of dreams and to develop a theory of a universal "collective unconscious mind," based on his observation that similar dream symbols occur in many different cultures.

Psychoanalytic theory holds that dreams reveal our infantile wishes in symbolic form. Recent theories have emphasized the role of dreams in our efforts to solve problems from waking life as we sleep. Dreams also provide evidence of the client's feelings for the therapist.

Although the meanings of some dream symbols are widely recognized (e.g., a long slender object is equated with a phallus), it is almost always wise to assume unique and multiple meanings for the content of any dream. Thus, a simple dream reported by a young woman of being chased by a threatening man could be understood on many levels—as a wish to be pursued, a flight from sexual responsibility, or a conflict about being "chaste." Further information from the client indicated that the man in the dream resembled her employer, an older married man whose first name was the same as that of her father's twin brother. Thus, a deeper analysis of the dream might eventually lead into her repressed wishes to sleep with her employer or even with her uncle or her father.

It should be noted that the interpretation of dreams and their usefulness for understanding hidden motivations or conflicts is a subject of debate. Indeed, there are some who view dreams as simply random neuronal discharges that have little relevance for understanding human behavior. Others suggest that, although dream content itself may be of limited value, the client's associations to (i.e., thoughts about) the content reveal a great deal about what he or she finds emotionally significant.

The Process of Psychodynamic Change

Lifting Repression

One of the fundamental assumptions of psychodynamic theory is that we handicap ourselves by banishing certain anxiety-arousing thoughts and feelings from our awareness and relegating them to the realm of the unconscious. This process of *repression* fosters the development of a great many psychological symptoms and irrational behaviors. A primary aim of psychodynamic treatment is to undo the repression that has taken place over many years, in order to give people access to material buried in the unconscious. When unconscious material is made conscious, decisions become more rational, and we cease to feel like the victims of feelings, thoughts, and behaviors that seem beyond our comprehension and control.

The lifting of repression in treatment occurs gradually. As it happens, clients remember matters that were previously inaccessible to them. Repressed wishes—often the unrealistic pleasure-seeking demands we had as small children—can be examined by our adult minds. By bringing adult reason and logic to bear, clients can lessen some of the anxiety, shame, and guilt connected with them. People can also abandon their ways of defending themselves against the recognition of these infantile wishes, freeing up energy to deal with the adult world more creatively and more effectively.

The Role of Regression

Regression (literally "to go backwards") denotes a tendency to return to more infantile or childish ways of thinking, feeling, and behaving. Regression may be quite healthy and productive, as when we engage in various forms of play, or when we allow ourselves to be cared for when we are ill. Regression is easily seen in young children—for example, when the toilet-trained youngster regresses to bed-wetting during a stressful time.

The therapeutic situation encourages regression by its very nature, for it stirs up old longings to be cared for by an all-powerful parent. When regression occurs, clients find themselves experiencing the therapist as they experienced important people during childhood. In fact, the client who is having a regressive reaction in therapy may literally feel like a small child in relation to the therapist and may speak in a childlike voice, make unrealistic demands for love and affection, and even insist that he or she is physically small and helpless. How a client reacts to the therapist during such periods of regression constitutes important data about the person's early experiences. It allows the therapist and the client to understand how such regressive experiences distort the client's perceptions of and responses to current life situations.

This requires considerable flexibility on the part of the client. While genuinely experiencing feelings of being a child, the client is asked to step back with the therapist and understand those feelings with the mind of an adult. After feeling like a child during the therapy hour, the client must be able to go back into the world and function as an adult.

Many people are not capable of this sort of flexible, reversible regression. More disturbed people (e.g., those with psychotic illnesses or severe personality disorders) are "stuck" in infantile modes of functioning in their daily lives. For them, further regression in psychotherapy is unnecessary and often dangerous. Other people, who function well in their daily lives, may have achieved their current level of functioning with great difficulty; their tenuous psychological equilibrium might be disrupted by a major regression in psychotherapy. The therapist must therefore constantly assess the client's capacity to tolerate regression, so that experiencing childhood emotions and behaviors does not overwhelm the client and interfere with the work of therapy.

Both the client's capacities to tolerate anxiety and frustration and the strength of the therapist-client alliance are important indicators of the client's ability to benefit from the experience of regression in therapy. The question of how much regression is useful, and for whom, continues to be a topic of heated debate among clinicians.

Interpretation and Working Through

Life events (past and present), dreams, associations, and the client's mode of relating to the therapist are all invaluable sources of data about how the client's mind works. It is the therapist's job not only to elicit this information, but to help the client find meaning in it. The therapist perceives connections between various aspects of the client's mental life and can offer tentative interpretations—the validity of which the therapist and client can then test out together. Through *interpretation*, the client gains some insight into the dynamic motivations that lead to persistent symptoms. Interpretation connects present thoughts, feelings, and behaviors with unconscious wishes and the defensive maneuvers the client uses to keep from recognizing those wishes.

Interpretations make the unthinkable thinkable. They are therefore bound to stir up anxiety and must be timed so that the client is more or less receptive to them. This usually involves waiting until the client has worked on a problem long enough that unconscious material is very close to awareness. Interpretation may also be necessary when the client's level of frustration is so great that it becomes difficult to continue the work of therapy unless the source of the frustration is clarified.

Ideally, a single interpretation of the origin of a symptom or behavior would bring about change and "cure." However, this is rarely the case. Intellectual understanding is not equivalent to emotional understanding and real integration of a new piece of knowledge. So, for example, a client might suddenly become aware of the roots of his phobia of horses, yet find that his fear persists.

Single interpretations are not enough to bring about change, because single bits of awareness are intertwined with many other patterns of reacting and thinking. In fact, any new piece of awareness that comes from an interpretation must be relearned and tested in new situations and in association with other experiences—it must be integrated more fully into the client's self-concept.

This process of rediscovering interpreted material in new contexts is known as *working through*. It involves amassing evidence to support the truth of some new piece of information—evidence that includes recovered memories, present life situations, and the relationship with the therapist. The same issue must be discussed repeatedly in therapy before the sort of insight comes about that involves genuine change. This process of validating new knowledge is one of the rate-limiting steps in psychotherapy and a major reason that psychotherapy takes longer than many people think it should.

Common Misconceptions About Psychodynamic Therapy

Among the most frequently voiced erroneous ideas about psychodynamic treatment—particularly psychoanalysis—are the following three:

Myth: Treatment uncovers instances of original childhood traumas that are the causes of symptoms in adult life. In fact, there are rarely single original traumatic events underlying psychological problems. People learn to behave as they do over many years by repeating behaviors in similar situations. The goal of treatment is to examine the client's current experiences in life and in the relationship with the therapist, and to demonstrate how old patterns of thinking, feeling, and behaving are still active in the client's current relationship to the world. Memories of the past simply confirm the continuity between present and past attitudes. Human behavior cannot be reduced to simple cause-and-effect explanations. So rather than playing detective and looking for the single childhood trauma that "caused" an adult symptom, the therapist looks for ways in which the client has repeatedly dealt with stressful experiences in maladaptive ways. We can almost never answer the question of why someone developed a symptom, any more than we can know why someone else with similar childhood experiences remains symptom-free in adult life.

Myth: The psychodynamic therapist must be a "blank screen" and not a real person in the therapy. Psychodynamic therapy involves very different degrees of self-disclosure on the part of the therapist, depending on the needs of the client. But all therapies rely on a considerable degree on the reactions of the therapist as a real person. The client needs this aspect of the relationship to highlight the ways he or she distorts this (and other) relationships.

Myth: Psychodynamic therapy makes the client unnecessarily dependent on the therapist. Regression in therapy can make the client feel as if he or she were a child relating to a powerful parent. However, this is only a temporary phase of treatment that helps the client see how new relationships become distorted by feelings from the past. In fact, psychodynamic therapy aims to give clients the skills to continue to understand their own mental life long after treatment has ended— i.e., to become *more* autonomous rather than less so.

Types of Psychodynamic Psychotherapy

The model of psychodynamic change described above serves as the basis for a variety of therapies. The most prominent of these will be described here briefly (Table 15-1).

Individual Psychotherapy
Psychoanalysis. Psychoanalysis was the original mode of treatment developed by Freud and his followers. It aims at a reorganization of character structure, with an emphasis on self-understanding and the correction of developmental lags. Symptom relief usually occurs as a result of this understanding but is not the immediate objective of the treatment. The client lies on a couch, while the analyst is seated behind the client and out of view. Free association, dream analysis, and the development and working through of transference distortions in the relationship with the analyst are the most salient features. Sessions are usually held four or five times a week, and a completed analysis generally takes three to five years; however, the

Table 15–1. Types of psychodynamic therapy.

Individual psychotherapy
  Psychoanalysis
  Exploratory psychotherapy
  Supportive psychotherapy
  Time-limited psychotherapy
Group psychotherapy
Couples therapy
Family treatment

length of treatment varies considerably with the nature of the problems being treated.

People in psychoanalysis must be able to tolerate a fair degree of frustration and ambiguity because of the lack of structure in the analytic situation. Analysis is therefore suitable for people who are at the healthier end of the spectrum of psychological disorders—people with neurotic conflicts and personality disorders of lesser severity. The usefulness of psychoanalysis in the treatment of severe personality disorders is questionable, and its use in schizophrenia and other psychotic illness is generally contraindicated.

Exploratory psychotherapy. Like psychoanalysis, exploratory psychotherapy aims at understanding motivations and unconscious forces that hamper daily living. However, exploratory psychotherapy focuses less on the analysis of infantile wishes and conflicts, and more on current life situations and dynamic patterns of dealing with others in the here and now. Analysis of transference remains a central feature, but transference reactions are often less intense than in analysis, where the therapist's relative inactivity allows such reactions to flower. The sort of temporary regression that is fostered in psychoanalysis is usually avoided in psychotherapy.

The client does not lie on a couch but sits in a chair, promoting a more "real" face-to-face interaction with the therapist. Sessions are usually held one to three times a week (occasionally more frequently), depending on the client's motivation and capacity to tolerate the intense feelings that are more likely to be stirred up when sessions are frequent. Treatment may last for several sessions, or several years, depending on the nature of the problem and the extent of the client's motivation. Medication may be used in combination with exploratory therapy if the client's symptoms indicate the need.

Exploratory psychotherapy is employed in the treatment of a wide range of psychiatric illnesses, including many psychotic conditions, depression, personality disorders, and neuroses. Clients must be motivated to understand their inner life and its manifestations in their dealings with the world. The major contraindication to exploratory psychotherapy is the inability to tolerate the exploration of feelings without having to act on them in destructive ways (e.g., suicidal behavior or violent acts toward others). The therapist must be alert to such adverse reactions in therapy, adjusting the frequency and intensity of sessions according to what the client can tolerate.

Supportive psychotherapy. Although all forms of psychodynamic therapy involve some measure of support, supportive therapy is distinct from exploratory work and psychoanalysis because its goal is not the development of insight, but the lessening of anxiety. The therapist does this through reassurance, advice, modification of social factors where possible, and the bolstering of the client's personal strengths and more adaptive defenses (see Chapter 4). The therapist is generally more active and more directive than in the other modalities.

One potential danger in doing supportive therapy is that it may foster a dependency relationship that is harmful and infantilizing rather than helpful. But some clients who have little interest in or capacity for achieving psychological insight can function much better in the world when "maintained" by a supportive relationship with a therapist. Supportive therapy generally occurs once a week or less, but at times it is carried out more frequently. Supportive treatment is indicated for those in need of temporary emotional support during a crisis, for those who are resistant to or too severely disturbed to respond to insight-oriented treatment, and for those who are not interested in changing their lives but simply in returning to a previous level of adjustment.

Time-limited psychotherapy. (This is also called *brief psychotherapy* and *short-term anxiety-provoking psychotherapy.*) Time-limited psychotherapy is a specific form of psychodynamic treatment developed as an alternative to more prolonged and more costly treatments. It is particularly useful when the demand for treatment exceeds available resources. The aim of time-limited therapy is to help the client understand the roots of and achieve some resolution of a particular emotional problem that is a source of acute distress. Rarely does the therapy touch on transference issues or character problems; instead it focuses on current life situations. Dependence and regression are actively discouraged.

The number of sessions is usually agreed upon at the outset of treatment (from eight to 20 or more), and there is an emphasis on personal autonomy and independent functioning throughout the course of therapy. The therapist works actively to maintain the focus of the sessions on a central issue that is identified by therapist and client at the outset of treatment. This often keeps the client's anxiety level relatively high throughout the treatment.

Clients who do well with this sort of treatment are generally the same ones who would profit from intensive insight-oriented work: people who function relatively well at work and in relationships, who can think in psychological terms, and who have a clear motivation to change. However, short-term therapy may in fact be more desirable than prolonged work for people who are in an acute crisis that has an easily identified focal issue, and who are interested in crisis resolution rather than a thorough exploration of themselves with the potential for a deeper restructuring of character.

Group Psychotherapy
The psychodynamic principles used in individual psychotherapy have been applied with considerable success in working with groups. Group therapy is a powerful treatment modality by itself, and it is also used effectively in conjunction with individual therapy for some clients. Both because of its therapeutic effects and because it is less costly than individual therapy, group therapy has been widely employed in many settings.

Groups vary greatly in structure and in the way meetings are run. Group membership may range from two or three to more than 15, but most groups have six to 10 members. Groups of this size are large enough for a sense of group identity to develop and for clear patterns of group interaction to emerge, but not so large as to lose sight of each individual's issues and needs. There is usually one leader, but co-leaders are not uncommon—often male and female coleaders to help elicit clients' transference feelings for parents. Groups generally meet once a week for 1½ hours, but sessions may be more or less frequent.

The goals of group therapy are primarily the same as those of individual therapy—self-understanding, self-acceptance, and the modification of behavior to enable the client to form more satisfying relationships. The tools used in group therapy are also similar, including the use of transference interpretations, associations, and even dream material. However, the very fact that several people with emotional difficulties come together with therapists in one room to discuss their lives opens up the possibility for a wider range of interactions than can take place between one client and one therapist.

Clients can provide each other with mutual validation of experiences, so that individuals feel less isolated by what they think are unique and unacceptable emotional difficulties. They also give one another advice, which is often less helpful in its content than in its demonstration of concern and caring. People who have felt like burdens to family and friends are able to experience being helpful to other group members as they offer support, insight, and reassurance in group meetings.

Groups are very effective in recapitulating family situations. Clients interact with group leaders and other group members as they once interacted with parents and siblings. Through interpretation, they can come to understand how they are distorting these current relationships. Group members can also learn social skills from one another—how to resolve conflict, how to be responsive to others, and how to be less judgmental of others' behavior. As members come to be more comfortable with one another, they can take risks and try out new behaviors that are too threatening to test out elsewhere (e.g., a client may begin to experiment with increased assertiveness). The group becomes a microcosm of larger social groups, and clients can learn how they operate in group situations (e.g., family and job) outside therapy.

Group therapy has been used for virtually all types of mental illness. It is particularly useful for people with personality disorders, whose character problems are obvious to others but not to them. Such people can often tolerate being confronted by their peers with evidence of their maladaptive behaviors better than they can tolerate confrontation by an authority figure like the group leader. Sociopaths, drug addicts, and alcoholics are among those who have benefited from such treatment. Group treatment is also used for people who are psychotic (e.g., schizophrenics). Group meetings with psychotic people are usually fairly structured and actively guided by the therapist, often focusing on specific tasks like the improvement of social skills.

Group therapy may be used alone or in conjunction with other forms of treatment (e.g., medication or individual therapy). People may be in group therapy for months or years, depending on their motivation. Groups may contain members with many different types of problems, or may be limited to people with a particular illness (e.g., alcoholism, manic-depressive illness). Groups are used for both outpatient therapy and inpatient work, and they are useful in such diverse settings as prisons and college health services.

Couples Therapy
Couples therapy deals with a partnership between two people and the problems that arise within this relationship. Formerly called "marital therapy," it is useful not only for married couples, but for heterosexual and homosexual couples who are living together or

committed to each other in some other fashion. Its usefulness has certainly extended beyond the bounds of the traditional institution of marriage.

Psychodynamic couples therapy focuses on the intrapsychic conflicts and dynamics of each member of the dyad, but only insofar as these issues affect the relationship. Therapy is aimed at facilitating communication within the couple, clarifying individual goals, and resolving conflicts where possible, and helping each member see how he or she distorts the relationship with the partner as a result of earlier life experiences with parents, siblings, and other important people. Couples therapy is not necessarily aimed at keeping the couple together, but at helping the couple to understand how the relationship works and does not work, and whether problems can be resolved.

Common issues dealt with in couples therapy are discrepancies in verbal and nonverbal communications between the partners, varying expectations of the relationship, and problems in sexual functioning. Sessions are usually held weekly, but may be more or less frequent. Couples therapy may be done in combination with individual therapy (for one or both partners) or may be used as the only treatment modality. Although treatment by a single therapist is common, couples treatment is also quite effectively carried out by two therapists of different sexes, since this may enable each member of the couple to feel that he or she has a same-sex "ally" to identify with in the therapy. Sessions are usually carried out with both partners present, but there may be individual sessions at the outset or at various times during the course of therapy, as issues arise that need one-on-one attention.

Contraindications to couples treatment are few, but include acute psychosis in one or both partners, obvious psychopathology in one or both partners that requires individual therapy before couples work can proceed, and the harboring of an "unexposable" secret by one partner.

Family Treatment

Family relationships have always been of intense interest to psychodynamic therapists, but the actual direct treatment of entire family units is a relatively new development in mental health care.

Dynamically oriented family therapy explores how family members interact during sessions with one or more therapists. The therapists observe patterns in styles of communication among family members, family patterns of becoming organized or disorganized in response to specific challenges, and roles and alliances adopted by various members. Families generally do not notice these patterns, because they are caught up in perpetuating them in order to maintain some equilibrium within the family unit. Family therapists not only observe behaviors that create disharmony and dysfunction in the family, but they also ask the family to step back and look at themselves as they have been unable to do in the past. Family therapy provides a setting in which the members often become more aware of how other members feel. As family members come to understand more about the consequences of their pathological behavior patterns, they have the possibility of changing behaviors and exploring more satisfying ways of dealing with one another.

Like group therapy, family therapy generally requires more activity by the therapist than does individual therapy. It may also require directive techniques aimed at realigning alliances, proposing alternative means of managing problems, and insisting upon the rights or needs of particular family members to be heard.

Family therapy is often carried out in conjunction with couples therapy and/or individual therapy for one or more family members. Sessions are generally held weekly. As in couples work, many family therapists work in pairs, both to model interactions between the therapists and to check with one another their perceptions of the family's style of behaving.

The Goals of Psychodynamic Treatment

People seek psychotherapy for a wide variety of problems. The specific therapeutic modalities and the intensity of their application are determined only after careful assessment of the client's needs. Each of the dynamic therapies seeks to increase the person's sense of self-acceptance and well-being, while improving his or her ability to obtain satisfaction in work and at play.

Two general categories of beneficial effect can be discerned in people who have undergone psychodynamic psychotherapy. The uncovering of unconscious sources of conflict acts to free people from the burden of irrational fears and inhibitions carried over from early life experiences. Further, it enables them to handle the stresses and conflicts of everyday life more effectively.

The second benefit is in the gradual shift in the person's view of self and others. The therapeutic relationship provides a unique opportunity for self-exposure and intimacy in a protected setting. At the same time, heightened awareness of the complexity and ambiguity of human interaction gradually replaces the "tunnel vision" and automatic behavior that often characterize people who seek this form of treatment. The result is a richer and deeper recognition of life's inherent difficulties and limitations, and the development of a more flexible repertoire of responses to these limitations.

BEHAVIOR THERAPY

Behavior therapy, or *behavior modification,* is an approach to the treatment of specific behavioral symptoms such as phobias, compulsions, anxiety, and speech disorders. Behavior therapy focuses on observable actions rather than inferred mental states, and it aims at eliminating maladaptive behaviors by means of techniques that are based largely on learning theory.

Behavior therapy begins with an analysis of the responses that cause the client distress or diminish his or her satisfaction and productivity. This analysis outlines the types of situations and reinforcing factors that have fostered and maintained the problematic behavior (e.g., stuttering). The next step consists of developing a detailed schedule of exercises for eliminating these behaviors and replacing them with more desirable ones. Among the most important forms of behavior therapy currently in use are systematic desensitization, flooding, positive reinforcement, extinction, and aversive conditioning (Table 15-2).

Systematic Desensitization

Systematic desensitization is widely used in modern mental health care. It is based on the premise that people can master anxiety-provoking situations by approaching those situations gradually and

Table 15–2. Models of behavior therapy.

Systematic desensitization
  Mastering anxiety-provoking situations by approaching them gradually
    and in a relaxed state that inhibits anxiety
Flooding
  Confronting the feared stimulus for prolonged periods until it is no
    longer frightening
Positive reinforcement
  Stengthening behavior and causing it to occur more frequently by
    rewarding it
Extinction
  Causing a behavior to diminish by not responding to it
Negative reinforcement
  Responding to an undesirable behavior with some means of punishment

---

while in a relaxed state that inhibits anxiety. Clients are first taught the technique of progressive relaxation, which consists of tensing major muscle groups and then relaxing them in a fixed order (e.g., beginning at the top of the head and working down). In the next step, the client and therapist determine which situations produce anxiety and construct a hierarchy of feared situations.

For example, in the case of a man who is afraid to fly in an airplane, the hierarchy would involve 10 to 12 scenes that might include buying a ticket, walking to the gate, entering the plane, taking off, and landing. These scenes are ordered according to how much anxiety they produce. The client then puts himself into a relaxed state, using progressive relaxation, and he is asked to vividly imagine the first scene while in his deeply relaxed state. He repeats the exercise for the first scene until he experiences only minimal anxiety, at which time he can move on to the next scene. The goal is to be able to imagine the most anxiety-provoking scene (e.g., the plane landing) while remaining calm. This inhibition of anxiety carries over into corresponding real-life situations. It is often helpful for the client to practice entering actual feared situations between treatment sessions, once the fears have been overcome in therapy.

Systematic desensitization is commonly used with great efficacy in treating phobias. It is also helpful to some people who have compulsive behaviors or a sexual dysfunction. It is less useful for more diffuse anxiety that is not specific to particular situations.

Flooding

Flooding is another approach to treating situation-specific anxiety. In flooding, clients confront the feared object or situation (e.g., a spider) at full intensity for prolonged periods of time until it is no longer frightening. The confrontation may be done by having the client imagine the frightening scene, but results are generally better when the exposure is to a real-life situation. This technique is less widely used than systematic desensitization, in part because it involves such a high degree of anxiety that many people do not tolerate it well.

Positive Reinforcement, Extinction, and Negative Reinforcement

The basic premise of *positive reinforcement* is that behavior will be strengthened and will occur more frequently if it is rewarded—e.g., with praise, increased attention from others, or the avoidance of pain. The theory behind *extinction* holds that a specific behavior will diminish if it is not responded to at all, and *negative reinforcement* involves responding to an undesirable behavior with some means of punishment.

You may see these principles put into use in constructing treatment programs for severely disturbed patients on hospital wards or in day-care facilities. You may, for example, work on an inpatient unit that has a *token economy*—a system in which patients earn tokens for adaptive, socially sanctioned behaviors and are fined for maladaptive ones. Patients may earn tokens for such activities as grooming themselves properly, cleaning rooms, or helping in group activities. They can then use the tokens to buy snacks, watch television, or take a trip off the hospital grounds (e.g., to a movie theater). They are fined tokens for such behavior as disrupting meetings, becoming physically abusive, or remaining isolated and uncommunicative. Such a system can be individually tailored to each patient's needs, to help him or her acquire the skills and behaviors that will promote better functioning and more autonomy. Such systems have also been useful in other communities, e.g., in treatment facilities for juvenile delinquents or the mentally retarded.

Aversive conditioning involves applying negative reinforcement to well-established behaviors. A maladaptive behavior is coupled with a noxious stimulus, so that the person experiences a motivational conflict between the desired behavior and the unpleasant consequences that go with it. For example, aversive conditioning has been used to treat alcoholism, by giving a person ethanol along with an emetic that produces severe nausea and vomiting. For many people, repeated administration of this treatment suppresses the desire to drink. Critics argue that this approach provides only a temporary solution to what is usually a chronic problem.

Aversive conditioning has also been used to treat people who want to change a homosexual orientation to a heterosexual one. While watching films or tapes of erotic homosexual scenes, the client concurrently receives either emetics that produce nausea and vomiting or mild electric shocks. The clients are then shown erotic heterosexual scenes, without concurrent noxious stimuli. This form of treatment has also been used to treat sexual perversions (see Chapter 11). Its use in changing the choice of sexual object from homosexual to heterosexual is quite controversial, and it has not been clearly demonstrated to be effective in achieving this goal.

In general, behavior therapy is very useful in treating relatively specific symptoms. It does not, however, address deeper psychological problems, such as those encountered among people with neurotic conflicts or personality disorders, nor is it the primary mode of treatment in any of the psychotic illnesses.

Every clinician should know about behavioral treatments and ideally should be able to practice some simple techniques.

HYPNOSIS

Hypnosis is neither a form of sleep nor a form of therapy. Rather, it is a particular type of concentration that is attentive, receptive, and quite focused. It is accompanied by diminished awareness of peripheral stimuli. You have undoubtedly experienced hypnotic or trance-like states—for example, in being so absorbed in a novel that you ignore what is going on around you and must reorient yourself to the environment when you stop reading.

In a treatment situation that employs hypnosis, the client allows the therapist to structure this form of intense concentration in a way that facilitates and accelerates the achievement of particular psychotherapeutic goals. Hypnosis is most often used for the relief of specific symptoms such as anxiety, insomnia, phobias, conversion reactions, and pain. It is also used to control habits—particularly smoking and overeating.

Essentially, treatment involves teaching people self-hypnosis techniques so that they can first put themselves into a trance-like state, and then use hypnotic suggestions that "restructure" their thinking about the problem being treated. For example, people who want to quit smoking are taught to put themselves into a trance-like state every few hours and at any time they crave a cigarette. In this state, they run through several points that are designed to reorient their thinking, such as, "Smoking damages my body. I need to take care of myself. I will not harm myself in this way." Similar suggestions for use under self-hypnosis can be designed by therapists and clients to ease anxiety, curb overeating, help overcome phobias, and lessen the psychological components of chronic pain.

Hypnosis has significant limitations as a therapeutic technique. It cannot, for example, treat more global difficulties, such as neurotic conflicts, psychotic illnesses, or personality disorders. Its usefulness even for the isolated symptoms mentioned above is questioned by some clinicians, who argue that symptom relief resulting from hypnotherapy is only temporary in many cases. Nevertheless, hypnosis continues to be a valuable tool in modern clinical practice when applied judiciously.

COGNITIVE THERAPY

Cognitive therapy is a relatively new mode of short-term psychotherapy specifically developed for the treatment of depression and anxiety. It is based on the premise that our moods and feelings are influenced by our thoughts, and that self-defeating and self-deprecating patterns of thinking foster dysphoric moods in many depressed people. By correcting these distorted ways of thinking, the cognitive therapist restructures depressed clients' views of themselves, the world, and the future—substituting more realistic, self-enhancing thoughts that reduce such painful feelings as anxiety, guilt, and hopelessness.

Cognitive therapists identify many common forms of cognitive distortion that foster depression. For example, a student who feels like a failure when she gets an A-minus instead of an A on an exam is using what cognitive therapists call "all-or-nothing thinking"; the worker who blames himself when the car breaks down and he is late for work is using "personalization." Cognitive distortions involve faulty interpretation of real events—usually in a way that casts the depressed person in a very negative light. These distortions often stem from self-defeating "silent assumptions" that depressed people harbor about themselves, such as, "I am worthless if I cannot do things perfectly."

Clients in cognitive therapy are asked to identify and write down negative thoughts—at first with the help of the therapist, and subsequently on their own. The therapist can then help the client identify the distortions in these thoughts and substitute more rational responses. The therapist also helps the client recognize self-defeating silent assumptions and exchange them for more realistic ones.

Cognitive therapy is a short-term treatment (often 10 to 15 sessions) that has been compared favorably with the use of the antidepressant drug imipramine in preliminary trials with depressed people. Its efficacy remains to be proven in large-scale controlled studies that are currently under way. Critics argue that negative thoughts do not cause painful feelings but result from them, and that changing one's thinking is not sufficient to bring about a lasting change of mood. These critics also argue that the real therapeutic factors in cognitive therapy are the trust, support, and rapport that are part of any good therapeutic relationship. Nevertheless, cognitive therapy may prove to be an effective, low-cost modality that could be used widely in the treatment of depression.

CLIENT-CENTERED PSYCHOTHERAPY

Client-centered psychotherapy is a form of treatment introduced by Carl Rogers. It is often referred to as "rogerian therapy." It is non-directive and emphasizes the importance of the relationship between client and therapist, as well as the client's right to self-determination. The therapist attempts to act as a catalyst to facilitate the client's emotional growth—ideally without imposing any of the therapist's views on the client. Clients verbalize their problems, and the client-centered therapist rephrases their words to reflect and clarify the feelings they are trying to express. The therapist must be genuine, must offer the client unconditional acceptance, and must provide accurate empathic understanding of the client's problems. When these three conditions are met, client-centered therapists believe that the client will have increased self-understanding and a greater capacity for adaptive behavior.

However, many clinicians have criticized rogerian therapy as not being useful for certain types of clients, particularly those with personality disorders. They argue that uncritical acceptance of the client can be undesirable, particularly when his or her behaviors are clearly maladaptive. (For example, the client with an antisocial personality disorder who steals to buy drugs must be confronted about such behavior.) Client-centered therapy is best suited for people with neurotic disturbances, who can benefit from an empathic and nonjudgmental relationship.

SUMMARY

The types of psychotherapy described above are but a few of the many forms of treatment developed in the past few decades. You have no doubt heard of a great many others—modalities such as gestalt therapy, transactional analysis, and emotive therapy. There are also many different schools of thought besides Freudian psychology within psychodynamic psychotherapy—including Jungian, Adlerian, and Sullivanian theories and techniques. A general survey of all these types of therapy is beyond the scope of this chapter. Rather, this discussion is meant to indicate the range of psychosocial treatments currently in use.

REFERENCES

Childress AR, Burns DD: The basics of cognitive therapy. Psychosomatics 22:1017-1027, 1981

Frank JD: General psychotherapy: the restoration of morale, in American Handbook of Psychiatry, vol 5. Edited by Arieti S. New York, Basic Books, 1975, pp 117-132

Frankel FH: Hypnosis: Trance as a Coping Mechanism. New York, Plenum Press, 1976

Fromm-Reichmann F: Principles of Intensive Psychotherapy. Chicago, University of Chicago Press, 1950

Greenson RR: The Technique and Practice of Psychoanalysis, vol 1. New York, International Universities Press, 1967

Kolb LC: Psychotherapy, in Modern Clinical Psychiatry, 9th ed. Philadelphia, WB Saunders, 1977, pp 767-804

Kovacs M: The efficacy of cognitive and behavior therapies for depression. Am J Psychiatry 137:1495-1501, 1980

Marks IM: Review of behavioral psychotherapy, I: obsessive-compulsive disorders. Am J Psychiatry 138:584-592, 1981

Marks IM: Review of behavioral psychotherapy, I: sexual disorders. Am J Psychiatry 138:750-756, 1981

Marmor J: Short-term dynamic psychotherapy. Am J Psychiatry 136:149-155, 1979

Minuchin SA: Families and Family Therapy. Cambridge, Mass, Harvard University Press, 1976

Strachey J: The nature of the therapeutic action of psychoanalysis. Int J Psychoanal 15:127-159, 1934

Wolpe J: Psychotherapy by Reciprocal Inhibition. Stanford, Calif, Stanford University Press, 1958

Wynne L: Some indications and contraindications for exploratroy family therapy, in Intensive Family Therapy. Edited by Boszermonyi-Nagy I, Framo J. Hoeber, 1965

Yalom ID: The Theory and Practice of Group Psychotherapy, 3rd ed. New York, Basic Books, 1985

Chapter 16

Somatic Therapies

The somatic therapies used in modern psychiatry consist of psychotropic drugs and electroconvulsive therapy (ECT). This chapter covers general principles of the pharmacologic treatment of mental disorders and the use of specific classes of psychotropic drugs. ECT is discussed briefly at the end of the chapter.

OF WHAT RELEVANCE IS PSYCHOPHARMACOLOGY TO NONPHYSICIANS?

Why should you bother to read a chapter on medication and ECT, if you do not prescribe these treatments? The answer may be obvious, but it is worth stating, if only to dispel the myth that the various mental health disciplines are separate entities that do not overlap.

You must learn about somatic therapies in psychiatry because many of your clients will need these treatments, and they will rely on you to be aware of them. In most cases, you will be the only person to whom a client comes for help. It is then your diagnostic skill and your familiarity with somatic treatments that will determine whether the client has access to this realm of mental health care. Many symptoms that are medication-responsive will go untreated unless you recognize the need to refer your client to a psychopharmacologist.

Your role in somatic therapy does not end with referral to a psychiatrist. You are likely to be the primary treater for many clients who take medication. They will see you more frequently than they see the prescribing physician. When side effects appear or adverse reactions to medication occur, you will be the first person to whom clients bring their concerns. You may be the only one to notice potentially dangerous medication effects; for example, incipient tardive dyskinesia, or a mild akathisia, or the mania precipitated by an antidepressant.

Finally, some clients must take medications over a period of months or even years. Those of you who have ever taken a 10-day course of prescribed medication know that it takes considerable diligence to comply with a regimen of two or three doses per day. Clients need support from you in order to be able to put up with the inconvenience and frustration of having to organize their lives around a medication regimen. In this respect, your understanding of somatic therapies and your willingness to talk about them will determine whether many of your clients take their medication. It is important that you and the prescribing physician remember that your role in determining the success or failure of somatic therapies is a critical one.

PSYCHOTROPIC MEDICATIONS

Psychotropic drugs are chemical agents that have an effect on the mind. Many mind-altering substances are abused in our society for "recreational" purposes. Only a minority of known psychotropic agents are actually useful in the treatment of mental disorders.

Why Are Psychotropic Drugs Used in Psychiatry?

The question is not an idle one. The media and popular literature have, at times, painted a rather gloomy picture of mental institutions in which patients are kept "spaced out" on large doses of medication. A few critics of our mental health care system argue that drugs deprive people of their right to be psychotic. The mention of major tranquilizers conjures up images of mind control and the repression of individual freedom.

Yet the advent of modern psychopharmacology in the last three decades has revolutionized the treatment of mental illness, giving millions of people relief from symptoms that are both frightening and crippling. Prior to the 1950s, there were few methods available for treating severely disturbed people. Seclusion behind locked doors and barred windows and the use of physical restraints were more common and more necessary than they are today. Treatment included "hydrotherapy," insulin shock, neurosurgery, and management with narcotics, barbiturates, and bromides. These have virtually disappeared from psychiatry, and for good reason. Mania, florid hallucinations, severe agitation, and life-threatening depression have all proved responsive to modern psychopharmacologic agents. Fewer people require long-term treatment behind locked doors, and it has been possible to return many of the chronically mentally ill and many treatment settings to the community.

The number of patients hospitalized in psychiatric facilities at any given time has been drastically reduced over the last 20 years. To be sure, this is due in part to our society's increased awareness of the detrimental effects of chronic institutionalization on human behavior, as well as to economic and political considerations. Also, new applications of group therapy techniques in day-care programs and outpatient clinics have proved effective in helping people live outside a structured inpatient setting. But much of the credit for this shift from inpatient to outpatient treatment must go to the use of psychotropic medications. They have not only proved effective in relieving acute psychotic symptoms, but they have also been useful in preventing recurrences and in stabilizing functioning over long periods of time.

We must temper this praise, however, with some perspective on the limitations of the psychotropic medications. In fact, they only alleviate symptoms—*they do not cure*. In this respect, their efficacy is limited to staving off some of the manifestations of major mental illness, without exerting any clearly definable, lasting effect on the underlying pathology. Also, many people do not respond to these medications, even when "classic" symptoms would predict a good response. The drugs carry side effects that range in severity from uncomfortable to dangerous, and all can be toxic. Finally, they are generally slow to work in at least one crucial respect—the antipsychotic effect of the major tranquilizers may take days or weeks to be evident, and the antidepressant effects of the tricyclics generally appear many days after the medication is begun.

What Do Psychotropic Medications Do?

It is useful to think of these drugs as falling into discrete groups. Each group of psychotropics alleviates a particular set of symptoms. They can generally be grouped as shown in Table 16-1.

The major groups of psychotropics—antipsychotic agents, antidepressants, and antimanic agents—have actions that are directed

Table 16–1. The types of psychotropic medications.

The major groups—act against specific symptoms of mental illness
    Antipsychotic agents
    Antidepressants
    Antimanic agents
Other classes—produce particular effects without regard to presence or
  absence of illness
    Antianxiety agents
    Psychomotor stimulants
    Sedative-hypnotics

---

against specific symptoms of mental illness. Unlike "uppers" or "downers," these drugs do not work through simple arousal or sedation, but through more specific effects. Normal subjects do not experience euphoria when they take antidepressants or depression when they take an antimanic drug, and they do not find their thought processes altered by the antipsychotics. If anything, the major psychotropic medications produce little more than sedation in normal subjects, but they can produce specific therapeutic effects in those who are ill.

The other classes of psychotropic medications are less specific in their actions. Antianxiety agents, psychomotor stimulants, and sedative-hypnotics produce similar effects in most people who use them, whether a mental illness is present or not. These drugs are of little value in treating psychosis and mood disorders. They are much more commonly abused than the major psychotropics.

A word about terminology is in order. The term *tranquilizer* is frequently used incorrectly to describe any sedating drug. There are two very different types of medications to which the term is correctly applied. *Major tranquilizers* are also called antipsychotic agents; their effects are both antipsychotic and sedating. This group includes drugs like chlorpromazine (Thorazine), trifluoperazine (Stelazine), and haloperidol (Haldol). *Minor tranquilizers* are the antianxiety agents, such as diazepam (Valium) and chlordiazepoxide (Librium), which alleviate anxiety but do not alleviate psychotic symptoms. Other sedating drugs (such as the barbiturates) are more accurately labeled *sedative-hypnotics*.

Appendix C lists many of the more common psychotropic medications, arranged by drug category. Appendix D arranges these medications by their brand names, followed by their corresponding generic names and category. When you hear a drug referred to by its brand name, you can use this table to quickly find its chemical name and major use in clinical practice.

PRINCIPLES OF PRESCRIBING
PSYCHOTROPIC MEDICATIONS

For every client you see, you must make a judgment as to whether pharmacotherapy is both warranted and prudent. This requires facts.

Clinical Evaluation

First, your clinical evaluation must be thorough. You must arrive at a tentative diagnosis based on the following factors.

A careful history. You should enlist the help of family members in getting a history if the client's reliability is questionable. In particular, a careful delineation of symptoms, previous treatments and responses, history of drug or alcohol abuse, family psychiatric history, medical history, and current medications is important.

A physical examination. A physician must assess the client's physical health and rule out underlying medical disorders that might mimic psychiatric illness. For outpatients, a routine examination done by the family physician in recent months will suffice if no medical problems are suspected.

Laboratory tests. These tests should include routine studies to rule out organic causes of psychiatric symptoms (e.g., hypothyroidism as the basis for depression) and may include special diagnostic tests to predict response to medication—e.g., measuring urinary 3-methoxy-4-hydroxyphenylethyleneglycol (MHPG) to predict response to various types of antidepressants. The routine laboratory work-up for each type of medication is discussed below.

A period of observation. When there is no acute problem (such as severe agitation or life-threatening behavior) that requires immediate use of medication, it is helpful to observe the client in a drug-free state for several days (or even several weeks) to see how symptoms change over time. This is particularly useful if there is some question about whether medication is likely to be helpful, or when there is confusion about the diagnosis. For example, a patient admitted to the hospital with a psychotic episode might not reveal that he has abused drugs. If a physician immediately administers an antipsychotic, the mistaken conclusion might be drawn that the medication alleviated a psychosis that would have abated of its own accord when the abused substance was cleared from the patient's body. Or an outpatient's depressive symptoms might improve dramatically after one or two meetings with a concerned therapist. If this person had been given antidepressants immediately, the effect would have been attributed to the medication, and the client might have been maintained on the drug unnecessarily. Another client's anxiety might mask an underlying psychosis. Such a person could easily be medicated incorrectly with an antianxiety agent before the disordered thinking became apparent.

Course of the Illness

You must know the expected course of the illness that has been diagnosed. Some psychiatric conditions are self-limiting (e.g., drug-induced psychosis). When it is safe to do so, it is always preferable to treat such cases conservatively and supportively until the illness runs its course.

Risks of Treatment

You must weigh the risks of not treating your client against the risks of the various forms of therapy available. Tricyclic antidepressants, for example, are highly lethal when taken in overdose; with suicidal people, this must always be taken into account. Major tranquilizers produce *tardive dyskinesia* (discussed below) in a minority of people, and this is generally unresponsive to treatment. Pharmacotherapy should never be undertaken lightly.

Choosing a Drug

Once the prescribing physician decides to prescribe psychotropic medication, he or she must determine which class of drug to use. This will depend on the diagnosis and the client's symptoms. But once it has been decided to use an antidepressant, or an antipsychotic, or an anxiolytic, there is a wide assortment of specific medications from which to choose. Within the broad groups of medications mentioned above, individual drugs differ very little in their ability to affect constellations of symptoms. Thus, the choice of which particular antipsychotic or anxiolytic to use will often be based on factors other than the symptoms you are trying to alleviate. These factors are discussed below.

Previous treatment response. The client's previous treatment response is an excellent indicator of what to try and what not to try. If something worked once, it is likely to work again. The converse is, of course, also true. Thus, if a client tells you that Haldol (haloperidol) was of no help in relieving his psychotic symptoms 10 years ago, it would be wise to avoid it now. If, however, he tells you that Loxitane (loxapine) was the only drug that took away his auditory hallucinations, and he suffers from the same symptom at present, loxapine is likely to be the best bet. This is, perhaps, stating the obvious. Yet too often we forget that we are often dealing with chronic conditions, that many clients have considerable prior experience with medication, and that they often know what has worked for them in the past. *Do not forget to ask.*

Medication histories of biological relatives. These can be invaluable in helping with this decision. Treatment response and side effects are strongly determined by genetic factors. So, for example, if a depressed client reports that her father was depressed and got better on imipramine (Tofranil), then imipramine would be a good first drug to use with her.

History of side effects. The client's history of side effects is equally important. No one is likely to take a medication that produces unbearable side effects. When you are dealing with someone who has been given a variety of antipsychotics in the past, find out which of those drugs were least unpleasant for the client to take.

The prescribing physician's familiarity with particular drugs. Familiarity with a particular drug is very important, including detailed knowledge of a drug's effects, side effects, and toxicity. This will affect the choices made by the prescribing physician.

Cost. The cost of the drug may be a factor, particularly if long-term treatment is required. Drug prices vary greatly according to the availability of generic forms and the extent of competition in the market. As a rule, newer drugs are more expensive.

Determining Drug Dosages

Unlike many other medications used in medical practice, there are no precise doses prescribed for most of the psychotropic drugs. Rather, there is a dosage range—often very broad—within which the physician must determine the amount that best meets the client's needs. And responses are highly individual. One person may require two, three, or even four times the amount of medication needed by another person of similar body weight in order to achieve similar therapeutic effects. Prescribing thus involves a process of fine tuning the therapy according to the symptoms and responses of the individual.

There is a high correlation between the severity of the target symptoms at which treatment is aimed and the minimum dosage that produces a favorable response. Severe symptoms will generally require higher dosages of medication, while mild symptoms are more likely to respond to dosages at the lower end of the therapeutic range. The most important considerations in determining drug dosages are *safety* and *therapeutic efficacy.*

Several of the antidepressants have a "therapeutic window"—a dosage range within which a therapeutic response is to be expected. Dosages that are outside the therapeutic window (i.e., too high or too low) are likely to have no effect or even adverse effects on the client. The antipsychotics have no such window, but they have an unspecified upper limit for safe and effective treatment. In such cases, the prescribing physician cannot rely solely on manufacturers' recommendations but must be particularly diligent about weighing the therapeutic effects against side effects in deciding how much medication is enough.

Administering Psychotropic Drugs

The two major routes of administration are oral and intramuscular. Intravenous administration of psychotropics generally takes place in well-controlled inpatient settings, often for research purposes. Most situations can be managed without intravenous medication.

Doses administered by injection are roughly two to four times as potent as the same doses taken by mouth. This is largely because the liver, which does the bulk of the body's work in metabolizing psychotropics, is bypassed by intravenous injection, so that the medication reaches the circulation directly.

Although the minor tranquilizers and some other sedating drugs are at times given by injection, the drugs most often given intramuscularly are the antipsychotics. Injection is used for the following reasons:

- To produce rapid relief of severe agitation and other symptoms that might pose a danger to the client or to others,
- If the client is unable or unwilling to take medication orally, and
- When oral absorption of the drug is thought to be poor.

The disadvantages of giving these medicines intramuscularly are the following:

• Some of them are painful (e.g., chlorpromazine) and may cause irritation at the site of injection, and
• Intramuscular injection may be seen by some severely disturbed people as an assault.

When used to control agitation, intramuscular medication is considered a chemical restraint. This raises important issues about the person's right to refuse treatment. A full discussion of the legal and ethical dilemmas involved in chemical restraint is beyond the scope of this chapter, but it should be noted that chemical restraint must be used only when the need is clear—i.e., to protect the client or others from harm when other means of treatment have failed to put the client and others out of danger. It must *never* be used as punishment.

In addition to chemical restraint, the most common situations in which intramuscular medication is used are 1) in emergency rooms, where people are in crisis and need rapid relief, and 2) in outpatient programs, when people who cannot comply with daily oral regimens are given *depot* forms of antipsychotic medication by injection every two to four weeks. (A depot medication is in a chemical form that is absorbed very slowly into the bloodstream from the muscle into which it has been injected. Because this occurs over days, weeks, or months, it eliminates the need for frequent doses of medication.)

Advising Your Clients About Medication

How you and the prescribing physician present the treatment plan to your client can make a great difference in the amount of cooperation you receive, particularly when prescribing psychotropic drugs. Not only is compliance important but, in most cases, the client must tell you whether or not the treatment is working. There are few independent laboratory measures of drug response with the psychotropics, so you and your client must agree on specific target symptoms that you are trying to alleviate, and then together you must evaluate whether, in fact, those symptoms have been affected by the drug.

When the client is confused, unreliable, or otherwise unable to comply with the regimen on his or her own, a responsible friend or relative should be included in the discussion of how the medicine is to be taken. Assure the client that you and the prescribing physician are available to talk about the medication when questions arise.

Especially at the beginning of drug treatment, it is important that staff members be available by telephone or in person so that the client is not left alone with distressing side effects or other unexpected adverse reactions. In explaining the treatment plan to the client, be sure that the following information is included.

What symptoms are being treated (target symptoms). People will expect medication to help all their psychiatric symptoms, and this is almost never the case. Your client must know which specific symptoms the drug treatment is aimed at and which symptoms the drug cannot be expected to alleviate.

For example, if an antidepressant is prescribed for a recently widowed woman with severe vegetative depression, she should be told that the medication could help her sleep better and perhaps increase her appetite, but that she will continue to feel sad about her husband's death and may mourn his loss for some time to come. If a client is receiving another form of therapy (e.g., psychotherapy) in addition to medication, be sure the client knows what each treatment is meant to accomplish. Too often, people assume incorrectly that drugs are panaceas, that the problem is all "chemical," and that there is no need to cooperate in other forms of therapy. Such assumptions set the stage for disillusionment in cases where the medication fails to cure everything that ails the person.

Side effects that might occur. Informing the client of possible side effects is tricky. You want your clients to have some idea of what to expect when they take medication, but they could be frightened by an endless list of horrible (and often quite remote) possibilities. Here, judgment is critical. It is generally useful to describe the most common side effects, and to explain how the client can handle them if they occur (e.g., "The medicine might make your mouth dry. Many people find that chewing gum or hard candy helps keep the mouth moist").

Possible toxic effects or other dangers. Again, it is wise to mention only those effects that are common. For example, if drowsiness or dizziness is a common side effect, then the client must be cautioned about driving a car. If the effects of alcohol are enhanced by the medication, then caution the client about even social drinking. And the client must be alerted to the warning signs and symptoms of drug toxicity (e.g., symptoms of lithium toxicity such as nausea, vomiting, diarrhea, and stupor).

Above all, let the patient know that you and the prescribing physician are available, and that it is important to share questions or problems with you as they arise. If clients feel that they ought not to bother you with their concerns about medication, they may suffer distressing side effects (e.g., impotence) without reporting these, or they may discontinue the medication without discussing their concerns with you first.

Managing the Side Effects

Virtually all psychotropic medications have side effects, but we have little way of predicting which people will be particularly sensitive to which medications. The management of side effects is crucial to the successful drug treatment of mental illness, because treatment is commonly necessary for months or years. Compliance depends upon the client's willingness and ability to tolerate the medication.

People often discontinue their medication without consulting a physician, most commonly because they believe that the drug is not helpful or that they no longer require it, because they cannot bear unpleasant side effects, or because they believe their discomfort is due to side effects when it is in fact due to the symptoms of their illness.

Side effects can be difficult to recognize. Psychotic individuals may report bizarre symptoms that are actually manifestations of their illness, or they may be uncommunicative and incapable of reporting side effects at all. In dealing with people who are in emotional distress and who have impaired cognition, the therapeutic alliance is particularly important. The following are some effective ways that you and the prescribing physician can work to minimize or eliminate side effects:

- Monitor the client's mental and physical status regularly, including frequent meetings with the client—and, where indicated, the family.
- Pay careful attention to all the client's complaints, even when they seem trivial.
- Work as a team with other people involved in the client's care— physicians, nurses, social workers, psychologists, and other mental health workers. Professionals who see the client in other settings may be able to give you much-needed information about your client's reactions to medication.

- The client should be taking the lowest dosage that produces the desired effect. Many side effects are related to dosage.
- Advise and reassure the client. Many clients are capable of tolerating a significant amount of discomfort and inconvenience, provided they know it is in their interest to do so, and that you are concerned and supportive.
- Use of adjunctive medication. Particularly in the case of antipsychotics, side effects can be effectively relieved by antiparkinsonian drugs (discussed below).
- Discontinue the medication and try another medication if side effects become intolerable.
- Frequently reevaluate the client's need for the medication. If drug regimens are not regularly reevaluated, drug maintenance may be prolonged unnecessarily.
- Avoid polypharmacy—the prescribing of many drugs concurrently for a client in the hope that something will work. Each medication should be carefully chosen and its effect rigorously and frequently evaluated.

Combining Psychotropic Drugs

As a rule, combining two or more drugs of the same basic type (i.e., two antipsychotics or two antianxiety agents) is not desirable. Rather than enhancing the desired therapeutic effect, such combinations generally result in an increased risk of toxicity, increased side effects, and little or no therapeutic advantage.

However, combinations of *different* types of drugs are often useful. Antipsychotics, antidepressants, lithium, and antianxiety agents are frequently used in combination. Ideally, drug combinations are prescribed as a result of—and not instead of—a careful diagnostic evaluation. When medications are added to a regimen with no rationale and no target symptoms in mind, the result is usually a muddled and sometimes dangerous treatment.

A cardinal rule in drug treatment: Whenever possible, do one thing at a time. Too often, a prescribing physician tries unsuccessfully to make several changes in the treatment regimen concurrently. The results can be quite confusing. For example, if the physician lowers the dosage of a client's antipsychotic medication and simultaneously increases the dosage of an antidepressant, the client may take a turn for the better or worse, but you will be unable to assess which medication change made the difference.

This is true not only for medications, but for other elements in a client's treatment as well. By making one change in a treatment regimen at a time, the treatment team will have a much better chance of understanding the effects of specific contributions to the client's treatment. For example, if the physician decides to lower the dosage of your client's antipsychotic medication just as the client is about to begin weekly psychotherapy with you, you may not know whether an increase in psychotic symptoms during the first weeks of therapy is due to the lowered dosage of the medication or to the stresses of forming a new relationship.

Failure of Drug Treatment

The four most likely possibilities if drug treatment does not seem to work are listed below:

- The wrong type of drug was selected.
- The correct drug was selected, but the wrong dosage was prescribed.
- The correct drug and dosage were selected, but the client has not yet been taking the drug long enough to produce a therapeutic effect.
- The treaters have not obtained the client's cooperation in taking the medication reliably.

When drug treatment appears to fail, do not give up. Consider the points noted above and try to determine whether any of these factors is responsible for the treatment failure. Also remember that individuals respond quite idiosyncratically to psychotropic medications—a client who does not benefit from one drug may respond well to a different drug in the same class.

Gather all the information you can from the client, family members, and other members of the treatment team, and then determine what changes can be made—one at a time and systematically—to try to achieve the desired therapeutic effect. If it is feasible, get an additional consultation, for two heads are often better than one.

The Treatment Team

Somatic therapy often goes on in conjunction with other forms of treatment. While a physician prescribes medication, others may be involved with the client in psychotherapy, behavior therapy, group work, rehabilitation activities, and a host of other treatment modalities. The physician must speak with other members of the treatment team and enlist their cooperation in the psychopharmacologic intervention, preferably before any new medication is prescribed. Similarly, other team members must keep the prescribing physician informed of new developments in their work with the client (e.g., when the frequency of psychotherapy sessions is increased or decreased).

There are several reason for this emphasis on communication within the treatment team. First, it make for good care. Those who do not prescribe medication must nevertheless know what to expect when such a treatment is introduced. They must know what side effects and adverse effects to watch for, and they must know the goals of the somatic treatment in order to help the client understand and comply with the plan. Second, the client must have the sense that members of the treatment team are coordinating their efforts—that the right hand knows what the left hand is doing. If the physician prescribes a potentially lethal drug for a suicidal client, everyone involved in the treatment must know the risks and benefits involved in this plan, so that the client's use of the drug and suicidal impulses can be carefully monitored.

Finally, physicians and other treaters should communicate with each other as a matter of professional courtesy. When members of a treatment team do not value each other's help and input, it is easy for treatment goals to be subtly sabotaged. This may happen out of anger, or out of ignorance of what another treater is trying to accomplish.

The following are some basic points to remember about your role as a member of a treatment team:

1. Keep yourself informed of what other treaters are doing. Ask questions. Remember: no question (e.g., about medication or a psychotherapy strategy) is too elementary.
2. Keep other treaters informed about your own work with a client, and share your observations about the client's responses to various interventions (e.g., reactions to a change in medication).
3. Consult with other treaters before you make major changes in a client's treatment regimen, and expect that other treaters will do the same.
4. If you are part of a treatment team in which this sort of communication is not occurring, meet with all concerned to discuss and remedy the problem. Otherwise, it is your client who will suffer.

The basic guidelines above for the use of psychotropic medications apply to each of the specific classes of drugs discussed in the following sections.

ANTIPSYCHOTIC MEDICATIONS

Antipsychotic medications are useful primarily in the treatment of thought disorders and, more acutely, to relieve severe agitation.

How Do They Work?

The mechanism of action of the antipsychotics is not completely understood. The areas of the brain most affected by these drugs are the reticular formation, basal ganglia, hypothalamus, and limbic system. At the cellular level, the drugs inhibit the transmission of nerve impulses in the central nervous system (CNS) by blocking the action of dopamine, a neurotransmitter, at post-synaptic receptor sites. It is not known whether this dopamine-blocking activity is the mechanism by which psychosis is ameliorated.

Whatever their mechanism of action, the antipsychotics have been shown in large-scale studies to be extremely effective against the symptoms of acute psychosis.

What Are the Indications for Using an Antipsychotic?

Several illnesses usually call for the use of an antipsychotic:

Schizophrenia. This is the major condition for which antipsychotics are indicated. They are used in the following ways:

- By intramuscular injection to control acute, severe psychotic agitation or excitement.
- Orally in daily doses to control acute episodes of illness (e.g., to treat the recurrence of auditory hallucinations).
- As maintenance therapy to prevent recurrent exacerbations, in daily oral doses or in intramuscular doses of depot medication every two to four weeks.

Manic-depressive illness. Manic excitement is alleviated by antipsychotics, which are often used in combination with lithium in cases of acute mania and then discontinued when mania abates. The efficacy of long-term maintenance therapy of manic-depressive illness with antipsychotics is unproved (see Chapter 6).

Amphetamine psychosis. Antipsychotics are the drugs of choice for amphetamine psychosis. They are used only so long as psychosis persists (see Chapter 12).

Drug-induced psychosis. If the drug cannot be identified, it is better in most cases to "talk the person down" than to use medication. However, if agitation is life-threatening, antipsychotics can be of great benefit. (Antipsychotics should not be used to treat psychosis known to be caused by anticholinergic drugs.)

Agitated or psychotic depression. Antipsychotics are very effective, often in combination with an antidepressant. The efficacy of antipsychotics in retarded depression is less clear.

Chronic brain syndromes. Syndromes that involve psychosis may be treated symptomatically with antipsychotics.

Anxiety. Antipsychotics are not the drugs of choice for anxiety. They should be used only when antianxiety or antidepressant agents have proved ineffective and the anxiety is incapacitating.

If one of the above-mentioned illnesses has been diagnosed, you must still determine whether the symptoms of the illness are likely to respond to an antipsychotic (Table 16-2). The symptoms that are most likely to respond are combativeness, hyperactivity, tension, hostility, hallucinations, sleeplessness, poor hygiene and self-care, acute delusions (of recent onset), and social isolation. The symptoms that are less likely to respond are lack of insight, poor judgment, impaired memory, disorientation, and chronic delusions.

Table 16–2. Responsiveness of symptoms to antipsychotic medications.

More likely to respond	Less likely to respond
Combativeness	Lack of insight
Hyperactivity	Poor judgment
Tension	Impaired memory
Hostility	Disorientation
Hallucinations	Chronic delusions
Sleeplessness	
Poor hygiene and self-care	
Acute delusions (of recent onset)	
Social isolation	

In considering the use of an antipsychotic, you must first arrive at a clear sense of what has caused the symptoms. Among those clients for whom antipsychotics are indicated diagnostically, you will find that the tense, hyperactive or hypoactive, obviously psychotic person is likely to improve with the drug. The individual whose level of activity is normal and who simply appears to be in a fog will be less likely to improve. Nevertheless, it is worth giving such people a trial of antipsychotic medication.

Before treating someone with an antipsychotic, the following basic work-up is indicated:

- History and physical examination;
- Blood pressure, both standing and reclining, to note baseline postural changes;
- Laboratory studies—complete blood count (including white blood cell count), liver function tests, urinalysis; and
- A baseline electrocardiogram (EKG) for people with any history of cardiac problems and anyone over 40 years old.

Types of Antipsychotic Medications

There are several pharmacologically distinct classes of antipsychotics, but all of them have similar therapeutic actions and all are about equally effective. There is no need to describe here in detail the different pharmacologic properties of these classes. Excellent discussions of the pharmacology of the antipsychotics can be found in the sources listed at the end of this chapter. Clinically, there are three important differences among the groups of antipsychotics, as described below.

Potency. Because the antipsychotics are of such different potencies, drug doses vary by a factor of up to 10^3. Thus, for example, if it takes 300 to 400 mg of chlorpromazine (Thorazine) to relieve a client's psychotic symptoms, it would take roughly 6 to 8 mg of haloperidol (Haldol) to achieve the same effect, as the potency of haloperidol is roughly 50 times that of chlorpromazine.

Side effects. The side effects, discussed below, vary greatly from one type of drug to another.

Client's idiosyncratic responses. Some people who do not respond well to a drug of one class respond satisfactorily to a drug that is chemically quite distinct.

Table 16–3. Equivalent doses of commonly used antipsychotic agents by chemical type (chlorpromazine = 100).

Generic name	Trade name	Potency relative to chlorpromazine
Phenothiazines		
Aliphatic		
Chlorpromazine	Thorazine	100
Piperdine		
Mesoridazine	Serentil	50
Piperacetazine	Quide	12
Thioridazine	Mellaril	100
Piperazine		
Acetophenazine	Tindal	20
Fluphenazine	Prolixin	2
Perphenazine	Trilafon	10
Trifluoperazine	Stelazine	5
Thioxanthenes		
Aliphatic		
Chlorprothixene	Taractan	65
Piperazine		
Thiothixene	Navane	5
Dibenzazepines		
Loxapine	Loxitane, Daxolin	15
Butyrophenones		
Haloperidol	Haldol	2
Indolones		
Molindone	Moban	10
Rauwolfia alkaloids		
Reserpine	Serpasil, etc. (generic)	1-2

Table 16-3 presents the most commonly used antipsychotic agents. They are listed according to their pharmacologic group. Their potencies are given relative to the potency of chlorpromazine (Thorazine).

Clinical applications of Table 16-3. This table can serve as a prescribing physician's "bible" for determining proper dosages of the antipsychotics. Essentially, the table helps the physician think of the dosage of any antipsychotic in terms of "chlorpromazine equivalents"—i.e., the strength of the dosage relative to an equivalent dosage of chlorpromazine.

Suppose, for example, that you want to treat an acutely psychotic young man with trifluoperazine (Stelazine). It has been determined that the minimum dosage of chlorpromazine that is likely to be effec-

tive in treating acute psychosis in a young adult is 400 mg orally per day. How much trifluoperazine (Stelazine) is the daily equivalent of 400 mg of chlorpromazine (CPZ)?
The arithmetic is simple:

$\dfrac{\text{Potency of drug X}}{\text{Potency of CPZ}}$	$\times$	Desired dose in CPZ equivalents	$=$	Desired dose of drug X
$\dfrac{5}{100}$	$\times$	400 mg	$=$	20 mg

As shown above, 400 mg of chlorpromazine equals 20 mg of trifluoperazine. Thus, the prescribing physician would want to give your patient at least 20 mg/day of trifluoperazine to adequately treat his condition.

If this psychotic man showed no improvement on trifluoperazine, even at increased doses, the prescribing physician would probably try another antipsychotic of a chemically different class, going back to the table to choose a drug like haloperidol or molindone. The initial dosage of the new drug would then be determined on the basis of its potency relative to chlorpromazine.

Side Effects

All antipsychotic agents carry side effects. You can expect to see side effects in most people treated with these drugs (Table 16-4).

Table 16–4. Side effects of antipsychotic medications.

Sedation	Postural hypotension
Extrapyramidal side effects (EPS)	Allergic or toxic side effects
Dystonia	Agranulocytosis
Parkinsonism	Dermatitis
Akathisia	Allergic hepatitis
Akinesia	Metabolic or endocrine side effects
Tardive dyskinesia	Toxic retinopathy
Lowered seizure threshold	EKG changes
Anticholinergic side effects	Retrograde ejaculation
Dry mouth	
Blurred vision	
Constipation	
Urinary retention	

Sedation. Sedation occurs in 80 percent of cases and usually lasts about one week. This may be a desired effect (for insomniacs), or it may be a problem (e.g., for students or for those who feel drowsy when driving an automobile). To treat sedation, the physician might lower the dosage, give the entire daily dose at bedtime, or use a less sedating drug.

Extrapyramidal side effects. Extrapyramidal side effects refer to disturbances in functioning of the extrapyramidal tracts of the nervous system. These side effects occur in 10 to 30 percent of cases. There are several types, as outlined below.

Dystonia (a state of abnormal muscle tension) occurs early in treatment, often within the first two days. Manifestations include spasms of the eye, face, neck, and back muscles, which can produce bodily contortions that are quite dramatic and frightening. However, dystonia is more commonly experienced as simple muscle stiffness. Acute dystonic reactions are easily and rapidly treated as described below. For recurrent dystonias, the prescribing physician will lower the dose, switch to another antipsychotic, or use antiparkinsonian medications prophylactically in conjunction with the antipsychotic.

Parkinsonism—a cluster of symptoms like those seen in Parkinson's disease—occurs generally within one to four weeks after treatment is begun. Symptoms include bradykinesia (decreased movement), shuffling gait, decreased energy, mask-like facial expression, and tremor. Parkinsonism is treatable by the same means as dystonias (see below).

Akathisia is very common and occurs within one to six weeks after treatment is begun. It involves restlessness, pacing, rocking, and an inability to sit still. It is often experienced as "jumpy legs." Akathisia is treatable with antiparkinsonian drugs, but it is easy to mistake for psychotic agitation; the physician must be careful not to mistreat it by raising the dosage of the antipsychotic.

Akinesia is relatively uncommon, but its late and insidious onset makes it easy to miss. It involves markedly decreased or absent body activity, which can be mistaken for a symptom of psychosis and wrongly treated by raising the dosage of the antipsychotic. Proper treatment involves lowering the dosage, switching to another drug, or using antiparkinsonian medication.

Tardive dyskinesia is the most ominous of the side effects of the antipsychotics. This syndrome develops late in treatment (after one to 20 years of maintenance therapy); it is estimated to occur in from 2 to 50 percent of chronic schizophrenics. It involves involuntary movement, including lip smacking and sucking, jaw movements, "flycatcher" tongue movements, writhing movements of the extremities, and occasional difficulty swallowing. Although many cases are irreversible, some do remit completely when antipsychotic medication is discontinued. Antiparkinsonian drugs are of no help in treatment and may increase the severity of the movement. The best (and probably the only) treatment for tardive dyskinesia is prevention, by using antipsychotics only when absolutely indicated and in the lowest effective doses, and by monitoring clients on antipsychotics frequently with trials off medication to assess their ongoing need for the drug. Obviously, the occasional discomfort and impairment caused by these involuntary movements (they are often mild and not noticed by the client) must be weighed against the client's psychotic illness in determining whether antipsychotic medication is warranted even when symptoms of tardive dyskinesia develop.

Lowered seizure threshold. Chlorpromazine in particular increases the likelihood of seizures in people who have preexisting seizure disorders. Therapy with antipsychotics must therefore be undertaken with caution (but is not contraindicated) with such clients.

Anticholinergic side effects. These are very common, usually mild, but somewhat annoying; they disappear within days or weeks. Dry mouth, blurred vision, rapid heart beat, nasal congestion, and constipation are the most frequent of such effects. Occasionally, the side effects are more severe, such as paralysis of the intestines or urinary retention. Clients must be screened for preexisting narrow-angle glaucoma, since antipsychotics can precipitate acute exacerbations of this condition, which may result in loss of eyesight.

Postural hypotension. This refers to a sudden and abnormally large drop in blood pressure that occurs when the subject stands up, and may result in fainting. It is particularly common in the elderly and must be monitored closely to prevent falling and possible trauma.

Allergic or toxic side effects. Although these are uncommon, you must be alert to their possible occurrence.

Agranulocytosis refers to a decrease or absence of white blood cells in the circulation. White blood cells are an essential element of the body's immune system and are necessary to fight infection. Agranulocytosis occurs in the first three to eight weeks of treatment in roughly one in 5,000 people taking chlorpromazine, and somewhat less commonly with other drugs in this class. Early manifestations are fever and sore throat that usually precede altered white blood cell count. It can be treated by stopping all medication and working to prevent infection.

Dermatitis, or skin rash, is common—not only an allergic reaction to the drug, but also as a result of drug-induced sensitivity to sunlight. People taking antipsychotics must be forewarned to use sun blockers, or they can be badly and dangerously sunburned.

Allergic hepatitis occurs chiefly with chlorpromazine (about one in 500 people) during the first four weeks of treatment. It is an inflammation of the liver manifested by jaundice (yellowing of the skin and the whites of the eyes). This is a benign condition that remits when the drug is stopped.

Metabolic or endocrine side effects. These very uncommon effects include weight gain, menstrual irregularity, abnormal production of breast milk and breast enlargement, high blood sugar, and elevated or decreased body temperature.

Toxic retinopathy. This condition, in which the retina of the eye is damaged, is caused only by thioridazine (Mellaril) in dosages of more than 800 mg per day.

EKG changes. Arrhythmias, T-wave inversions, and changes in the QRS interval are relatively rare, but they are more common with thioridazine (Mellaril) than with other antipsychotics.

Retrograde ejaculation. This refers to the ejaculation of semen up into the man's urinary bladder instead of out of the penis through the urethra. It is a painful condition that is primarily caused by thioridazine (Mellaril), so other antipsychotic agents are recommended in treating men for whom this might be a problem.

Treatment of Extrapyramidal Side Effects

Dystonias, parkinsonism, akathisia, and akinesia are all responsive to antiparkinsonian drugs. The most commonly used drugs in the treatment of extrapyramidal side effects are listed below:

Diphenhydramine (Benadryl) is an antihistamine that is very safe, not prone to being abused, and useful in acute dystonias since intravenous administration brings relief within minutes. It can be given orally, intravenously, or intramuscularly. Sedation and pronounced anticholinergic effects make this drug less desirable for treating extrapyramidal side effects on a long-term basis. The usual dosage is 25-50 mg intramuscularly or intravenously for acute dystonia, and 25-50 mg orally every four to six hours to prevent recurrent dystonic episodes.

Benztropine mesylate (Cogentin) is an antiparkinsonian drug that is very effective for acute and long-term treatment of extrapyramidal side effects. The usual dosage is 1-2 mg orally one to three times a day as needed to prevent extrapyramidal side effects. Cogentin may be used on a long-term basis and is also available in intramuscular and intravenous forms (in doses of 0.5-2 mg) for treatment of acute reactions.

Trihexyphenidyl (Artane), another antiparkinsonian drug, is quite similar to Cogentin. Many people find it less sedating than either Cogentin or Benadryl and therefore more suitable for long-term treatment. The usual dosage is 2 mg orally one to three times a day.

Lorazepam (Ativan) has been found effective in treating akathisia, but at this time it has not been formally approved by the U.S. Food and Drug Administration (FDA) for this purpose. Generally, a dosage of 0.5-2.0 mg orally two or three times a day is sufficient.

If the client requires an antiparkinsonian drug for side effects, continue the drug for one to three months and then taper it off to determine whether it is still required. A majority of people will have become "acclimated" to the antipsychotic and will not exhibit their previous side effects when the antiparkinsonian drug is discontinued. However, a significant number of clients require antiparkinsonian therapy for as long as they take the antipsychotic.

Note that some people experience a "high" from Cogentin and Artane, and some may abuse these drugs when the side effects are no longer present.

Use During Pregnancy

The antipsychotics have not been shown to cause an increased incidence of congenital malformations in the fetus when taken by the mother during pregnancy. Nevertheless, it is advisable to avoid administering them if possible, at least during the first trimester, unless psychotic symptoms are clearly evident and require control. The medications are excreted in breast milk and should therefore be avoided if possible while a client is breastfeeding a child.

Drug Interactions

Some drugs that interact with the antipsychotics include the following.

- The efficacy of *oral anticoagulants* is decreased by phenothiazines.
- *Antacids* may decrease the absorption of antipsychotic medications.
- The phenothiazines potentiate (exaggerate) the effects of *antihistamines, antihypertensives, central nervous system depressants* (e.g., alcohol), *oral hypoglycemics*, and *succinylcholine*.
- A *scopolamine* overdose (e.g., Compoz, Sominex) or the use of *diuretics* in combination with the phenothiazines can cause a hypotensive crisis (a precipitous drop in blood pressure).

Choosing an Antipsychotic

Since they are all of roughly equal efficacy, how does the prescribing physician decide which antipsychotic to use for a particular individual?

Rely on the client's history. If your client has had antipsychotic medication in the past, find out which drugs worked and which did not.

Consider compliance. When working with an outpatient who cannot reliably take daily oral medication, the prescribing physician must consider giving depot fluphenazine by intramuscular injection every two to four weeks. Fluphenazine is one of the only antipsychotics available in this long-acting form.

Decide which side effects are least likely to be troublesome to the client. Since all antipsychotics carry side effects, one set must be weighed against another. In most cases, the choice is between low-potency drugs, which have primarily anticholinergic and sedating effects, and high-potency drugs, which are less sedating but more likely to cause extrapyramidal reactions (dystonias, parkinsonism, and akathisia). For a severely agitated individual who cannot sleep well, you might deliberately choose a more sedating (low-potency) drug like chlorpromazine (Thorazine) because sedation would be desirable. Paranoid clients might be particularly frightened by muscle spasm (dystonia), so a high-potency drug might be avoided, or given along with prophylactic antiparkinsonian medication. For a college student who is studying for examinations, a low-potency antipsychotic might cause too much drowsiness and blurred vision, whereas a high-potency drug like haloperidol (Haldol) would not compromise his or her studying capacity.

Table 16-5 lists some of the most commonly used antipsychotics, showing the degree to which they cause sedation and/or extrapyramidal side effects.

Table 16–5. Commonly used antipsychotics, their relative potencies, and their sedating and extrapyramidal effects.

Generic name	Trade name	Relative potency	Sedation hypo-tension	EPS
Phenothiazines				
Aliphatic				
Chlorpromazine	Thorazine	100	+ + +	+ +
Piperidine				
Thioridazine	Mellaril	100	+ + +/+ +	+
Piperazine				
Fluphenazine	Prolixin	2	+	+ + +
Perphenazine	Trilafon	10	+	+ + +
Trifluoperazine	Stelazine	5	+	+ + +
Thioxanthenes				
Aliphatic				
Chlorprothixene	Taractan	65	+ +	+ +
Piperazine				
Thiothixene	Navane	5	+	+ + +
Dibenzazepines				
Loxapine	Loxitane	15	+ +	+ + +
Butyrophenones				
Haloperidol	Haldol	2	+	+ + +
Indolones				
Molindone	Moban	10	+	+ +

Prescribing the Antipsychotics

Once an antipsychotic is chosen, how is it prescribed?

Emergencies. Severely combative, aggressive, and destructive psychotic people can be rapidly and effectively treated with repeated intramuscular injections of an antipsychotic to decrease excitement and to protect the client and others from harm. (This is known as "rapid neuroleptization.") Before such a treatment is used with a client who is unknown (e.g., in a hospital emergency room), the following conditions, which might be obscured or worsened by the administration of an antipsychotic, must be ruled out:

- Head injuries,
- Space-occupying intracranial lesions (e.g., a subdural hematoma, or blood clot, pressing on the brain),
- Epilepsy,
- Severe hypotension or hypertension,

- Intoxication with drugs that have anticholinergic effects, and
- Imbalance of serum electrolytes (sodium, potassium).

If none of these conditions is present, any one of the anti-psychotics listed below may be used via intramuscular injection (initial doses are suggested, along with an acceptable dosage range):

- Haloperidol (Haldol): 2 mg (range, 1-10 mg)
- Perphenazine (Trilafon): 10 mg (range, 4-30 mg)
- Fluphenazine HCl (Prolixin HCl): 2.5 mg (range, 1-25 mg)
- Trifluoperazine (Stelazine): 5 mg (range, 1-10 mg)
- Thiothixene (Navane): 5 mg (range, 4-30 mg)

The end point of this rapid neuroleptization is a decrease in excitement, and the process is commonly continued until the person falls asleep. To achieve this, the dose may be repeated every hour (even every 30 minutes if excitement is severe). Intramuscular doses can be safely repeated as long as there is no significant drop in blood pressure. Frequent monitoring of blood pressure is essential during this treatment.

There is an ongoing argument in the psychiatric literature as to whether rapid neuroleptization is more effective than a single intramuscular injection followed by oral medication.

Acute psychosis. For clients who are acutely psychotic but who do not exhibit severe agitation, rapid neuroleptization is not necessary. Instead, the physician should begin with oral doses of the medication, starting at a subtherapeutic dosage and increasing it gradually until the desired effect is achieved or until the side effects become intolerable and some adjustment must be made. The phases of acute treatment, when effective, are likely to be as follows:

- *One to five days*—Excitement and hyperactivity disappear, and the client becomes more cooperative.
- *Two days to two months*—The client's thought disorder persists but he or she functions better in daily living.
- *One to six weeks (or more)*—Ameliorization of the client's thought disorder.

Acute psychosis responds to a minimum of 300-400 mg per day of chlorpromazine (or the equivalent dose of another drug) in most healthy people. The average dosages required for the acutely psychotic individual range from 400 to 900 mg a day orally. How quickly this dosage is reached will depend on the person's size (larger people often require higher dosages), age (the elderly generally require lower dosages), and history (tolerance of high dosages in the past permits rapid increase in the dosage). For young, healthy individuals who have had no prior experience with antipsychotics, it is best to start with 100 mg per day and increase the dosage over several days as rapidly as it is tolerated.

How high is too high? The dosage of an antipsychotic can be increased to fairly high levels to achieve the desired result if the side effects are tolerable, but daily dosages above 1,500/mg orally do not often result in additional improvement. (However, a few people improve on dosages of up to 4,000 mg orally per day.)

The antipsychotics have very long half-lives—i.e., they are eliminated from the body slowly and are long-acting. Thus, the entire daily dosage may be given at one time to achieve continuous antipsychotic effects, if the client can comply more easily with a once-a-day regimen.

Maintenance therapy. Once the client has been stabilized on an antipsychotic, how long does treatment continue? The answer is not clear. Chronic therapy with an antipsychotic carries significant risks, particularly the risk of tardive dyskinesia. Thus, maintenance therapy should only be used if there is a clear indication that the client requires such treatment.

Acute drug-induced psychoses generally remit rapidly; prolonged antipsychotic treatment is not necessary. Mania is treated acutely with antipsychotics, but most manic-depressive clients need not be continued on antipsychotics once the acute psychosis has cleared and they are stabilized on lithium.

A client who suffers a first psychotic episode of unknown etiology (particularly an adolescent) must be tapered off the medication after several weeks to several months of successful drug treatment, so that the ongoing need for medication can be assessed. Such a person may never have a subsequent psychotic break and should not be medicated indefinitely.

Maintenance therapy is required for chronic conditions in which psychosis recurs within weeks or months after treatment is stopped. Most people who fall into this category are chronic schizophrenics, schizoaffectives, and those manic-depressives who do not remain symptom-free on lithium alone. About 40 to 60 percent of people who are diagnosed as chronic schizophrenics have relapses within six months after antipsychotic treatment is stopped. For these people, long-term maintenance has been shown to decrease their rates of relapse and rehospitalization.

Even the most chronically ill people (i.e., those with a history of multiple psychotic episodes and multiple hospitalizations) should be given occasional closely supervised trials off medication to be sure that treatment is not being prolonged unnecessarily.

Long-term maintenance dosages of antipsychotics can usually be lowered to 20 to 50 percent of the dosage required during the acute psychotic episode. There is no standard maintenance dosage, so it must be arrived at by monitoring symptoms carefully and determining the lowest dosage at which target symptoms are kept in abeyance.

If treatment seems ineffective, consider whether the dosage is adequate and whether the client is taking the drug. If the client shows no response to an adequate dosage of medication after two weeks of treatment, it is useful to try another medication. Lack of response to one antipsychotic does not imply that the person will not respond to another.

ANTIDEPRESSANTS

Drugs that alleviate and prevent depression have proved invaluable in the treatment of mood disorders. These drugs fall into two major classes—the tricyclic antidepressants (TCAs) and tricyclic-like medications, and the monoamine oxidase inhibitors (MAOIs). These medications, along with electroconvulsive therapy (ECT), are the most effective somatic therapies now available for the treatment of certain types of depression. Stimulants, such as amphetamine, were once widely used in elevating the depressed person's mood, but since the advent of these more effective and more specific antidepressant agents, mood elevators are no longer the treatment of choice.

As was mentioned in Chapter 6, the causes, symptoms, and clinical courses of various depressive syndromes are quite varied. No one treatment is uniformly effective for all types of depression, and the antidepressants are not panaceas. Nevertheless, a majority of people with severe depression do respond favorably to antidepressants, and many who do not respond to one drug will respond to another or to ECT.

Psychotherapy or Medication

This choice is not an either-or proposition. Many advocates of medication argue that drugs work more rapidly than psychotherapy to alleviate depression, and that they are more cost-effective. Psychotherapists counter that medication interferes with effective treatment since it allows clients to attribute a "chemical" cause to their difficulties and thereby avoid important intrapsychic and interpersonal issues that have fostered the depression.

In fact, medications and psychotherapy work in complementary ways—the medication alleviates many of the physiological symptoms of the illness, while psychotherapy helps to ease emotional pain and promote more effective functioning in the world. Outpatient studies of mild depression have shown the combination of psychotherapy and pharmacotherapy to be more effective than either treatment alone.

Which depressed people are most likely to benefit from an antidepressant? Two factors should be considered in answering this question: the symptoms and the syndromes, as shown in Table 16-6. The depressive symptoms most likely to be alleviated by antidepressant medication are the *vegetative signs:* appetite disturbance and weight loss, sleep disturbance (especially early morning awakening), decreased energy, decreased sexual drive, psychomotor agitation or retardation, and diurnal mood variation (depression worse in the morning).

The symptoms less likely to respond to antidepressants are those that are the more *subjective* and *psychological signs:* demoralization, low self-esteem, hopelessness, and helplessness. Such feelings are more responsive to psychotherapeutic interventions.

Table 16–6. Responsiveness of symptoms and syndromes to antidepressant medications.

More likely to respond	Less likely to respond
Symptoms	
Appetite disturbance and weight loss	Demoralization
Sleep disturbance	Low self-esteem
Decreased energy	Hopelessness
Decreased sexual energy	Helplessness
Psychomotor agitation or retardation	
Diurnal mood variation	
Syndromes	
Major depressive episodes	Dysthymic disorder
Agitated depression	Personality disorder

The depressive syndromes *most likely to respond* to antidepressants include vegetative signs and discrete episodes of illness that seem to have a life of their own. Discrete episodes of depression have a clear time of onset, as opposed to more "characterologic" depression, which the client regards as having always been present. *Major depressive episodes* ("endogenous depression") are not greatly influenced by changes in the person's environment or by specific social or therapeutic interactions; they generally include vegetative signs. *Agitated depression* ("involutional melancholia") is common in people over 45 years of age and is characterized by pacing, hand-wringing, hair-pulling, and vocal expressions of psychic pain. Antipsychotics and ECT are also particularly useful in these cases.

The syndromes *less likely to respond* to antidepressants are those that have no clear onset or discrete episodes, but that have a clear relationship to environmental events (i.e., the client's wife has left him) and minimal vegetative disturbance. These include *dysthymic disorder* that has been present for at least two years in adults and is characterized by longstanding feelings of hopelessness, inadequacy, and low self-esteem without prominent physiologic disturbance, and *personality disorders* in which depression is a concomitant of longstanding interpersonal difficulties and chronically impaired functioning. For example, people with borderline personality disorder often complain of depression and may even report sleep and appetite disturbance, but these symptoms are often the direct result of the underlying personality disorder and current life events. Such difficulties are not resolved by pharmacotherapy.

Syndromes that are generally self-limiting do not require antidepressant therapy. *Reactive depression* due to severe environmental stress includes, for example, grief reactions after the death or loss of a loved one. Support, psychotherapy, and brief symptomatic treatment (e.g., with antianxiety agents) usually suffice. *Drug-induced depression* (e.g., depression caused by the antihypertensive reserpine) is usually resolved when the offending drug is discontinued. *Depression secondary to physical illness* generally resolves when the underlying physical condition improves (e.g., anemia, hypothyroidism).

Syndromes that are not "pure" depressive syndromes are sometimes responsive to antidepressant treatment. These include *manic-depressive illness* and *schizoaffective disorders*. Although lithium treatment is more common and generally more effective on a long-term basis, antidepressants can be useful in treating the acute depressive phases of manic-depressive illness. A word of caution, however: since antidepressants can precipitate mania, they must be used judiciously with people who are prone to manic episodes. For schizoaffective disorders, antipsychotics and antidepressants are often used in combination when people manifest features of both affective illness and schizophrenia. Again, antidepressants must be used with caution since they exacerbate psychosis in some cases.

In cases of depression that are not clear cut—when symptomatology is not clearly vegetative—the decision to medicate or not to medicate remains a matter of clinical judgment. Most clinicians agree that it is best to try antidepressants when there is a reasonable possibility that the drug could be of benefit to the client and when a trial of the medication can be carried out safely.

Dexamethasone Suppression Test

As the discussion above suggests, there is some disagreement over which people are likely to respond to antidepressants. In the past few years, much publicity has been given to the dexamethasone suppression test (DST), which promised to be a definitive biochemical test for depression that would enable clinicians to reliably sort out those depressed people who would respond to antidepressant therapy from those who would not. Since you are likely to encounter the DST in your work, a brief discussion of this new laboratory study is provided here.

The development of the DST began with the observation that many depressed people had elevated serum cortisol levels and poor regulation of adrenocorticotropin (ACTH) production. Cortisol is a steroid that is normally produced by the adrenal gland to regulate a variety of metabolic processes in the body. ACTH is a hormone made by the pituitary gland that stimulates cortisol production. In turn, ACTH production is regulated by the hypothalamus. In normal people who are given a small dose of dexamethasone (a synthetic steroid), the body's production of cortisol (a natural steroid) will automatically be suppressed over the next 24 hours. However, in some depressed people given the same oral dose of dexamethasone, cortisol production is only partly suppressed or recovers too early, suggesting an abnormality in the regulation of hormone production somewhere in the body's regulatory system—i.e., in the hypothalamus, the pituitary, or the adrenal gland.

The DST is given as follows: 1 mg of dexamethasone is given orally at 11 P.M., and venous blood is drawn for cortisol assays at 8 A.M., 4 P.M., and/or 11 P.M. the following day (in outpatients, the test is usually limited to a 4 P.M. sample). The DST is considered abnormal if any of the samples shows a plasma cortisol level above 4.5–5.0 mg/dl. The test costs $25 to $50 for each blood sample assayed.

Investigators have reported that 90 percent of people who have abnormal ("positive") DSTs have melancholic or endogenous depression—a high rate of specificity for this test. Ideally the DST could help clinicians establish or rule out the presence of endogenous depression if the clinical findings were equivocal. However, the test is not particularly sensitive, for only about 50 percent of people who are diagnosed clinically as suffering from major depression have abnormal DST responses; the rest are not identified by this screening measure.

To complicate matters, many medical conditions other than depressive illness can give false-positive DSTs, including Cushing's disease, liver disease, pregnancy, and drug use (e.g., alcohol, phenytoin, carbamazepine, or sedatives). New research suggests that the DST may not specifically identify people who are endogenously depressed, but may also be positive in some cases of mania, acute psychosis, chronic schizophrenia, stroke, and dementia.

The DST has not been shown to be superior to clinical findings in predicting whether someone will respond to antidepressant therapy, nor has it proved helpful to clinicians in choosing particular medications for treating depression. Some psychiatrists use serial DSTs to measure an individual's response to treatment, but it has not been shown that this technique for monitoring improvement is more reliable than one's clinical judgment. Therefore, the diagnostic interview continues to be the most accurate tool available for the diagnosis and treatment of depression that is responsive to somatic therapy, and the DST remains of greater research interest than clinical utility.

Clinical Evaluation

Before a client is started on an antidepressant, it is important to collect certain data that might influence the choice of treatment (Table 16-7).

History
When taking a history, pay particular attention to the following:

- *Current medications:* Drugs like reserpine, methyldopa, stimulants, oral contraceptives, alcohol, marijuana, and other drugs of abuse can cause depression.
- *Family history:* A family history of depressive episodes that were responsive to medication is a good predictor of response in your client. Note which drugs alleviated depression in relatives, because drug responsiveness, like depression itself, has genetic determinants, and what worked for the parent or grandparent is likely to work for the grandchild as well. If there is a family history of

Table 16–7. Medical work-up for antidepressant therapy.

Medical history
   Current medical conditions
   Current medications
   Family history

Physical examination

Baseline laboratory studies
   Complete blood count with differential
   Routine blood chemistry—SMA-12
   Thyroid function tests (T3, T4, TSH)
   Urinalysis

EKG (if client over 40 or any history of cardiac symptoms)

mania, proceed with caution in using antidepressants, because they can precipitate mania in those who have an underlying bipolar illness.

- *Current medical conditions:* Cardiac problems are particularly important to elucidate, given the side effects of the antidepressants (discussed below). Question the client carefully about a history of congestive heart failure, heart attacks, arrhythmias, and postural hypotension. Other problems to screen out include prostatic enlargement (antidepressants can cause obstruction of the urinary tract and urinary retention) and narrow-angle glaucoma (antidepressants can precipitate acute exacerbations and result in loss of eyesight).

- *Suicidal ideation:* This is a tricky problem, since many depressed people are prone to suicidal ideation and attempts. Tricyclics are highly lethal in overdose; the lethal dose is only 10 to 30 times the daily therapeutic dosage. MAOIs can interact with certain tyramine-containing foods (discussed below) to cause severe hypertension, resulting in stroke and death. For suicidal people, prescribing must be done with care. Prescriptions for outpatients can be written weekly or even every few days if necessary as a sign to the client of the treatment team's concern and attention. Severely suicidal people can be treated in the hospital to prevent overdose in the initial phases of treatment.

Physical Examination
Baseline laboratory studies. The following laboratory studies are useful in ruling out an underlying medical illness which causes depression:

- Complete blood count with differential cell count,
- Routine blood chemistries (serum sodium and potassium, blood sugar, blood urea nitrogen, etc.),
- Thyroid function tests (T3, T4, and TSH), and
- Urinalysis

Tricyclics and Related Drugs

The tricyclic antidepressants (TCAs) and tricyclic-like compounds constitute the treatment of choice for most depressions. Except in a limited number of cases for which ECT is more clearly indicated, the tricyclics should be the first treatment considered in somatic therapy for depressed people.

Despite considerable research, we do not know how these drugs alleviate depression. As was discussed in Chapter 6 (Affective Disorders), some depressed people have been found to have low CNS levels of the neurotransmitters *serotonin* and *norepinephrine* in the central nervous system (CNS). The tricyclics affect the concentration of these neurotransmitters at nerve synapses in the CNS by blocking their reuptake by presynaptic neurons, thus increasing their availability at the junctions between neurons. It has been hypothesized that this *neurotransmitter effect* is the mechanism by which the drugs alleviate depression, but the data supporting this theory are equivocal.

Clinically, it is useful to know which TCAs increase CNS levels of serotonin and which increase levels of norepinephrine, because a client whose depressive symptoms do not respond to one drug may respond to a drug of the other type; see Table 16-8 for the characteristics of the commonly used antidepressants.

The tricyclic antidepressants. Imipramine (Tofranil) and *amitriptyline* (Elavil) are the oldest and best studied of the tricyclic antidepressants. They are still the most widely prescribed TCAs, but newer drugs with fewer side effects are beginning to be used extensively in clinical practice. Amitriptyline is quite sedating and has predominantly serotonergic effects; it is therefore useful in treating people who have sleep difficulties. Imipramine is less sedating and primarily noradrenergic in its effects.

Desipramine (Norpramin) is a demethylated metabolite of imipramine; it is thus "purer" in its noradrenergic effect. It has fewer anticholinergic side effects (dry mouth, blurred vision, constipation) than the other TCAs and is therefore quite useful for sensitive clients. *Nortriptyline* (Aventyl) is another demethylated metabolite of amitriptyline. *Protriptyline* (Vivactyl) has little in the way of sedative proper-

Table 16–8. The commonly used tricyclic and related antidepressants and their characteristics.

Generic name	Trade name	Chemical group	Noradrenergic or serotonergic	Daily dosage range (mg)	Comments
Dibenzocycloheptadienes					
Amitriptyline	Elavil and others	Tricyclic	Mostly serotonergic	75-300	Sedating
Nortriptyline	Aventyl	Tricyclic	Both	40-100	Demethylated metabolite of amitriptyline
Protriptyline	Vivactyl	Tricyclic	Both	15-60	Least sedating tricyclic
Dibenzazepines					
Imipramine	Tofranil and others	Tricyclic	Mostly noradrenergic	75-300	Oldest, most widely studied
Desipramine	Norpramin, Pertofrane	Tricyclic	Noradrenegic	75-300	Demethylated metabolite of imipramine; least anticholinergic
Dibenzoxepines					
Doxepin	Sinequan, Adapin	Tricyclic	Both	75-300	Very sedating; least cardiotoxic
Dibenzoxazepines					
Amoxapine	Asendin	Tricyclic	Both	200-300	Rapid onset of action
Dibenzo-bicyclo-octadienes					
Maprotiline	Ludiomil	Tetracyclic	Noradrenegic	150-200	May have more rapid onset of action
Triazolopyridines					
Trazodone	Desyrel	Triazole	Serotonergic	200-300	Little cardiotoxicity, some antianxiety effects

ties and is therefore useful for patients who would find sedation unpleasant. *Doxepin* (Sinequan) has two major advantages: few anticholinergic side effects and very little effect on the heart. It is useful for people with cardiac rhythm disturbances and other cardiac abnormalities.

Tricyclic-like compounds. Many new antidepressant agents that are related to the tricyclics have recently come onto the market or are under investigation. *Amoxapine* (Asendin) is related both to the tricyclics and to the dibenzazepine group of antipsychotics. It has both antidepressant and sedating properties, and its onset of action is more rapid than that of the tricyclics (often as little as four to seven days). There is some concern that amoxapine carries a risk of tardive dyskinesia because of its chemical similarities to the antipsychotics. *Maprotiline* (Ludiomil) is a tetracyclic antidepressant that has mild anticholinergic and sedating side effects. Its antianxiety properties are questionable. *Trazodone* (Desyrel) is chemically distinct from all other available antidepressants. It has proved quite effective in alleviating depressive symptoms. It has very few anticholinergic and cardiovascular side effects, and suicide by trazodone overdose has been relatively uncommon. You will hear about other TCA-related compounds in clinical use, as new ones are continually being developed.

Side Effects
Autonomic, primarily anticholinergic effects. These are quite common and are to be expected in most people. They include dry mouth, blurred vision, and constipation—all of which resolve spontaneously or with symptomatic treatment. Sweating may also occur. Postural hypotension may be more serious than the effects mentioned above. The person may have to make slower changes in posture or wear elastic stockings. Less common anticholinergic effects include urinary retention, paralytic ileus (paralysis of the intestines), and the acute exacerbation of narrow-angle glaucoma.

Central nervous system effects. CNS effects include agitation, fine tremor, angry states, mania, schizophrenic excitement, and the exacerbation of latent psychosis. Some people report sudden falls and balance problems. Sedation is a property of many of the TCAs; TCA-induced drowsiness may be unpleasant or welcome, depending on the client's symptoms.

Cardiovascular effects. Cardiovascular effects are more common in overdose than at therapeutic levels, but the TCAs can cause palpitations (unusually forceful or erratic heartbeats) and direct depression of the heart muscle. Since the TCAs exert an effect on the heart rhythm, they must be used with great caution in people who have rhythm disturbances or a history of recent heart attack. A thorough cardiac evaluation is essential for people who have cardiac symptoms or a history of cardiac illness.

Drug interactions. Drug interactions include potentiation of the effects of quinidine and antagonism of the antihypertensive effects of guanethidine. TCAs can also cause severe toxic reactions when given in combination with MAOIs, although this is questioned by some clinicians. In shifting someone from TCA treatment to an MAOI, it is necessary to wait one to three weeks after the TCA is discontinued before beginning the MAOI.

Overdose. An overdose results in cardiac arrhythmias, convulsions, increased deep tendon reflexes, confusion, coma, and death. The lethal dose of most TCAs is relatively low—roughly 10 to 30 times the daily therapeutic dosage.

Prescribing Regimen
The usual regimen followed by the prescribing physician is outlined below:

- Begin with a low dose.
- Raise the dosage slowly to within the recommended effective dosage range or until side effects prohibit further dosage increases. A typical daily dosage for someone starting on imipramine would be as follows:

Day 1	50 mg
Days 2-4	75 mg
Days 5-10	100 mg
Days 11-16	150 mg

Similar regimens are suitable for most of the other TCAs. Doses may be divided (often two or three times per day) to lessen side effects, but a single daily dose is acceptable and may make the client's compliance easier to obtain.

- Obtain a serum drug level if possible to help in adjusting medication to a proper therapeutic dosage. The plasma levels shown in

Table 16–9. Plasma levels associated with maximal therapeutic response to tricyclic antidepressants.

Drug	Plasma level (ng/ml)
Nortriptyline	50–170
Imipramine (+ desipramine)	>200
Desipramine	40–160
Amitriptyline (+ nortriptyline)	>160
Doxepin (+ desmethyldoxepin)	>100

Table 16-9 have been associated with maximum therapeutic response. For drugs whose therapuetic levels have not been established, raise the dosage to the upper limits of the recommended therapeutic range, as long as no intolerable side effects develop.

• Wait at least three weeks after the client is receiving an adequate dosage to evaluate therapeutic effects. If no therapeutic response occurs after three to four weeks, raise the dosage of the TCA or switch to a TCA of a different chemical group.

Continuing therapy. Once the initial depressive symptoms have remitted, how long should one continue antidepressant therapy? Studies have demonstrated that people are least likely to have a relapse of depressive symptoms if they are treated continuously for seven to eight months after an acute depressive episode. Medication can then be tapered off and discontinued over a week to 10 days. If depressive symptoms recur, the drug is then reinstated.

Maintenance therapy. Which people need long-term maintenance on an antidepressant? This is not an easy question to answer. Some people have one episode of depression and never experience a recurrence. For them, maintenance therapy is unnecessary. Other people have recurrent depressive episodes, but so infrequently (e.g., every 10 years) that maintenance therapy is not warranted. On the basis of large follow-up studies, it appears that people who have two depressive episodes within five years are likely to experience recurrences. For such people, preventive treatment of depressive episodes is recommended.

Monoamine Oxidase Inhibitors

The monoamine oxidase inhibitors (MAOIs) block the action of the enzyme monoamine oxidase, which breaks down norepinephrine within nerve cells. By inhibiting the action of monoamine oxidase, the MAOIs increase the concentration of norepinephrine at receptor sites, and this is believed to be related to their antidepressant action.

MAOIs are clearly second-line drugs in treating depression for two major reasons: 1) their clinical efficacy is less than (or at best equal to) that of the TCAs in most controlled trials, and 2) their side effects are particularly dangerous. They are clearly not to be used by non-specialists, and they should normally only be used when other treatment modalities (ECT, TCAs) have failed or are contraindicated. The available MAOIs are shown in Table 16-10.

Table 16–10. Available MAOIs and their average dosages.

Generic name	Trade name	Average daily dosage (mg)
Hydrazides		
Isocarboxazid	Marplan	10–30
Phenelzine	Nardil	45–75
Nonhydrazide		
Tranylcypromine	Parnate	20–40

Some clinicians report that MAOIs are more effective than TCAs in atypical depressions—e.g., for people who are more depressed in the evening, people with multiple somatic complaints, and people with phobic anxiety states. However, the TCAs remain the drugs of first choice for most forms of depression.

Side effects and adverse effects. The major side effects of the MAOIs are *hypertensive crisis* and *interactions with other drugs*.

Hypertensive crisis (a sudden, dramatic increase in blood pressure) is perhaps the most widely known side effect of the MAOIs. It occurs primarily when the client on an MAOI eats foods that contain the substance tyramine. Such foods are numerous and include certain types of cheese, wine, beer, pickled herring, chicken livers, cream, chocolate, and yogurt. Hypertensive crisis can result in severe headache, stroke, and death. A client taking an MAOI must be able to comply with a diet that involves the strict avoidance of a number of foods.

The drugs with which MAOIs interact are too numerous to list here, but the major ones include cold and sinus remedies, pain killers, amphetamines, alcohol, narcotics, diuretics, antihypertensives, and hypoglycemics. The combination of these drugs with an MAOI can cause severe hypertension, hypotension, or central nervous system depression.

The lethal dose of an MAOI is relatively low—six to 10 times the average daily dosage. Thus, the potential for suicide by means of overdose or by the abuse of tyramine-containing foods is high.

These drugs are not to be used in combination with TCAs, except in special cases under the close supervision of a psychopharmacologist.

LITHIUM

As early as 1949, the antimanic properties of the lithium ion were described in the literature (Cade 1949). By 1970, lithium carbonate was approved for clinical use in the United States. It has been a mainstay in the treatment of manic-depressive illness ever since. Lithium has been shown to be effective against the symptoms of acute mania, as well as in preventing recurrent episodes of affective illness during long-term maintenance.

We do not know how lithium works, nor have we located its site of action. Its physical, chemical, and biological properties are similar to those of sodium. However, it crosses cell membranes slowly, and a therapeutic response is not generally achieved until five to 10 days after treatment is begun.

Uses

Acute manic episodes. Lithium has been shown to be effective in controlling acute mania in roughly 80 percent of people within one to two weeks after treatment is begun. During the "lag period" between the start of treatment and the beginning of the therapeutic effect of the drug, clinicians usually "cover" the person with an antipsychotic to control agitation and diminish psychosis.

Bipolar illness (maintenance therapy). Lithium has proved effective in preventing severe relapses of both manic and depressive episodes in bipolar illness. It appears to diminish both the severity of the episodes and the frequency of recurrence.

Recurrent unipolar depression (maintenance therapy). Studies have shown lithium to be as effective as imipramine in preventing recurrent depressive episodes in people with unipolar depression. Although the TCAs are currently the treatment of choice for prevention of depressive episodes, increasing attention is being paid to the benefits of lithium for this purpose. However, FDA has not yet approved the use of lithium in unipolar depression. There is no conclusive evidence supporting the efficacy of lithium in relieving acute depressive episodes.

Schizoaffective disorder. Lithium is of limited use in treating this illness, since the affective features are atypical and mixed with features that are more characteristic of schizophrenia. Antipsychotics are the treatment of choice in schizoaffective disorder, but lithium is often added to the regimen when an antipsychotic alone does not sufficiently ameliorate the symptoms or prevent recurrent exacerbations.

Other uses. Much research is being done on other psychiatric conditions that may be responsive to lithium. Various cyclic mood disturbances are under consideration, along with impulse disorders, other aggressive states, and unstable personality disorders. It appears that a family history of affective illness and/or a favorable response to lithium in some family member favors a therapeutic response in people with a variety of atypical mood disorders.

Effects

Although lithium takes away the subjective experience of being "high" and ameliorates manic psychosis and excitement, it has almost no effect on normal people. Many people liken taking lithium to the experience of taking an aspirin. There is little or no sedation, and no appreciable effect on thinking or motor activities in the nonmanic person. Nevertheless, people who have manic-depressive illness often dislike the drug because it takes away the euphoria that is a subjectively pleasant aspect of mania.

Lithium is given orally, and is rapidly absorbed into the bloodstream. It reaches peak levels in one to three hours after ingestion. It is distributed throughout the body and is eliminated by the kidneys. Normal kidney function is essential, and kidney functioning must be monitored throughout treatment. The rate of lithium excretion by the kidney may vary as a result of several factors. Most notably, as sodium intake decreases, lithium retention by the kidney increases. Thus, such variables as diet, the use of diuretics, and the rate of perspiration can significantly affect blood levels of lithium and even result in lithium toxicity.

Side Effects

The *early side effects* of lithium treatment, which are very common and usually subside within a few days, include the following:

- Gastrointestinal distress, including nausea, vomiting, diarrhea, stomach pain;
- Muscle weakness and the subjective experience of being dazed or tired;
- Hand tremor (a fine tremor, in contrast to the more coarse tremor of parkinsonism); and
- Increased thirst and frequency of urination.

The later side effects include the following:

- Persistent hand tremor;
- Increased thirst and frequency of urination that may be severe and persistent (which can be treated by stopping the drug or by carefully adding concurrent treatment with a thiazide diuretic [paradoxical effect]);
- Weight gain and/or edema (retention of fluid by the body);
- Precipitation of latent hypothyroidism or swelling and malfunction of the thyroid gland (nontoxic goiter);
- Leukocytosis ($\sim$15,000/mm^3), an increased white blood cell count that occurs commonly and is relatively benign;
- EKG changes (common), including T-wave depression and widened QRS complexes; and
- Kidney abnormalities. A small proportion of people develop kidney damage (interstitial nephritis), which is manifested by increased thirst, frequent urination, and difficulty in concentrating urine, resulting in loss of large quantities of body water. To prevent such irreversible kidney damage, it is wise to monitor people on lithium maintenance by measuring their serum creatinine levels at three- to six-month intervals; any severe increase in the frequency of urination should be carefully evaluated.

Lithium Poisoning

Lithium toxicity is common. It occurs when the amount of lithium in the bloodstream is as little as 50 percent above therapeutic levels. Mild lithium toxicity can be reversed simply by omitting several doses and then beginning again at a lower dosage when the serum lithium level has fallen to within a nontoxic range and toxic symptoms have remitted. Severe toxicity must be managed in the hospital, usually by osmotic diuresis.

Common causes of an elevated serum lithium level are listed below:

- Overdose,
- Sodium or fluid loss (e.g., sweating, vomiting, diarrhea), and
- Concurrent medical illnesses.

A client who contracts even a minor illness should let the prescribing physician know immediately and refrain from taking lithium if he or she experiences vomiting or diarrhea. The level of lithium in the blood should be measured at such times to reassess the dosage.

It is important that both you and your client be aware of the signs of lithium toxicity (Table 16-11).

Table 16–11. The signs of lithium toxicity.

Early signs	Late signs
Slurred speech	Impaired consciousness—
Drowsiness	somnolence, confusion, stupor
Muscle weakness	Hypertonic muscles and
Coarse tremor and muscle twitching	fasciculations (muscle twitching)
Loss of appetite	Increased deep tendon reflexes
Vomiting and diarrhea	Hyperextension of arms and legs
Ataxia (loss of muscle coordination)	Seizures
Confusion	Coma
	Death

Clinical Evaluation

Before a client is started on lithium, the following evaluations must be completed.

Medical History and Physical Examination
The prescribing physician must be sure to elicit any history of kidney, cardiovascular, or thyroid disease. Other possible contraindications include the need for a low-salt diet, the use of diuretics, chronic diarrhea, organic brain syndromes, and old age or severe debilitation. Any of these require caution in prescribing lithium.

Baseline Laboratory Tests
Baseline laboratory tests should include the following:

- Blood urea nitrogen, creatinine, and urinalysis to assess kidney function. The usefulness of other baseline kidney function tests (e.g., 24-hour creatinine clearance) is debatable.

- White blood cell count, since an increased white blood cell count is common in the course of therapy.
- Thyroid function tests (T3, T4, and TSH). Decreased thyroid functioning can occur during treatment.
- Electrolytes, especially sodium. This is most useful if the person is suspected of being dehydrated.
- EKG, for people with cardiac symptoms, men over age 35, and women who are postmenopausal.
- Liver function tests and serum glucose test, for people who may have liver ailments or who have a history of alcoholism or hypoglycemia (low blood sugar).

Follow-Up Laboratory Studies for Lithium Maintenance

During maintenance therapy with lithium, the following studies should be performed periodically as indicated:

- Lithium level every one to two months,
- Serum creatinine every three months, and
- White blood cell count, T3, T4, TSH, and urinalysis every six to 12 months.

Any unexplained change in the client's lithium level should prompt the prescribing physician to retest the serum lithium level and serum sodium level and to repeat any other studies that seem indicated.

Administration

Lithium comes in three oral forms: regular lithium carbonate (Eskalith, Lithane), a slow-release form of lithium carbonate (Lithobid), and a liquid form, lithium citrate (Cibalith-S). The first is the most commonly used preparation; it comes in 300-mg capsules. Lithium is always given in divided doses, generally two or three times daily (the slow-release form can be given twice a day). Dosages are individually determined for each person according to his or her serum level of lithium. Therapeutic blood levels are generally 1.2 to 1.5 mEq/liter in acute mania, and 0.8 to 1.2 mEq/liter for long-term maintenance. Note that samples for determining blood levels are drawn about 12 hours after the last dose of medication (usually before the first dose in the morning), because blood levels are artificially high in the hours immediately following ingestion.

Acute mania. Treatment usually begins with a dose of 900 to 1200 mg of lithium carbonate per day (less in small or elderly people).

Serum levels are measured every two to three days, raising the dosage until serum levels reach 1.5 mEq/liter or until signs of toxicity develop. Some people require as little as 300 mg per day to reach a therapeutic level, while others require as much as 3600 mg per day. After one to two weeks, when mania subsides, it is usually necessary to lower the dosage, since the client will no longer require as much medication and may become toxic. A level of 0.8-1.2 mEq/liter will usually suffice for maintenance beyond the acute manic phase.

Maintenance. Many clinicians believe lithium is more effective in the prevention of manic and depressive episodes than in the acute treatment of mania. Lithium has been clearly demonstrated to decrease both the severity and the frequency with which mania and depression recur.

Who is a candidate for lithium maintenance? Only those people who have a history of *recurrent* manic and depressive episodes. Those who have suffered a first episode may be taken off lithium and observed, since subsequent attacks may never occur or may not recur for many years.

Lithium maintenance involves careful monitoring of blood levels (monthly, or at least bimonthly) to prevent toxicity. Most people can be maintained on 600-1800 mg per day to achieve a blood level of 0.8-1.2 mEq/liter.

Toxic blood levels range from mild toxicity at 1.5 to 2.0 mEq/liter, to a potentially lethal condition at 4.0 mEq/liter or greater. *Blood levels should be checked immediately whenever the dosage is adjusted, when signs of toxicity develop, when hypomanic symptoms occur, and when any but the most trivial illness develops.*

ANTIANXIETY AGENTS

Anxiety is everywhere. It is a symptom we have all experienced. In many cases, it is quite adaptive to the situations in which we find ourselves. However, anxiety can become so overwhelming that it is incapacitating and leaves people unable to carry on with their daily lives. This has prompted an age-old search for drugs that alleviate anxiety.

Virtually any sedating drug will diminish the effects of acute anxiety, but many sedatives (e.g., the barbiturates) significantly impair a person's ability to think, to perceive and react to stimuli rapidly, and to exercise normal motor skills. Many sedatives are also highly addictive, are widely abused, and have such low lethal doses that suicide with these agents is common.

The antianxiety agents are among the most frequently prescribed drugs in medicine, primarily because the demand for relief from anxiety is great, and because antianxiety agents are safer than sedative-hypnotics. They cause less impairment of cognitive and motor functioning, addiction is relatively uncommon, and they are much less lethal when taken in overdose.

The two major classes of antianxiety agents are the *benzodiazepines* and the *glycerol derivatives*. The benzodiazepines are the safer and more commonly used of these two classes.

Antianxiety agents do not cure anxiety, they only alleviate it temporarily. Thus, these agents are not the primary treatment of choice for any psychiatric disorder. They are most clearly indicated for *short-term* treatment of transient forms of anxiety. Since most people tolerate anxiety without becoming dysfunctional, antianxiety agents are indicated only when the client becomes in some way disabled by his or her distress.

Why the emphasis on short-term treatment, and only when the anxiety is disabling? First, because the drugs are not without hazards, especially when given for long periods of time. People soon become tolerant to the antianxiety, euphoriant, and disinhibiting effects of the drugs and are likely to abuse them to achieve the desired effects as tolerance develops. Psychological dependency and physical addiction thus become hazards in long-term treatment.

Second, antianxiety agents mask the symptom instead of treating the disease. Physicians who prescribe these medications as substitutes for time, concern, and support do their clients a disservice. Particularly in the case of neurotic and personality-disordered people, psychotherapy is generally more useful than antianxiety medication.

Uses

The following are the major psychiatric disorders for which treatment with antianxiety agents is indicated:

Acute situational anxiety. Particularly when anxiety lies in the anticipation of some dreaded situation, these agents provide temporary relief. An important use is in relieving anxiety secondary to physical illness and prior to surgical procedures.

Phobic disorders and panic attacks. Antianxiety agents do not treat the primary problem in either of these cases, but they do alleviate the concomitant anxiety and are useful in conjunction with other types of therapy, such as antidepressants and behavior modification (see Chapter 8).

Dysthymic disorder. Antianxiety agents are of limited usefulness on a short-term basis when acute anxiety temporarily impairs functioning. Their use can, however, impede the progress of psychotherapy by masking symptoms and allowing the client to assume that medication will cure everything.

Drug withdrawal syndromes. The substitution of benzodiazepines for the abused drug is an effective means of withdrawal from some agents, particularly alcohol.

Organic brain syndromes. Antianxiety agents can reduce dangerous hyperactivity and excitement, such as in LSD hallucinosis and Alzheimer's disease.

Extrapyramidal side effects. Antianxiety agents are useful in treating extrapyramidal side effects, particularly akathisia, caused by antipsychotics.

Antianxiety agents are less useful in somatoform disorders (they are of no use in conversion hysteria), personality disorders, and severe primary affective disorders. They are of little use in schizophrenia and other psychoses.

The Benzodiazepines

The benzodiazepines are the most commonly used antianxiety agents—so common, in fact, that Valium and Librium have become household words. The benzodiazepines have been shown to be effective against acute anxiety, to have relatively few adverse effects, to have few interactions with other drugs, and to be freer from serious dependency problems than other sedating agents. The nine benzodiazepines currently licensed for use in the United States for the treatment of anxiety and insomnia are shown in Table 16-12.

All the benzodiazepines have similar effects, as described below.

Disinhibition. The benzodiazepines block conditioned fear and avoidance responses. This may be why the benzodiazepines cause increased hostility and aggressive behavior in some people.

Sedation. All the benzodiazepines are sedating. Although flurazepam (Dalmane) is highly touted for its usefulness as a hypnotic, studies have shown flurazepam to have no significant advantage over other benzodiazepines in producing sleep. People on benzodiazepines must be cautioned about driving and about the use of

Table 16–12. Characteristics of the benzodiazepines.

Generic name	Trade name	Duration of action	Average daily dosage (mg)	Comments
Chlordiazepoxide	Librium and others	Long acting	15–100	Muscle-relaxant properties
Diazepam	Valium	Long acting	6–30	
Clorazepate	Tranxene, Azene	Long acting	15–60	
Prazepam	Centrax, Verstran	Long acting	20–60	
Flurazepam	Dalmane	Long acting	15–30	Used primarily at bedtime for sleep
Halazepam	Paxipam	Long acting	60–160	
Lorazepam	Ativan	Short acting	2–6	Used to treat akathisia
Oxazepam	Serax	Short acting	30–120	
Alprazolam	Xanax	Short acting	0.75–1.5	Possible antidepressant effect and efficacy in panic disorders
Clonazepam	Clonopin	Long acting	1.5–20	Prevention of petit mal, akinetic, and minor motor seizures

alcohol (the sedative effects of the benzodiazepines are greatly enhanced by alcohol).

Anticonvulsant activity. Some benzodiazepines are used effectively in the treatment (diazepam) and prevention (clonazepam) of seizures.

Muscle relaxant. The efficacy of the benzodiazepines in relieving muscle spasm and tension has been the subject of debate, and the results of controlled studies are equivocal.

Because their effects are essentially the same, the major clinical difference among these drugs is in their duration of action. Long-acting compounds (Table 16-12) are cleared from the body more slowly and can build up to high levels in the bloodstream when taken over days or weeks. Since the antianxiety effects of long-acting agents last about as long as those of the short-acting compounds, the long-acting agents must be given in frequent divided doses, despite their slow elimination from the body. Long-acting agents are metabolized and eliminated particularly slowly in people who have liver disease and in elderly men. Short-acting agents may have an advantage over long-acting ones in that, since they are more rapidly cleared from the body, they do not exert effects on the central nervous system much beyond the period of desired sedation and disinhibition.

Administering Benzodiazepines

Benzodiazepines may be given orally, intramuscularly, or intravenously. Most medication is given in oral form, often in an outpatient population. However, the medication can be given intramuscularly for agitation when indicated. Diazepam (Valium) and chlordiazepoxide (Librium) are slowly and sometimes incompletely absorbed into the bloodstream when given intramuscularly. Intravenous administration is usually reserved for acute seizure activity because one complication of this route of administration is respiratory depression or arrest.

Oral benzodiazepines are very safe, since it is virtually impossible to commit suicide by using one of these drugs alone. However, they can be lethal when taken in combination with alcohol or other central nervous system depressants.

Benzodiazepines versus antipsychotics. Both types of medication are given for excitement and agitation. However, benzodiazepines have no antipsychotic effect and may at times worsen psychosis.

Antipsychotics are generally used when psychosis is present, or when panic is overwhelming and unmanageable by other means. Benzodiazepines are indicated for most nonpsychotic forms of anxiety, since they do not cause extrapyramidal side effects and carry no risk of tardive dyskinesia. In this respect they are safer than antipsychotics. Most nonpsychotic anxious people find antipsychotics overly sedating and subjectively unpleasant.

Benzodiazepines versus barbiturates. Both are sedatives, but benzodiazepines are safer because they are 1) less addictive; 2) less sedating, causing less drowsiness and incoordination; 3) less lethal in overdose; and 4) less disinhibiting. Although barbiturates are still prescribed by some physicians to treat agitation and anxiety, they are clearly not as desirable as the benzodiazepines for this purpose and ought to be avoided if possible.

Glycerol Derivatives

Glycerol derivatives are a class of minor tranquilizers that were developed prior to the advent of the benzodiazepines (Table 16-13). They are as effective against anxiety, but they are much less safe than the benzodiazepines. Like the barbiturates, the glycerol derivatives cause excessive drowsiness and loss of coordination, produce tolerance more rapidly, have greater potential for addiction, and are lethal at relatively low doses.

Meprobamate is particularly lethal in relatively low doses. Its use in suicide attempts is therefore a hazard of treatment. Tybamate has a shorter duration of action and causes fewer side effects than meprobamate. The most common side effects of these drugs are *hypotension* (low blood pressure) and *allergic reactions* (particularly skin rashes).

The glycerol derivatives are generally less desirable agents in the treatment of anxiety than the benzodiazepines. One exception may be in pregnancy, since meprobamate is thought to be safer for use by pregnant women than the benzodiazepines.

Table 16–13. The glycerol derivatives.

Generic name	Trade name	Duration of action	Average daily dosage (mg)
Meprobamate	Equanil, Miltown	Long acting	800–3200
Tybamate	Solacen, Tybatran	Short acting	500–1500

ELECTROCONVULSIVE THERAPY

Electroconvulsive therapy (also known as ECT or "shock therapy") may well be the most wrongly maligned treatment in medicine. Popular literature has depicted ECT as a repressive and cruel procedure. In one state, groups have even worked to outlaw it. Oddly enough, ECT is one of the most humane and most efficacious treatments available in mental health care. Its "bad press" stems largely from outdated information about how ECT is administered and from public concerns about the authoritarian aspects of the mental health system.

ECT involves the induction of a grand mal seizure by means of an electrical pulse through the brain. Each treatment consists of the induction of one seizure while the person is under anesthesia, and a course of ECT consists of several such treatments.

Uses

Endogenous depression (major depressive episodes). ECT is a uniquely advantageous treatment for major depressive episodes, since it works much more quickly than antidepressants to relieve symptoms (often within a few days); it is safer for many frail, elderly people who have histories of heart disease; and it is probably more effective than TCAs in depression that is accompanied by paranoid or somatic delusions. Major depressive episodes accompanied by severe vegetative disturbances respond remarkably well, with an improvement rate of 80-90 percent. ECT is effective for many severely depressed people who do not respond to medication. However, it is contraindicated in "neurotic" or "characterologic" depression (i.e., dysthymic disorder), which can be worsened by such treatment.

Acute mania. ECT has been shown to be as effective in treating acute mania as in treating severe depression. Particularly for manic patients who are at risk of harming or exhausting themselves, ECT can give rapid relief.

Schizophrenia. The efficacy of ECT in schizophrenia is a matter of controversy, but acutely ill nonchronic schizophrenics tend to respond to ECT as well as they do to antipsychotics, while chronic schizophrenics tend to do less well with either ECT or antipsychotics. ECT is often used when other treatments have failed with schizophrenics.

Other disorders have not responded well to ECT, although the treatment has been tried in a wide variety of illnesses.

How Does ECT Work?

As with the other somatic therapies in psychiatry, we do not know the mechanism by which ECT exerts its therapeutic effects. The hypotheses put forward to explain its mode of action are too numerous to list here, but one interesting observation is that ECT increases the rate of norepinephrine turnover in the central nervous system.

Administration

ECT was initially given to people who were awake and not premedicated. This made the subjects quite fearful prior to the procedure and created an increased risk of fractures and dislocations due to violent movement during the seizure itself. Most ECT is now given with three types of medication prior to the treatment: 1) atropine to block vagal nerve stimulation caused by ECT and to reduce oral and nasal secretions, 2) general anesthesia with a short-acting barbiturate (e.g., methohexital sodium) to reduce discomfort, and 3) a depolarizing muscle relaxant (e.g., succinylcholine) to eliminate complications of the convulsion itself.

ECT is either *bilateral* or *unilateral*. That is, the two scalp electrodes that deliver the seizure-inducing electrical stimulus are either placed over separate cerebral hemispheres or over the same (usually the nondominant) cerebral hemisphere. Although there is some evidence that unilateral ECT causes less subsequent memory loss than bilateral ECT, unilateral ECT may not be as effective as bilateral ECT.

When the person is fully anesthetized, the electrical stimulus is applied, usually 70 to 110 volts for 0.1 to 0.5 seconds at an amperage ranging from 200 to 1600 milliamperes. The tonic phase of the seizure begins immediately and lasts for about 10 seconds. Respiration returns to normal within a minute or two, and the person gradually recovers from the postconvulsive coma. The anesthetist administers oxygen to the subject during the procedure to prevent brain anoxia.

The number of ECT treatments needed for each person is gauged individually according to the therapeutic response. Depressed people usually require an average of six to 10 treatments, while schizophrenics often require between 10 and 20 treatments. Treatments are commonly given three or four times a week (roughly every other day); however, some clinicians have used ECT seven days per week, and others have experimented with giving more than one treatment in the same day.

When the person has apparently achieved a maximal response— i.e., when successive treatments yield no further beneficial effect—it is prudent to give two or three additional treatments to help prevent early relapse.

Preparations for Performing ECT

Obtain informed consent. Explain the reasons for selecting this treatment, as well as the anticipated benefits and potential risks of ECT.

Medical history and physical examination. Pay particular attention to any history of cardiovascular disease, which may increase the risks involved in ECT. Severe high blood pressure may require increased medication to minimize the possibility of a stroke during ECT. People with musculoskeletal injuries may require additional muscle relaxants during the procedure. The only absolute contraindication to ECT is a brain tumor that causes increased intracranial pressure, since ECT also causes a transient increase in intracranial pressure and might cause herniation of the brain out of the skull. A history of recent treatment with catecholamine-depleting drugs (e.g., reserpine) is also a contraindication. ECT is particularly useful for elderly people, who frequently have cardiac and other major medical problems. The clinician must judge whether the risks of ECT are greater than the risks of allowing severe depression and agitation to go untreated. Often, ECT carries the lesser risk, and the person's response to treatment can be life-saving.

Laboratory work-up. Routine blood chemistries, complete blood count, urinalysis, chest x-ray, spinal x-ray, EKG, and electroencephalograph (EEG).

Pretreatment regimen. If possible, all medications should be discontinued shortly before and during the course of ECT. If this is impossible, the dosages should be reduced as much as possible, particularly for drugs that have cardiovascular effects or side effects. Lithium should not be used concurrently with ECT, since there is evidence of increased neurotoxicity with this combination. The person should take nothing by mouth for eight hours before treatment to reduce the risk of vomiting and aspiration (inhalation of vomitus).

Side Effects

The most common side effects of ECT are shown in Table 16-14 and described below.

Table 16–14. Common side effects of ECT.

Most common
Memory loss
Headaches
Muscle aches
Less common
Weight gain
Amenorrhea (loss of menstrual periods)
Increase in permeability of the blood-brain barrier
Systemic hypertension
Apnea (respiratory arrest)
Cardiac arrhythmias

- *Memory loss.* The acute brain syndrome that follows ECT is the most common and most widely publicized of its side effects. This syndrome consists of a confused state, variable intellectual impairment, and amnesia that may persist for several months following a course of treatment. The amnesia involves both memory for recent events (retrograde) and difficulty in retaining newly learned information (anterograde). The amnesia gradually lessens over the weeks following treatment and resolves completely in six to nine months. People who have received unilateral ECT tend to complain less of memory impairment than those who received bilateral ECT. The question of whether memory impairment persists beyond a few months is unresolved, but controlled studies have failed to show any permanent memory loss or cognitive impairment in people who receive a normal course of ECT.
- *Headaches,* which are responsive to aspirin.
- *Muscle aches,* which are transient.

The less common side effects of ECT include the following:

- *Weight gain,* possibly due to treatment of anorexia.
- *Amenorrhea* (loss of menses) or other menstrual changes, lasting up to several months.
- *Transient increased permeability of the blood-brain barrier,* which may alter the effects of certain drugs.
- *Marked systemic hypertension* (high blood pressure), which occurs as a part of the generalized seizure.
- *Apnea* (respiratory arrest) following treatments (respiratory support should always be available).

- *Cardiac arrhythmias*, primarily premature ventricular contractions mediated through vagal hyperactivity that occur during the brief period of slowed heart beat that normally follows the seizure. This should be prevented by the use of atropine, but cardiac arrests do very rarely occur during treatment, and resuscitation equipment must be on hand.

Risks Versus Benefits

Obviously, ECT is not an innocuous procedure, if only because of the risks inherent in the use of general anesthesia. Although death due to cardiac arrest occurs in fewer than one in 10,000 treatments, it also constitutes an important risk. And memory impairment can be disconcerting and even frightening.

Yet ECT is the most effective treatment available for serious endogenous depression, and its onset of action is much more rapid than that of any of the antidepressants or lithium. Large-scale studies have shown 1) that the risks of ECT are significantly lower than the risks of untreated severe depression and 2) that ECT is particularly effective in lowering the rates of death from suicide and the total number of deaths among severely depressed people.

ECT is most clearly indicated under the following circumstances:

- In certain types of severe depression, such as when depression is accompanied by somatic delusions.
- When other treatments for depression are likely to be more toxic to the client, such as in frail, elderly people who have severe heart disease.
- When depression is life-threatening, as with actively suicidal people—and when rapid remission is of the utmost importance.

The risks of not using this relatively safe treatment must be weighed carefully. Unfortunately, ECT's bad press has at times made client acceptance of the procedure a problem. In such cases, other forms of treatment (e.g., TCAs) may be tried first, and ECT used as a last resort.

REFERENCES

Abramowicz M (ed): Medical Letter on Drugs and Therapeutics. New Rochelle, NY, Medical Letter, Inc (A bimonthly publication of new information on all aspects of medication.)

Appleton WS, Davis JM: Practical Clinical Psychopharmacology, 2nd ed. Baltimore, Williams and Wilkins, 1980

Ayd FJ Jr (ed): International Drug Therapy Newsletter. Baltimore, Ayd Medical Communications (A monthly newsletter containing information on new research and use of psychotropic drugs.)

Baldessarini RJ: Chemotherapy in Psychiatry. Cambridge, Mass, Harvard University Press, 1977

Bassuk E, Schoonover S, Gelenberg A (eds): The Practitioner's Guide to Psychoactive Drugs. New York, Plenum Press, 1983

Cade JFJ: Lithium salts in the treatment of psychotic excitement. Med J Aust 2:349-352, 1949

Crook T, Cohen GD (eds): Physicians' Handbook on Psychotherapeutic Drug Use in the Aged. New Canaan, Conn, Mark Powley Associates, 1981

Goodman LS, Gilman A (eds): The Pharmacological Basis of Therapeutics, 7th ed. New York, Macmillan, 1985

Shader RI (ed): Manual of Psychiatric Therapeutics. Boston, Mass, Little, Brown, 1975

Shader RI, Greenblatt D, Ciraulo DA: Benzodiazepine treatment of specific anxiety states. Psychiatric Annals 11:16-20, 1981

Squire LP, Chace PM: Memory function six to nine months after electroconvulsive therapy. Arch Gen Psychiatry 32:1557-1564, 1975

Weiner RD: The psychiatric use of electrically induced seizures. Am J Psychiatry 136:1507-1517, 1979

Appendix A

Sample Psychiatric Evaluation

The following is an example of an initial psychiatric evaluation summary of the kind described in Chapter 3. Each psychiatric facility has its own format for such write-ups, and you should follow the form used in the particular institution in which you work. This sample will give you a general idea of how these summaries are done. It is an outpatient evaluation; you may find that inpatient write-ups are more detailed.

HOSPITAL OUTPATIENT CLINIC EVALUATION SUMMARY AND TREATMENT PLAN

Patient: Doe, John

Evaluator: Mary Smith, Psychology Interm

Date: October 20, 1986

Identifying Data:

Mr. Doe is a 25-year-old single man who is a third-year law student at Eastern University. He lives by himself in an apartment in Boston and was referred to the Clinic by a friend who had been in treatment here two years ago.

Chief Complaint:

"I feel all screwed up. . . .I've got so many decisions to make in the next few months and all I'm doing is getting high."

History of Present Problem:

Mr. Doe dates his current difficulties as beginning three months ago, when he broke up with the woman with whom he had been living for the past year. The woman, Joan, moved out, and "had been dissatisfied with me because she said I wasn't giving her enough." In addition, in the last eight weeks he has had increased distress from a duodenal ulcer (first diagnosed in 1977). He is being treated for this medical problem by Dr. Michael Jones, internist.

The patient is "worried and indecisive" about his future. He expects to graduate from law school this May but is pessimistic about finding a job. He is also indecisive about what legal area he would like to work in. He worries that he won't pass his bar exams this summer.

Mr. Doe reports awakening at 4:00 A.M. after four hours of sleep most every day for the past two months and is unable to get back to sleep. He feels more depressed in the early morning. He has been smoking two or three marijuana joints per day over the past eight months, and states he feels more able to handle day-to-day responsibilities when he is high. Mr. Doe reports not feeling hungry in recent weeks, and he has lost 12 pounds in two months. At times he has had vague thoughts of suicide but has no plans to hurt himself and no history of self-destructive behavior. He reports frequent periods of weeping when he is alone and thinks of the loss of Joan. He notes a loss of interest in his schoolwork and in sports, and a general feeling of lethargy when he is not high. He is unable to reduce his use of marijuana, even though he states he wishes to do so. He denies any previous history of depressive symptoms, and denies any history of euphoria, increased activity, or disordered thinking. He has had no previous psychiatric treatment.

Past History:

Mr. Doe is the only child born to parents of Scottish descent. Father, age 52, is a high school graduate and a machinist at a firm in Boston where he has been employed for the past 28 years. Mother, age 50, is employed as a part-time secretary, and has been working on a part-time basis since the patient was 12 years old. Both mother and father are "hard workers." He continues to see parents at their home for dinner about once a month.

His earliest memory is at age four, when he felt "very frightened and alone" during a hospitalization for a tonsillectomy. During preschool and latency years, patient and father often went on camping trips together and he reports feeling closer to father. As a child, Mr. Doe received some instruction in the Presbyterian Church, but says religion was never that important in his life.

In elementary school and high school, Mr. Doe always received above-average grades. He paid great attention to detail in all his school assignments and at times was ridiculed by his peers for his overzealousness. In elementary school he was friendly with several boys, and was very active in Little League baseball and Boy Scouts. Mr. Doe began to date girls at age 16. He had several brief heterosexual relationships that ended as a result of his being "overbearing, demanding, and too controlling." He notes that he relates to women in this way when he finds himself getting "too close."

In college, he remained very devoted to his studies, often preferring to study rather than to take part in social activities. He received his B.A. in English from Boston University in 1982 and hoped to gain admission to a prestigious law school. In college he received only average grades despite considerable effort, and was "disappointed" that he was unable to gain admission to a more prestigious law school. Both parents, especially father, always took great pride in Mr. Doe's academic achievements. Mr. Doe is the first college graduate in his extended family.

Family Psychiatric History:

Positive for depression: maternal grandfather suffered one episode of depression at age 65, which the patient believes resolved during a brief psychiatric hospitalization that included "shock treatments".

No other family history of affective illness, psychosis, or drug or alcohol abuse.

Medical History:

Negative except for duodenal ulcer (see above). Internist's report has been requested and will be forthcoming. Patient currently takes antacids infrequently, as needed for gastrointestinal discomfort, but no other prescribed or over-the-counter medications.

Drug and Alcohol History:

Marijuana use as noted above. Also drinks four or five beers per week. No other current drug use. Experimented with LSD and "mushrooms" on several occasions in college.

Mental Status:

Mr. Doe presented as a neatly dressed man who looked his stated age of 25. He made little eye contact throughout the interview, and appeared mildly anxious. Speech was clear, normal in rate, and somewhat monotonous in tone. He reported feeling "down in the dumps" and appeared sad, but affect varied little with thought content. He showed no evidence of a thought disorder, and no perceptual distortions. He reported vague suicidal ideation without any plan for harming himself, and denied any homicidal ideation. He was alert and oriented to time, place, and person. Concentration (digit span), memory, and judgment appeared to be within normal limits, as was his ability to interpret proverbs abstractly. He related to the interviewer in a formal and deferential manner.

Formulation:

Mr. Doe presents with a history of depression including anhedonia, lethargy, early morning awakening, and anorexia with weight loss over the past two months. He also reports continuous heavy marijuana use over the past eight months. In recent weeks he has experienced difficulty doing his schoolwork and has lost interest in his usual social and recreational activities. All of this has occurred subsequent to losing his girlfriend and as he faces graduation from law school.

His clear depressive symptomatology over the past two months is complicated by marijuana abuse, and the extent to which cannabis has exacerbated his loss of motivation is unclear. A positive family history of affective disorder, as well as the presence of vegetative signs, suggest a significant biological component to this depressive episode and possible responsiveness to antidepressant medication.

His current symptoms occur in the context of more chronic emotional difficulties, particularly indecisiveness, difficulties with intimacy, and concerns about his own adequacy and self-worth. He is accustomed to being an achiever, and sees himself as falling short of his high standards for performance. The loss of his girlfriend and his fears about finding employment as graduation nears seem to have precipitated the present crisis. His usual obsessional defenses (intellectualization, isolation of affect), "self-medication" with cannabis, and his highly organized and somewhat rigid style of dealing with the world have not been successful in warding off his current depression.

Mr. Doe suffers from vegetative symptoms of depression, apparently precipitated by recent environmental stresses. He also reports long-standing emotional difficulties that impair his work and social life. Given this picture, a combination of psychotherapy and pharmacotherapy may be an effective treatment plan. Career counseling might help to alleviate some of his anxiety about future employment. It will be important to keep Dr. Jones informed of the patient's treatment, in order to coordinate Mr. Doe's medical and psychiatric care.

Diagnosis:

Axis I	296.20	Major depression, Single Episode
	304.31	Cannabis dependence, continuous
Axis II		Obsessive-compulsive traits
Axis III		Duodenal ulcer
Axis IV		Psychosocial stressors

    a.   recent loss of girfriend
    b.   increased academic pressures
    c.   fear of being unable to find employment as an attorney after graduation

Severity: 4-moderate

Axis V   Highest level of adaptive functioning past year: 3-Good

Treatment Plan:

1. Once weekly individual psychotherapy to focus on patient's substance abuse, career and academic concerns, and difficulty in maintaining gratifying interpersonal relationships.

2. Referral for psychopharmacology consultation to assess suitability for treatment with antidepressant medication.

3. Referral to counselor at Career Planning Bureau at Eastern University to assist him in his job search.

4. Obtain patient's written permission to speak with Michael Jones, M.D., regarding psychiatric and medical treatment.

Mary Smith, Psychology Intern

Frieda Mason, M.D., Supervisor

Appendix B

Table of Commonly Abused Drugs

Class	Trade Name* (or Source)	Street Names
Narcotic analgesics		
morphine	morphine sulfate	dope, M, Miss Emma, morpho, white stuff
heroin	none	H, hard stuff, horse, junk, skag, smack
hydromorphone	Dilaudid	lords
oxymorphone	Numorphan	blues
meperidine	Demerol	
methadone hydrochloride	Dolophine	dollys, amidone
pentazocine	Talwin	
tincture of opium	paregoric	PG, licorice
cough preparations with codeine	elixir Terpin Hydrate	schoolboy, blue velvet
	Robitussin A-C	Robby
hydrocodone	Hycodan	
oxycodone	Percodan	

*Many of these drugs are sold under a variety of trade names; only one or two popular examples are used for each.

Source: *A Psychiatric Glossary*, 5th ed. Washington, D.C., American Psychiatric Association, 1980, pp. 58–62.

Class	Trade Name* (or Source)	Street Names
Nonnarcotic analgesics (*continued*)		
propoxyphene	Darvon	
Barbiturates		barbs, candy, dolls, goofers, peanuts, sleeping pills
amobarbital	Amytal	blue angels, bluebirds, blue devils, blues, lily
pentobarbital	Nembutal	nebbies, yellow bullets, yellow dolls
secobarbital	Seconal	pink lady, red devils, reds, seccy, pinks
phenobarbital	Luminal	phennies, purple hearts
amobarbital/secobarbital	Tuinal	Christmas trees, double trouble, rainbows, tooies
Other Sedative Hypnotics		
chloral hydrate	Noctec	
ethchlorvynol	Placidyl	
flurazepam	Dalmane	
glutethimide	Doriden	CIBA's
methaqualone	Quaalude	sopors
methyprylon	Noludar	
paraldehyde	Paral	
scopolamine	Sominex	truth serum
Muscle relaxants		
meprobamate	Miltown	
Anxiolytics		
chlordiazepoxide	Librium	
diazepam	Valium	
oxazepam	Serax	
chlorprothixene	Taractan	

*Many of these drugs are sold under a variety of trade names; only a single popular example is used for each.

Class	Trade Name* (or Source)	Street Names
Central nervous system stimulants		
d, di amphetamine	Biphetamine	black beauties
amphetamine sulfate	Benzedrine	A's, beans, bennies, cartwheels, crossroads, jelly beans, hearts, peaches, whites
amphetamine sulfate/ amobarbital	Dexamyl	greenies
dextroamphetamine sulfate	Dexedrine	brownies, Christmas trees, dexies, hearts, wakeups
methamphetamine hydrochloride	Methedrine	bombit, crank, crystal, meth, speed
methylphenidate hydrochloride	Ritalin	
cocaine	cocaine	bernies, big C, coke, flake, happy dust, ice, snow
Drugs with hallucinogenic properties		
d lysergic acid diethylamide (LSD)	synthetic derivative (ergot fungus)	acid, pink wedges, sandos, sugar cubes, LSD
psilocin/psilocybin	mushroom (psilocybe mexicana)	business man's acid, magic, mushroom
dimethyltryptamine (DMT)	synthetic	DMT, DET, DPT
morning glory seeds	bindweed (rivea corymbosa)	flower power, heavenly blue, pearly gates
mescaline	peyote cactus	barf tea, big chief, buttons, cactus, mesc

*Many of these drugs are sold under a variety of trade names; only a single popular example is used for each.

Class	Trade Name* (or Source)	Street Names
Drugs with hallucinogenic properties (*continued*)		
methyldimethoxy-amphetamine (DOM)	synthetic (derivative)	STP
myristicin	nutmeg	MMDA
muscarine	mushroom (amanita muscaria)	fly
phencyclidine	Sernyl	angel dust, dust, PCP, peace pills
Tetrahydrocannabinols		
marijuana	cannabis sativa (leaves, flowers)	grass, hay, joints, Mary Jane, pot, reefer, rope, smoke, tea, weed, Acapulco gold, Panama red
hashish	cannabis sativa, resin	
Volatile Solvents and Gases		
benzine	gasoline	
toluol	glue vapor	
carbon tetrachloride	cleaning fluid	
naphtha	cleaning fluid	scrubwoman's kick
amyl nitrite	amyl nitrite	amys, pears, snappers, poppers
nitrous oxide	nitrous oxide	laughing gas, nitrous

*Many of these drugs are sold under a variety of trade names; only a single popular example is used for each.

Appendix C

Some Common
Psychotropic Medications

(Classified by type)

Type of Medication	Generic Name	Trade Name*
Antianxiety	lorazepam	Activan
	clorazepate	Azene, Tranxene
	prazepam	Centrax, Verstran
	clonazepam	Clonopin
	flurazepam	Dalmane
	meprobamate	Equanil, Miltown
	chlordiazepoxide	Librium
	halazepam	Paxipam
	oxazepam	Serax
	tybamate	Solacen, Tybatran
	diazepam	Valium
	alprazolam	Xanax
Antidepressant	doxepin	Adapin, Sinequan
	amoxapine	Asendin
	nortriptyline	Aventyl
	trazodone	Desyrel
	amitriptyline	Elavil

*Many of these drugs are sold under a variety of trade names; only one or two popular examples are used for each.

Type of Medication	Generic Name	Trade Name*
Antidepressant (continued)	maprotiline	Ludiomil
	isocarboxazid	Marplan
	phenelzine	Nardil
	desipramine	Norpramin, Pertofrane
	tranylcypromine	Parnate
	imipramine	Tofranil
	protriptyline	Vivactil
Antimanic	lithium citrate	Cibalith-S
	lithium carbonate	Eskalith, Lithane
Antipsychotic	loxapine	Loxitane
	haloperidol	Haldol
	thioridazine	Mellaril
	molindone	Moban
	thiothixene	Navane
	fluphenazine	Prolixin
	piperacetazine	Quide
	mesoridazine	Serentil
	reserpine	Serpasil
	trifluoperazine	Stelazine
	chlorprothixene	Taractan
	chlorpromazine	Thorazine
	acetophenazine	Tindal
	perphenazine	Trilafon
Anticonvulsant	carbamezepine	Tegretol

*Many of these drugs are sold under a variety of trade names; only one or two popular examples are used for each.

Appendix D

Some Common Trade Names
of Psychotropic Medications

Trade Name	Generic Name	Type of Medication
Adapin	doxepin	Antidepressant
Asendin	amoxapine	Antidepressant
Ativan	lorazepam	Antianxiety
Aventyl	nortriptyline	Antidepressant
Azene	clorazepate	Antianxiety
Centrax	prazepam	Antianxiety
Cibalith-S	lithium citrate	Antimanic
Clonopin	clonazepam	Antianxiety
Dalmane	flurazepam	Antianxiety
Daxolin	loxapine	Antipsychotic
Desyrel	trazodone	Antidepressant
Elavil	amitriptyline	Antidepressant
Equanil	meprobamate	Antianxiety
Eskalith	lithium carbonate	Antimanic
Haldol	haloperidol	Antipsychotic
Librium	chlordiazepoxide	Antianxiety
Lithane	lithium carbonate	Antimanic
Loxitane	loxapine	Antipsychotic

Trade Name	Generic Name	Type of Medication
Ludiomil	maprotiline	Antidepressant
Marplan	isocarboxazid	Antidepressant
Mellaril	thioridazine	Antipsychotic
Miltown	meprobamate	Antianxiety
Moban	molindone	Antipsychotic
Nardil	phenelzine	Antidepressant
Navane	thiothixene	Antipsychotic
Norpramin	desipramine	Antidepressant
Parnate	tranylcypromine	Antidepressant
Paxipam	halazepam	Antianxiety
Pertofrane	desipramine	Antidepressant
Prolixin	fluphenazine	Antipsychotic
Quide	piperacetazine	Antipsychotic
Serax	oxazepam	Antianxiety
Serentil	mesoridazine	Antipsychotic
Serpasil	reserpine	Antipsychotic
Sinequan	doxepin	Antidepressant
Solacen	tybamate	Antianxiety
Stelazine	trifluoperazine	Antipsychotic
Taractan	chlorprothixene	Antipsychotic
Tegretol	carbamezepine	Anticonvulsant
Thorazine	chlorpromazine	Antipsychotic
Tindal	acetophenazine	Antipsychotic
Tofranil	imipramine	Antidepressant
Tranxene	clorazepate	Antianxiety
Trilafon	perphenazine	Antipsychotic
Tybatran	tybamate	Antianxiety
Valium	diazepam	Antianxiety
Verstran	prazepam	Antianxiety
Vivactyl	protriptyline	Antidepressant
Xanax	alprazolam	Antianxiety

Index

All pages numbers in **bold type**
refer to tables in the text.